Ask Your Pharmacist

Ask Your Pharmacist

A Leading Pharmacist Answers Your Most Frequently Asked Questions

Lisa M. Chavis, R.Ph.

St. Martin's Press ☙ New York

www.stmartins.com

Book design by Richard Oriolo

LIBRARY OF CONGRESS CATALOGING-IN-PUBLICATION DATA

Chavis, Lisa M.
   Ask your pharmacist : a leading pharmacist answers your most frequently asked questions / Lisa M. Chavis.—1st U.S. ed.
      p.   cm.
   Includes bibliographical references and index.
   ISBN 0-312-26554-9
   1. Drugs—Popular works.   2. Pharmacy—Popular works.
   I. Title.

RS158 .C48 2001
615'.1—dc21

                                                    2001019151

First Edition: July 2001

10   9   8   7   6   5   4   3   2   1

The book *Ask Your Pharmacist* is dedicated to Cheryl MacDonald,
who patiently organized, edited, cajoled, encouraged, and
finally sighed with relief when the
last question was answered.
Thanks to my best friend!

Contents

FOUR

Coughs, Colds, Flu, and Sore Throats: That Favorite Time of Year   104

Bronchitis ▪ Common Cold ▪ Coughs ▪ Flu ▪ Sinusitis ▪ Sore Throat

FIVE

Embarrassing Questions: "Could You, Er, Tell Me, Um, What to Do About . . . ?   124

Bad Breath ▪ Constipation ▪ Crab Lice ▪ Dandruff ▪ Diarrhea ▪ Excessive Hair Growth ▪ Gas ▪ Hemorrhoids ▪ Scabies ▪ Sweating ▪ Urinary Incontinence

SIX

Taking Care of Your Eyes and Ears: "The Better to See and Hear You With, My Dear"   153

Allergic Conjunctivitis ▪ Cataracts ▪ Dry Eyes ▪ Ear Infections ▪ Earwax ▪ Eyesight Correction ▪ Flying and Ear Discomfort ▪ Pinkeye ▪ Swimmer's Ear ▪ Tinnitus or Ringing in the Ears

SEVEN

Lips, Gums, and Teeth: "Smile Pretty!"   174

Canker Sores ▪ Cold Sores and Fever Blisters ▪ Fluoride Supplements ▪ Gingivitis ▪ Lip-Balm Addiction ▪ Toothache ▪ Tooth Whiteners

EIGHT

Legs, Feet, and Toes: Stand Up for Those Tootsies   189

Athlete's Foot ▪ Blisters ▪ Bunions ▪ Corns and Calluses ▪ Diabetic Foot Care ▪ Gout ▪ Ingrown Toenails ▪ Intermittent Claudication ▪ Leg Cramps ▪ Plantar Fasciitis ▪ Plantar Warts ▪ Restless-Leg Syndrome ▪ Toenail Fungus ▪ Varicose Veins

Acknowledgments

To my agent, Sheryl Fullerton, for her persistence, patience, and persuasiveness. It was her vision of *Ask Your Pharmacist* that brought this project to reality.

To my editor, Heather Jackson, for her insight, organization, and humor—all while facing the challenges of new motherhood.

To my mother, Paula Chavis, for being my *favorite* pharmacy patient. Love you, Mom!

To three pharmacists I have had the opportunity to know over the years; I respect their friendship and dedication immeasurably: Sandy Fandetti, Bob Brillon, and Eric McPherson.

I would also like to acknowledge each of the thousands of pharmacists who every day look up from counting prescriptions with a smile when a patient asks, "Could you help me with this problem?" Pharmacy is a profession the public trusts—thanks to all of YOU!

Ask Your Pharmacist

Introduction

AFTER WATCHING COUNTLESS patients standing bewildered in front of the over-the-counter medicine aisles, I felt that there had to be a better way. Common questions like "What do I take for . . . ?" "Can I take this with . . . ?" "Does this work as well as that one?" were asked again and again. While it would be wonderful if there were always a trusted pharmacist accessible whenever such questions are asked, often that just isn't possible. So, with your questions and concerns in mind, *Ask Your Pharmacist* and "The Drug Lady" came into being.

How to Make the Best Use of *Ask Your Pharmacist*

This book is divided into chapters that each deal with a specific set of symptoms or conditions. For example, in chapter 1 you'll find a wealth of information on "Aches and Pains." From "Athletic Injuries" to "Shingles," the question-and-answer format presents a quick and easy way to find that topic of interest.

Each question about a symptom or condition has several treatment options. Whether you are interested in a more natural or complementary treatment, an over-the-counter medicine, or a specific prescription regimen, you'll find it all here.

Along the way, you'll find plenty of entries under the header "The Drug Lady Recommends. . . ." These are snippets of pharmaceutical advice that cover everything from how to save money on your medicines to the best choice for controlling embarrassing gas. Specific products are also mentioned to help you find exactly what is recommended.

Looking for a particular product by brand name? How about by its generic name? What if you simply need information on a medical term? Here's how to quickly find the information you need. Within each answer, *you'll see brand-name prescription drugs or brands of over-the-counter products written like this.* *Generic or chemical names are written like this.* **Medical terms with more information available in the glossary are found in this style.** Here's that key again:

- Brand-name medicines and products: *bold italics*
- Generic or chemical names: *plain italics*
- Medical terms: **boldface roman type**

Also, if you don't see what you're looking for right away, head to the back of the book. Here you'll find an Index, a Resources listing for additional information, Family and New Baby First-Aid Kits, and a great Glossary to help make sense of the sometimes confusing "pharmacy-speak."

But don't worry—I wouldn't give you all that information without having some fun too. Interspersed among the questions are "HUMOR PILLS." These are anecdotes and jokes taken directly from pharmacists and other medical professionals. Many are from stories passed down from health-care professionals, and some I think my friends must have made up: Incidents like those just couldn't occur in a pharmacy—could they? You'll have to decide, but I think you'll enjoy these bits from the lighter side of medicine. They say that laughter is the best medicine and I'm inclined to agree!

Why an *Ask Your Pharmacist* Book?

I have had the opportunity, as a columnist and a practicing pharmacist, to witness an incredible resurgence of consumer interest in medicines and better health. From answering consumer questions in the written and interactive media, to standing behind a counter dispensing medicines, certain common concerns have come up year after year. *Ask Your Pharmacist* was written to answer these questions.

Meet your own personal pharmacist:

The Drug Lady. She'll be your guide through the wonderful world of medicines. She'll answer your questions about medicine choices and the best way to take charge of your health. Enjoy the journey and never be afraid to *Ask Your Pharmacist.*

So, how can this book help you? Here are just a few ways:

- ▧ Few of us ever have all of our questions answered when we leave the doctor's office. Maybe there are time constraints, you are not feeling well, or you are trying to keep the children together for the trip home, but there always seems to be one more question that pops into your head just as you're driving away.

- ▧ Each of life's changes—new babies, children, teenagers, pregnancy, middle age, menopause, serious illness, and becoming older—brings with it new challenges and many questions. *Ask Your Pharmacist* is a volume that touches upon each of these events and attempts to make them a little more understandable.

- ▧ You do have options for health care. Whether it involves an over-the-counter medicine or a natural herb supplement to complement our standard health-care regimen, we like to know what our choices are. Good information about those choices is your best ally.

So Who Is "The Drug Lady"?

The name came from a dear customer who would always come into the pharmacy looking for his "Drug Lady" to answer his questions about medicines. He always said his doctor didn't have the time, and the books he read didn't explain things in terms he could understand. It is because of him and others like him that this book idea was born. It may not always be easy to stay healthy, but now you've got your very own pharmacist to go to whenever a question comes up. Chances are, you'll find what you're looking for and maybe even a little more.

The Drug Lady Disclaimer

I care about your health very much; that's why it's so important to me that you *do not* use the information contained in this book to diagnose and treat your own medical conditions. Being sick can be a very scary thing—this book is designed to help give you more information to back up what your doctor tells you.

The Drug Lady Recommendations

I'm a practicing pharmacist with a background in community pharmacy, drug information, natural medicine, and women's health. I have answered countless consumer questions via the Internet at the on-line pharmacy drugstore.com, through my weekly column "Ask Your Pharmacist," and from behind a pharmacy counter, so I have a good idea of what most patients are looking for. My goal is for you to find exactly what you need after reading each section. With that in mind, you will find many specific product recommendations. Most of my product recommendations come from people just like you who have tried different brands and like one or the other better. I've also talked with other pharmacists and asked which particular products their customers prefer. Balancing all of those recommendations with products that show a solid scientific background, I have chosen those that represent a good example of what is available in most pharmacies.

My recommendations don't come from any type of sponsorship or any bias other than my own. If I try a product and like it a lot, or think that it serves a really neat purpose, I'll let you know about it. Thank you for giving me an opportunity to share my knowledge with you!

Aches and Pains: "Oh, My Aching Body!"

Athletic Injuries ▦ Backache ▦ Fibromyalgia ▦ Headache and Migraines ▦ Osteoarthritis (see Chapter 10) ▦ Rheumatoid Arthritis (see Chapter 10) ▦ Shingles ▦ Sprains and Strains

WHEN OUR BODIES are in pain, the whole world feels out of balance. It's difficult to concentrate on anything more than simply making the pain disappear as fast as possible. Often we must learn which non-drug therapies, over-the-counter products, and prescription drugs best manage the pain. If you're thinking, "I don't want to manage it, I want to wrap it up and toss it out with the garbage"—that is certainly understandable. But some chronic conditions like **arthritis** and **migraine headaches** require us to take a different approach because, unfortunately, the pain cannot be eliminated altogether.

Pain is near-constant, making common life activities very difficult. Incorporating a variety of treatments into pain management allows us to learn to use the whole body to overcome the mental and physical stress that the hurtful condition brings. Let's look at some of these painful conditions and see which treatments seem to work best.

Athletic Injuries

Q. *I have two sons who play most of the sports offered at their school. How can I best treat sports injuries that may happen?*

A. Your worry is not only common but also well founded. Each school year there are over one million injuries reported just from playing high-school football—and that number doesn't take into account those kids who are hit by baseballs or tear their knees while scrambling for a basketball rebound. The information provided here can help them avoid many of these injuries. You'll also be better prepared just in case someone comes home with a swollen ankle from a misplaced soccer kick.

What Are Some Common Athletic Injuries?

There are as many different athletic injuries as there are sports. Injuries to the body from sports almost always involve either the bones, or the muscles, ligaments, tendons, and tissues surrounding the bones. Here are a few of the more common athletic injuries and their physiological explanations:

Dislocation. Dislocation is the painful stretching and sometimes tearing of a ligament that holds two bones together in a joint (such as a shoulder or a thumb). Often during hard physical contact, bones that are normally safely in a joint are abruptly popped out of joint. They either go back into their proper sockets on their own or must be manually (and painfully) put back into place.

Muscle cramps. When we ask our muscles to perform at peak efficiency, they obey. That is, until the muscle runs out of necessary minerals or fluids. The muscle gives a last great contraction, but can't stretch out again. Ouch! A muscle cramp just occurred.

Shin splints. As any runner knows, the constant slamming of your foot against a hard surface creates stress on the muscles. The muscles involved in shin splints are located on either side of the shinbone. Small tears over time create pain whenever the person walks, runs, or jogs.

Sprains and Strains. When you **sprain,** say, your ankle, you stretch the ligaments that connect bone to bone along a joint. A **strain,** in contrast, involves the muscle itself. The muscle may be stretched, or even torn. **(See "Sprains and Strains," page 25.)**

Tendonitis. When you use one muscle a great deal, the tendon often pays the price. The tendon connects the muscle to the bone, so it must take the force of the muscle each and every time the muscle expands and contracts. Tendons don't have the blood supply that muscles do, so the healing time for inflamed tendons (tendonitis) is much longer.

Tendons and Ligaments

Many people, athletes included, have difficulty distinguishing what it is that tendons and ligaments do. While both are tough, fibrous tissues that you want to take very good care of, they connect to different parts of your body. Tendons handle the stress from a muscle, while ligaments control the big-bone movements. Here is an easy way to remember this:

- Tendons connect muscle to bone (TMB—tendon/muscle/bone).
- Ligaments connect bone to bone (LBB—ligament/bone/bone).

Tennis elbow. Small but progressive tears in the muscles and tendons that connect the wrist to the elbow are to blame for tennis elbow. Muscles are able to heal faster, but the tendons and ligaments may stay inflamed for weeks.

How Are Athletic Injuries Treated?

Unfortunately, even with the best conditioning, injuries occur. In treating athletic injuries from minor muscle cramps to complete dislocations, the key is prompt medical attention.

The Drug Lady Recommends...

If your children are participating in school athletics, it is a good idea to come to a practice or two to size up the situation. Sports-injury experts say that a large number of injuries could be prevented if a few rules were followed. At your child's athletic events, make sure that

▨ your child is playing with others of his/her level of physical strength or development.

▨ proper stretching and conditioning methods are emphasized; warmer muscles are less likely to be hurt.

▨ children are encouraged to listen to their bodies; if something hurts, the adults in charge or their peers should get them to stop immediately.

Non-drug treatments

No athlete in training ever likes to hear this, but when most sports injuries occur, the best treatment is to rest the affected body part and give it time to heal. Contrary to what you may think, massage may not always be a good idea. It can be wonderful for releasing tight muscle cramps, but if the muscle or tendon is injured, massage may cause further injury. A better choice is hot-tub therapy for sore muscles. It provides heat, to bring blood into the muscles, and the water jets stimulate muscles without requiring them to exert effort.

Many sports-injury professionals recommend the "RICE" treatment for both **sprains** and **strains**. No, this does not involve sitting down and eating a bowl of rice after you hurt yourself. "RICE" is an easy way to remember what to do without having to go find this book:

R: **rest.** Stop all activity and rest the affected muscle, ligament, or tendon.

I: **ice.** Put ice on the hurt area immediately.

C: **compression.** Put a snug elastic bandage on the hurt part of the body.

E: **elevation.** If the injury involves the lower extremities, put your feet or legs up, slightly higher than your hips. Stay off your feet as much as possible, as gravity causes blood to pool around the injured area and swelling will be greater. You should follow the RICE method as soon as possible, preferably right after the injury occurs and certainly within the first 24 hours. After 24–48 hours (or when the swelling has gone down), you can use heat to help increase circulation to the injured tissue and make muscle movement less rusty.

Antioxidants, like *vitamin E* and *vitamin C,* show promise as protectants against muscle damage during heavy workouts. Adding a multivitamin with extra E and C to your daily routine is an easy way to take care of this nicely.

OTC treatments

Pain-relieving rubs like **Ben-Gay** or **Icy Hot** work by a method called counterirritation. Counterirritation causes a mild inflammation in the area of skin above where the muscle pain originates. The theory is that this irritation crowds out the feeling of deeper muscle pain. The active ingredient, *methyl salicylate,* is the most commonly used counterirritant. When these rubs are applied directly to the sore muscle area, the nerve endings are stimulated and a feeling of warmth quickly appears. Blood flow increases to the muscle tissue and a warm/cool sensation on the skin provides the feeling that the pain is less intense. *Menthol* and *camphor* are milder counterirritants that provide a cooling sensation to the skin. These don't actually help heal the muscle, but they do relieve the pain a bit.

Anti-inflammatory medicines may help a great deal in bringing down painful joint, muscle, or tendon inflammation. *Aspirin, ibuprofen, ketoprofen,* and *naproxen* are classified as **non-steroidal anti-inflammatory drugs,** or **NSAIDS** for short. The characteristics of these drugs are that they bring down swelling (inflammation) commonly associated with muscle, tendon, and joint pain. NSAIDs also interfere with the body's sensation of pain, effectively decreasing the way pain is felt. Look for brand names like **Aleve** (*naproxen sodium*), **Orudis KT** (*ketoprofen*), or **Motrin IB** (*ibuprofen*) for fast muscle-pain relief. House brands (or generics) of these medicines work just as well and may save you quite a bit of money. Take these with food as they can cause stomach upset.

It's also a good idea to keep hot and cold packs around the house, as well as a supply of bandages, braces, and splints to ease the pain of those bumps and bruises acquired during the sports seasons.

Bandages, Braces, or Splints?

Bandages are for covering a wound; they protect against bacterial infection and from bumping into objects that would hurt an open wound. For small cuts or scrapes, a *Band-Aid* works fine.

Bandages should be changed often. To keep bandaged fingers and toes dry, look for waterproof bandage covers or latex gloves.

Braces can be used to support a weak area of the body, like your ankle or knee, for instance. Many athletes put on a brace, both to protect themselves and to support the site of an old injury. Wrist braces by *Futuro* are a way for carpal-tunnel-syndrome sufferers to find some relief and prevent further damage. Back and waist braces are a must for those who do heavy lifting and need to give their back muscles some assistance. Fitting a brace requires taking body measurements of the area and using the package guide to determine which size is most appropriate. Taking a tape measure with you to the store isn't a bad idea. This will avoid having to return or exchange the brace if it doesn't fit.

Splints are used to completely immobilize an area of the body when moving it could cause further injury. Broken arms are immediately put into splints until a cast can be made. Splints are great for small appendages like broken fingers or toes. Finger splints, found in your local drugstore, are usually made of metal or hard plastic and can be taped for extra support. In a pinch you can even make one out of a plastic spoon and some athletic tape.

Prescription treatments

If the athletic injury results in severe pain, or for pain lasting longer than forty-eight hours, it is a good idea to have it checked by a doctor right away. While it may be a minor **sprain** or a bruise, it might also be a broken bone that must be set.

Your doctor may prescribe a pain medication, like *Vicodin,* which contains a combination of pain relievers: *acetaminophen* and the stronger narcotic *hydrocodone*. Muscle relaxants, like **Flexeril** (*cyclobenzaprine*) may also be called for. These medicines can make you very sleepy and groggy, so use care when doing any activities that require concentration, like driving or operating heavy machinery.

Muscle pain that persists, or tendons that become irritated and inflamed, may be treated with prescription corticosteroids, like *methylprednisolone,* which can bring down the swelling and quickly relieve the pain. Corticosteroids can cause stomach upset, so be sure to take them with food—and exactly as prescribed by the doctor.

Backache

Q. *My back aches constantly. I do some light lifting at work, which hurts, and picking up my two-year-old daughter can be very painful. Also, I stand up most of the day. I've been to the doctor and he says there's nothing physically wrong, just to take an over-the-counter painkiller. Which one is the best?*

A. It certainly sounds like you have a busy life! The constant pain of a backache is often enough to take the joy out of everyday events, and that's not good with a two-year-old to play with and care for. Let's find out what drug treatments seem to work best—and even explore ways to stop the pain without taking medication.

What Causes a Backache?

A backache can be a sign of a serious problem or simply the body's way of saying, "Take it easy for a while." We depend on our back muscles for everything from support in sitting to lifting a bag of groceries. If you've already been to the doctor and ruled out a more serious medical problem, maybe it's time to find the source of your aches.

Backache can be caused by many factors, including weight gain, weak abdominal muscles, poor posture, or lack of exercise. Combine those factors with standing all day and the strain of sudden lifting (like picking up and hugging your little daughter) and you often get back pain.

How Are Backaches Treated?

Non-drug treatments

One of your first (and ongoing) steps should be to very gently stretch and strengthen your abdominal muscles. This will provide the back with the muscle support it needs to carry its everyday load without strain. Try some abdominal crunches every morning when you get out of bed. These are easy: Lie flat on the floor on your back, pulling your knees up to a comfortable bent position, with your feet flat on the floor. Cross your hands over your chest or abdomen and *gently* lift your head and chest up to your knees for a count of three, then slowly roll back down. Start slowly and gradually until the number of repetitions you can do is twenty or more at one sitting. You will be surprised at how quickly your stomach muscles are able to support your frame without strain or pain.

Before you go off to the pharmacy aisle to stock up on pain relievers, you may want to try moist heat on the aching area of the back, or a nice warm bath with *Epsom salts,* sprinkled with *lavender* or *St. John's wort* **aromatherapy** oils. These provide a relaxing time-out from a sometimes hectic lifestyle. It has been shown that many people respond as well to these forms of relaxation as they do to medicines. It certainly won't hurt to give them a try! If your schedule doesn't permit the luxury of these "complementary" healing methods or if you're still skeptical, there is still quite a bit to choose from in the pain-reliever category.

OTC treatments

There are many types of pain relievers and it seems that more brands are being produced each day. *Aspirin, acetaminophen, ibuprofen, ketoprofen,* and *naproxen* are the main staples of the over-the-counter analgesic (or pain-reliever) category. They are not, however, equally effective for your specific back pain.

Acetaminophen is effective as a pain reliever for muscle and backaches and may be easier on your stomach, but it has no ability to bring down painful inflammation or swelling. Acetaminophen and alcohol don't mix well, either. There is a danger of liver damage for those who take acetaminophen and consume more than three alcoholic beverages a day.

Only *aspirin, ibuprofen, ketoprofen,* and *naproxen* are classified as non-steroidal anti-inflammatory drugs or NSAIDS for short. These drugs have the characteristic of bringing down swelling (inflammation) commonly associated with tendon, muscle, and joint pain. NSAIDS also help to decrease the body's sensation of pain by blocking chemicals called prostaglandins. Using NSAIDS for long periods of time may cause stomach irritation and even lead to stomach and GI bleeding. Taking these medications with food may prevent both stomach upset and possible ulcers. Look for brands like **Aleve** (*naproxen sodium*) with twice-a-day dosing (once every 12 hours). Now in your busy day you only need remember to eat at 12-hour intervals!

Prescription treatments

If these OTC medications don't help your back pain, I would advise going back to your doctor or another physician for a second opinion. There are muscle relaxants (like *cyclobenzaprine*) or pain relievers (like **Vicodin**) that may be prescribed. For severe pain, your doctor may try to treat the pain with a direct injection of a steroid into the painful area. In cases that fail to respond to all drug therapy, surgery may be required.

The Drug Lady Recommends . . .

Before turning to prescription muscle relaxants or painkillers that may leave you groggy and feeling "spaced out," you might want to try a chiropractor. These health practitioners are specially trained in the adjustment and realignment of the back. Chiropractors spend many years perfecting their therapy and often can find exactly where some forms of back pain originate and move the body back into the proper alignment for relief. This therapy isn't appropriate for every type of back pain, but it may be an alternative to consider. After speaking with your doctor, of course.

Fibromyalgia

Q. *After many months of pain, my wife was diagnosed with fibromyalgia. We don't know much about it. Are there any effective treatments? Can it be cured?*

A. The pain your wife is experiencing is shared with nearly six million other people, mostly women between the ages of twenty-five and forty-five. Medical science often has a unique way of working: Trace a disease to a cause, then find a cure for that cause. But because we don't know exactly what causes fibromyalgia, there is little available in the way of a cure. That doesn't mean the symptoms can't be treated and eased, but this pain will probably be with her for some time. The good news is that there is no long-term damage caused by this condition and with proper treatment the symptoms can be decreased a great deal.

What Is Fibromyalgia?

This condition of muscle pain, stiffness, and fatigue very closely resembles **chronic fatigue syndrome** (CFS). The pain may be in the form of a deep ache or a burning sensation. Certain areas of the body, like the rib cage, the back, and muscles at the back of the head, may be sensitive and painful to the touch. Other symptoms that may accompany fibromyalgia are the inability to sleep (insomnia), depression, swollen glands, and abdominal pain. Some of those who suffer from this condition notice that certain smells, bright lights, or loud noises seem to make it worse. As of yet there is no known cause for fibromyalgia; the scientific community has speculated on everything from poor circulation to a condition where chemicals in the brain slowly change form, causing intense muscle and joint inflammation.

Diagnosis is made by referring to a list of eighteen regions of the body—such as the second rib, base of the neck, or the middle of the knee—and determining where muscles, tendons, or bones are tender or painful. If eleven of the eighteen areas are checked, the doctor diagnoses fibromyalgia.

What Are the Treatments for Fibromyalgia?

Non-drug treatments

One of the most effective non-drug treatments for fibromyalgia is low-intensity aerobic exercise because of its ability to increase the mobility of muscles and joints. Exercise releases endorphins (chemicals in the brain), which decrease a person's sensitivity to pain. First, try exercises that are easy on the joints, like swimming and water aerobics. As your ability to do this without pain increases, walking and riding a bicycle can be incorporated into your daily activities. Starting slowly is fine. Try five minutes every other day until you can increase to twenty to thirty minutes at least four times a week. Remember, the more the joints and muscles are used, the better they feel.

Several clinical studies have shown some improvement of fibromyalgia symptoms with increased intakes of certain vitamins and minerals. Unfortunately, not all of these studies were officially double-blind, to ensure consistent results; I offer their general results with the caution that you keep in mind they may not work for everyone. You may try one, or try all together, as each has been shown to have some beneficial effect for the individuals surveyed.

- The combination of *magnesium* and *malic acid*—in the concentration of 300–600 mg elemental magnesium and 1,200–2,400 mg malic acid—taken daily for eight weeks, showed a decrease in muscle pain.
- *Vitamin E* in a daily dose of 100–300 IU may provide muscle-pain relief for some individuals.
- Studies have also shown that some fibromyalgia sufferers have lower-than-normal levels of *vitamin B-1* (also known as *thiamine*). Knowing this, it certainly wouldn't hurt to add a B complex to your daily vitamin regimen.

Meditation is often a good alternative to medication. Stress-relieving **aromatherapy,** gentle massage, and soothing heat all go a long way to help

The Drug Lady Recommends...

Several of my customers have found some relief from the pain, stiffness, and depression of fibromyalgia using the natural supplement *SAM-e.* SAM-e comes from the amino acid *methionine.* Its given name is *S-adenosyl-l-methione,* but we're much happier with the SAM-e ("sammy") nickname. It seems to work at the chemical level where it competes with certain substances called **prostaglandins** that regulate our sensation of pain. Reports also show that results can be seen in as little as ten days, taking 400 to 1,600 mg daily. However, if you have a history of manic depression, this supplement can actually bring on a manic phase.

ease the discomfort of fibromyalgia. Avoid alcohol and caffeine as these may cause the symptoms to become worse.

OTC treatments

Unfortunately, over-the-counter pain medicines like **Tylenol** (*acetaminophen*) or anti-inflammatory medicines (like *ibuprofen*) generally are not very effective in the long term for easing the pain of fibromyalgia. The greatest lessening of the pain is just after each dose, but for most, the effects are not long-lasting.

Prescription treatments

When the pain of fibromyalgia becomes severe or debilitating, your doctor may prescribe a shot of a corticosteroid with or without a numbing anesthetic. This steroid shot is directed right into the area that is most tender. The swelling and tenderness go away very quickly, but the relief is only temporary.

Often a sleeping pill (like **Ambien**) or an antianxiety medicine (like **Xanax**) is necessary to allow full rest and relaxation. Antidepressants, like **Prozac** or **Paxil,** are also being used to treat the depression often found with fibromyalgia. Talk to your doctor about whether any of these options might work for your particular situation.

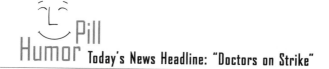

Doctors at a hospital in Brooklyn, New York, have gone on strike. Hospital officials say they will find out what the doctors' demands are as soon as they can get a pharmacist over there to read the picket signs.

Headache and Migraines

Q. *One of my regular customers steps to the counter looking as though she's been run over by a large truck. "I have a massive headache and would trade my BMW for some relief. What will help?"*

A. When the pounding of a headache won't stop, nothing else matters. The pain that surrounds the brain is often hard to predict. There are many types of headaches and just as many causes. Since the beginning of time, headaches have baffled medical science. It's difficult to function when you're at the mercy of such blinding pain, but there is hope.

What Causes a Headache?

Luckily, most headaches we experience are of the "primary" variety. This means that they occur more commonly and are not usually associated with any major illness, like a brain tumor or infection. Now that I have you worrying that every time your head aches, you might have a brain tumor, relax. In only about one percent of cases are headaches the sign of a serious condition like meningitis, stroke, or tumors. A primary headache is probably nothing more than your body's response to anxiety, anger, distress, or even sitting in the same position at your computer terminal all day long. The muscles at the base of the neck and back of the head tighten up, causing a dull, steady ache; that's the **tension headache**. Many people say that it feels as though a tight cord has been tied around their foreheads. However it's described, one thing is for sure—it hurts!

Of course, there are other types of headaches. A radiating pain that often starts from behind the eyes and extends down to the jaw and chin characterizes the **cluster headache.** Add to that a flushed face, sweating, watery eyes, and congestion, and you are in a pretty miserable condition—especially since this type of headache can last for fifteen to ninety minutes and can occur in "clusters" up to several times a day. Ouch!

Sinus headaches are a result of the buildup of pressure in the sinus cavity behind the eyes. Allergies or infections can cause this sinus pressure and a headache is often one of the first signs that trouble is brewing.

The vascular (or blood-vessel) headache's most common manifestation is the **migraine headache.** Anyone who has ever experienced a true migraine speaks of the "anticipation event," the feeling or an aura (like a strange sensation) just before being blindsided by the pain. Soon after, the sufferer is unable to endure bright light or any type of loud noise. Nausea and vomiting result from the blinding, pulsating pain, which can last from two hours to three days. Medical science agrees that migraines are caused by an unexpected and strong dilation of the blood vessels leading to the brain. As you can imagine, this can be especially disabling whenever it occurs, whether at work or while enjoying an afternoon in the park.

The Drug Lady Recommends . . .

Please note that if any type of headache occurs more than two or three times a month, it's time to see a doctor. Besides ruling out a deeper condition (remember that brain tumor we talked about earlier?), the headache sufferer is missing out on some very advanced medicines available to stop the pain. Over 90 percent of those with headache pain find relief either with prescription or non-prescription medications.

How Are Headaches Treated?

Non-drug treatments

Acupressure in the headache points, like the web between your thumb and first finger, can bring relief for some headache sufferers. Pinching gently on this area, called "the Hoku point," for several seconds is thought to ease the tightened nerve pathway. Pregnant women are advised *not* to use this method as some cases of early labor have been reported.

Aromatherapy with *lavender* has been shown to be successful with both tension and migraine headaches. Sinus-headache sufferers react better to the smell of *eucalyptus.*

The herb *feverfew* has been shown to be effective for many migraine sufferers. Two 125 mg capsules with a minimum content of 0.2 percent of the active ingredient *parthenilide* may be taken at the first sign of a headache. However, this herb is quite powerful and has been associated with rebound migraines (headaches that come fast and furious on the heels of the original migraine) that are more extreme than the original headache. Use this herb carefully and only as directed.

Some headaches have been linked to food. Certain foods known to trigger a headache include aged cheese, red wine, and monosodium glutamate (MSG, often used in Chinese restaurant cooking), chocolate, and smoked meats. You may want to eliminate these foods entirely from your diet to see whether you experience a decrease in the frequency and/or intensity of your headaches.

OTC treatments

If you've tried the more natural products to no avail and have now dragged yourself into the nearest pharmacy, you want to know what will give the fastest and most complete relief. There are quite a few products on the market, but with a blazing headache, the last thing you want to do is pull out a magnifying glass and try to read the ingredient labels.

The foundation of headache relief for many years has been *aspirin.* It is available in countless brands, in several strengths, and with coatings to protect the stomach. The recommended dosage is two 325 mg tablets every four hours, or two 500 mg tablets every six hours. There are even some extended-release forms of aspirin that can give relief for up to eight hours with just one dose. When it was found that *caffeine* worked well in combination with aspirin to constrict blood vessels, many different brands with this combination appeared on the market.

For those individuals who can't tolerate aspirin at all, **Tylenol** (*acetaminophen*) has proven invaluable for headaches. The dosage is similar to

The Drug Lady Recommends . . .

Today's combination products like *Excedrin* or *Goody Powders* pack a good punch against a pounding headache. They contain the three pain relievers *aspirin, acetaminophen,* and *caffeine* in a single dosage. *Excedrin Migraine* has even received FDA approval for use with migraine headaches. Check your labels closely, though, before you spend extra money. The same ingredients and strengths are in the regular *Excedrin Extra Strength* (and many house generics) that aren't advertised specifically for migraines.

that of aspirin, with strengths available from infant drops to an extended-release 650 mg caplet.

Also on the over-the-counter headache market are the over-the-counter anti-inflammatory drugs. Names you'll commonly see are **Motrin IB** or **Advil** (*ibuprofen*), **Orudis KT** (*ketoprofen*), and **Aleve** (*naproxen sodium*). These work by bringing down inflammation and releasing a bit of pressure in your aching head. They can cause stomach upset unless taken with food, but last longer and thus can be taken at longer intervals, i.e., every six to twelve hours, rather than every four.

Prescription treatments

When the problem becomes more than just a nuisance, headache specialists recommend keeping a daily log of the time, the strength, other symptoms, and the degree to which you are disabled. This will help your doctor make a more complete diagnosis and speed you toward relief. Headaches don't have to control your life.

Of course there are also other types of headaches requiring medication that's a little heavier than the over-the-counter shelves can provide. Severe migraines fall into this category—and it's a mistake for these sufferers not to seek medical attention.

Treating Migraines

Before the headache starts . . .

If you regularly experience migraines, you know you'd much rather stop them before they start. There are several drugs prescribed as "pro-phylactic agents," meaning that they stop the pain before it ever begins. Some beta-blockers (like *propranolol*), calcium-channel blockers (like *verapamil*), and antidepressants (like *amitriptyline*) are being used success-fully. Your doctor can tell you which ones might be right for your specific condition.

After the headache has begun . . .

Some of the older prescription drugs like **Cafergot** (*ergotamine* and *caffeine*) or **Midrin** (a combination of *isometheptene, dichloraphenazone, and acetaminophen*) are useful in stopping a migraine once it has begun. These combinations work by constricting the blood vessels and aiming for a certain spot in the brain where the headache originates.

Imitrex (*sumatriptan*) takes this spot selection one step further. When injected, this drug can eliminate all aspects of a migraine within fifteen minutes. Studies have shown that the pain leaves within two hours in 80 to 90 percent of all sufferers. Sumatriptan goes right for the receptors in the brain that are responsible for the pain—a very effective operation!

If you would rather avoid needles, there are certainly other prescrip-tion medicines to choose from (including **Imitrex**) that are available in tablet form. Other medicines in this same family include **Zomig** (*zol-mitriptan*), **Maxalt** (*rizatriptan*), and **Amerge** (*naratriptan*). Discuss your options with your doctor.

One side effect of these medications is a possibly serious constriction of the blood vessels surrounding the heart. So for those of you with coro-nary disease, diabetes, or even high cholesterol, these drugs should be used *only* under very close physician supervision.

Osteoarthritis

(See Chapter 10, page 255.)

Rheumatoid Arthritis

(See Chapter 10, page 259.)

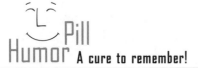

Pill Humor A cure to remember!

A fellow with a bad cough comes into the pharmacy, walks up to the counter, and asks for the pharmacist. A young clerk tells him the pharmacist is not available. The man asks the fellow if he can recommend anything for his cough.

The busy clerk points him to the shelf and the customer picks up a bottle. The customer takes a big swig, then, after a few minutes, with no apparent relief, he takes another, and another.

In a short while the pharmacist returns and sees his old friend, the customer with the cough, sitting quietly on a bench outside of the pharmacy. He says to his clerk that he has never seen the fellow so quiet before and wonders if he is okay.

The clerk tells the pharmacist the story of his transaction. The pharmacist looks at the shelf and angrily reprimands the clerk for pointing to the laxatives instead of the cough syrup.

The clerk timidly reminds the pharmacist that whatever the mode, the medication was effective. The pharmacist replies, "Not exactly. Now he's just afraid to cough!"

Shingles

Q. *My grandma has been suffering with the pain of shingles for several days. I've heard all kinds of things about what causes them. Is there something we can ask the doctor for to stop this pain? Is it contagious? What can she do to prevent the shingles from recurring?*

A. Your grandma has an infection caused by a tiny virus called the *varicella zoster* virus (VZV, for short). VZV is from the very same herpes family that causes chicken pox. This virus found a home deep in your grandmother's nerve cells, probably when she was first exposed to chicken pox as a child. VZV lies dormant and quiet in the nerve cells until triggered by a major stress like illness or an operation. When the virus wakes up, the painful rash we call shingles occurs.

What Are Shingles?

Shingles are most commonly seen as a band of painful, blisterlike skin eruptions on one side of the body. The band usually follows a specific nerve tract affected by the virus and the first symptoms to appear are a burning or prickling sensation. The rash of fluid-filled blisters follows in two to three days as the virus makes its way to the skin surface. Typically the rash worsens over the next three to five days as the blisters break open. The healing process of the blisters can take as long as two to three weeks before the skin clears up completely.

While cases of someone "catching" the shingles virus from an infected person are rare, it is possible. Children who have never had chicken pox are especially at risk.

Very often after a bout of shingles, there is residual pain along the nerve tract, which is known as **post-herpetic neuralgia** (**PHN**). This pain can persist for months or even years after the rash has disappeared. PHN is a very painful condition with no known cure. The over-the-counter remedies listed below may ease the pain somewhat, but often a doctor is needed to prescribe medication for the pain. Early antiviral treatment of shingles has been shown to be effective in lessening the chance that PHN will develop.

How Are Shingles Treated?

Non-drug treatments

After a trip to the doctor for antiviral medicine, you may ease the pain by applying cool, wet compresses to the blisters. Bathing or sponging off in cool water also can give temporary relief.

Because the urge to scratch is sometimes irresistible, it is a good idea to cut fingernails as short as possible to avoid scarring and further infection from scratches.

Vitamin B-12 injections are a more natural approach to pain relief for shingles. Many people find relief from these shots when over-the-counter remedies haven't been effective.

Licorice gel from your health food store applied directly to the skin also has been shown to bring a cooling sensation, along with minor pain relief.

OTC treatments

As the blisters of shingles begin to burst and ooze, *calamine lotion* can be used as a drying agent. However, this does not help the pain nor will it speed healing. With over-the-counter care for the pain of shingles, the aim is to bring down the inflammation and thus ease discomfort. Anti-inflammatory drugs such as **Motrin** or **Advil** (*ibuprofen*) or **Aleve** (*naproxen sodium*) can be helpful, but—as always—be sure to take them with food to avoid stomach upset.

The Drug Lady Recommends . . .

Capsaicin cream, or ointment from the cayenne-pepper plant, provides relief from the intense "pins and needles" pain of shingles or PHN. Apply the cream (brand name **Zostrix**) three to four times daily for best results. Something to be aware of: Some individuals don't notice an effect for up to two weeks. That's a long time to be in pain, so if this doesn't work within the first few days, ask the doctor for something else until the *capsaicin* kicks in. Also, to be sure the cream doesn't linger on your hands, use gloves or rinse with vinegar to remove all traces of the pepper-based product.

Prescription treatments

Just a few years ago, the best treatment for shingles was no treatment—just wait it out. Now, with the new antiviral medications on the market, treatment can begin as soon as the condition is diagnosed. Early treatment is very important to decrease the chances of nerve damage and post-shingles pain.

Early (within the first three days) use of antiviral medicines like **Zovirax** (*acyclovir*), **Famvir** (*famciclovir*), and **Valtrex** (*valacyclovir*) has been shown to cut the duration of a shingles attack in half. In some cases a pain medication like **Vicodin** (*hydrocodone/acetaminophen*) also may be added until the rash has subsided.

Sprains and Strains

Q. *My daughter plays soccer and is always coming home with some type of ankle or knee injury. I can't always tell what she's got and I can't easily find the answer in my home medical books. Could you tell me the difference between a sprain and a strain? On which injury do you use heat? . . . cold?*

A. This one always confused me too! When you or someone in your family has hurt themselves with either a sprain or a strain, the last thing you need is to have to read a medical textbook to figure out what works best. Following is a quick breakdown of what hurts and why and how to treat it.

What Are Sprains and Strains?

A **sprain** involves the ligaments around a joint. With a sprain, you stretch the ligaments that connect bone to bone along a joint. This area will often start swelling very quickly and a bruise may appear.

A **strain** involves the muscle itself. The muscle may be stretched, or even torn. Strains can involve major muscle groups or the tendons that attach the muscle to the bone. You'll know these by the sharp pain and tenderness at the spot of the injury. Bruising and swelling are generally minimal.

How Are Sprains and Strains Treated?

Non-drug treatments

Resting the area as soon as the injury occurs will prevent more damage. For the first twenty-four hours, remember the RICE treatment: Rest. Ice. Compression. Elevation. After twenty-four to forty-eight hours, warm soaks help increase blood circulation and loosen tight muscles.

Ice or Heat?

Many sports-injury professionals recommend the RICE treatment for both **sprains** and **strains**. RICE refers to

R: **rest** (the injured body part). Crutches for legs and slings for arms are excellent for immobilizing and resting the injury.

I: **ice** (apply packs on the injury). Alternate ten minutes on and ten off to bring down swelling.

C: **compression** (apply a close-fitting elastic bandage). An elastic bandage, like *Ace* or *Spandex*, may hurt a bit, but it will control swelling.

E: **elevation** (prop up the body part to decrease blood flow). Less fluid pools in the injured tissue, so swelling and inflammation are lessened.

These steps should be done within the first twenty-four hours after the injury. Rest, ice, compression, and elevation all help reduce painful swelling of the injured tissue. After the first twenty-four hours, heat may be used to help increase circulation to the injured tissue, which makes stiff muscles move more easily.

OTC treatments

Anti-inflammatories (like *ibuprofen, aspirin, ketoprofen,* or *naproxen sodium*) help a great deal in bringing down painful joint, muscle, or tendon inflammation. These can be irritating to the stomach, so be sure to take them with a meal or a snack.

The Drug Lady Recommends . . .

If you're not fond of taking pills or (like me) forget to take them every four to six hours, try the over-the-counter product called *Aleve*. It contains *naproxen sodium* as its powerful anti-inflammatory ingredient and, most important, it has to be taken only every twelve hours. It should be taken with food and a big glass of water to lessen stomach upset. Long-term use may cause GI irritation and even stomach ulcers, so be certain the stomach is coated with food or antacids and only use for short-term pain relief.

Prescription treatments

If the initial pain or swelling doesn't get better after three days or if you aren't able to put any weight on the area at all, it is a good idea to give the doctor a call. There may be a more serious injury that only X rays will show.

Your doctor may prescribe a pain medication, like **Vicodin,** that contains a combination of pain relievers: *acetaminophen* and the stronger narcotic *hydrocodone*. Muscle relaxants, like **Flexeril** (*cyclobenzaprine*) or **Soma** (*carisoprodol*), may also be prescribed for short-term use. These prescription medicines can make you very sleepy and groggy, so use care when doing any activities that require concentration, like driving or operating heavy machinery.

Allergic Reactions: Sniffles, Sneezes, and Unbearable Itches

Bee Stings and Anaphylactic Shock ▦ Drug Allergies ▦ Eye Allergies ▦ Food Allergies ▦ Hay Fever ▦ Hives ▦ Latex Allergies

OFTEN WE FORGET just how interdependent we are with the world around us. That is, until our bodies begin having allergic reactions to the very things we need to live—like substances in the air or in food. An allergy is the body's attempt to fight off a perceived threat in the form of an **allergen.** Allergens can be anything—animal fur, cottonwood seedpods, egg yolks, drugs, even the microscopic proteins deep inside a rubber tree. In an allergic reaction the body's immune system reacts intensely to substances that normally would help rather than hurt.

The immune system is set up with an extensive force of guards called "mast cells" that prevent attack by foreign substances. When we are exposed to something they detect as harmful, the mast cells explode. These tiny explosions release a chemical called **histamine** into the body and an allergic reaction follows.

Allergies are specific to the person having them; they are not contagious and usually only arise when one is exposed to the allergen. You can have an allergy to just about anything in your environment, but the most common ones involve insect bites; substances we ingest, like drugs or food; things we wear, such as latex products; or allergens introduced through our eyes, skin, or noses. Let's look at some of the best ways to deal with each type of allergy.

Bee Stings and Anaphylactic Shock

Q. *My son was stung by a bee while we were camping last year. He started to swell up all over and had a difficult time breathing. We saw a doctor in the emergency room who gave him a shot and wrote a prescription for an EpiPen. She said to only use it in case of an emergency. What kind of emergency? Do we give it to our son before we go camping or after another bee sting?*

A. Bee stings (or those from yellow jackets, hornets, and fire ants) typically cause quite a bit of pain, but in some people, like your son, the reaction is much stronger than just discomfort. Over one million Americans are allergic enough to these stings—a condition called anaphylactic shock—to require a trip to the emergency room.

What Is Anaphylactic Shock?

Anaphylactic shock is a very serious allergic reaction that occurs almost immediately after your body comes into contact with something to which it is allergic. Bee stings can cause an anaphylactic reaction, but other substances can too—penicillins, sulfa drugs, seafood, and vaccines that are made from horse serums. All of these substances act as allergens.

When your body comes in contact with an allergen that it perceives as an attacker, the blood vessels immediately begin leaking fluid into the surrounding tissues to flush it out. In severe reactions, this tremendous fluid release from your blood vessels can cause blood pressure to drop quickly. Very low blood pressure means that not enough oxygen can get to your brain, heart, and other important organs, so your body goes into **shock.**

The seriousness of an anaphylactic reaction cannot be overemphasized; its effects can include kidney failure, brain damage, or even death. If, after exposure to a possible allergen such as an insect bite or sting, you feel faint, break out in hives (see "Hives," page 44), have difficulty breathing, find that your lips and tongue are swelling and your skin is becoming pale and damp, or become confused and feel you might lose consciousness, call 911 immediately!

Once you have had an anaphylactic reaction, you have to be very cautious about insect bites in the future. The **EpiPen,** prescribed by the doctor, is an anaphylaxis kit to be used if or when you are bitten again and seem to be suffering a serious allergic reaction. The medicine inside the kit opens up airways, helping you to breathe until you can get medical help. An anaphylactic reaction may never occur again, but the odds of recurrence are greater after one severe reaction, and it is better to be prepared.

If your reaction to a bee sting isn't quite serious enough to warrant an

EpiPen

An *EpiPen* is one of several brands of anaphylaxis kits. Its pen-shaped injection system is easy to use and makes it popular with both youngsters and nervous adults. There are two types of EpiPen, the regular (for adults) and the *EpiPen Jr.* (for children up to 33 lbs). Each type has a premeasured and preloaded amount of *epinephrine* (adrenaline). You simply uncap the pen, put the black tip on your thigh, push firmly, and hold for a count of ten. Then you call for additional medical help. According to the company that makes EpiPen, the best spot for an injection is on the outside of the thigh and it can be done through light clothes with no problem. It is a good idea to practice this series of steps with your children (without administering the actual injection) so they are familiar with how to do this in case of emergency.

EpiPen, there are other options to minimize the discomfort from those pesky bites.

How Are Bee Stings Treated?

Non-drug treatments

If the stinger is still visible, scrape it from the skin with a knife or a fingernail, using care to remove it entirely. Getting the stinger out as quickly as possible removes the source of the allergen and decreases the swelling and redness. Next, put ice on the sting area to bring down the swelling. Try to avoid rubbing the area, since this will spread the bee's venom.

Some experts claim that a paste of meat tenderizer and water put directly on the sting will help the pain and itch. This makes sense because meat tenderizer contains an enzyme called *papain* that breaks down proteins like bee venom. If this paste is applied early enough, it can break down the poison before your body has a chance to mount a full-scale allergic reaction.

OTC treatments

There are always opportunities for bees or other insects to sting you when you're on an outdoor adventure, even if the adventure is just hanging out in the backyard. Here are a few items to always have close by:

- Chewable antihistamines, like **Benadryl** (*diphenhydramine*), are easy to carry in a camping pack or to keep in the glovebox of your car. (Remember that these can make you very sleepy.)
- **Tylenol** (*acetaminophen*) in either liquid or tablet form can be used to relieve the pain and discomfort of the sting.
- *Calamine lotion* or non-prescription *hydrocortisone* creams may also help the itching. (For a more complete list of items for the "Family First-Aid Kit," see appendix A, page 343.)

Prescription treatments

If the bee sting provokes a serious **anaphylactic reaction,** like swelling or extreme itching and redness, the doctor will prescribe an anaphylaxis

The Drug Lady Recommends . . .

If you or someone in your family has a history of allergic reactions, it is very important to always carry a small anaphylactic kit (like *EpiPen* or *Ana-Kit*) for the "just in case" situations. It is also a good idea to carry a *MedicAlert* card or wear *MedicAlert* jewelry if you have a history of anaphylactic reactions.

kit. This kit (*EpiPen* or *Ani-Kit*) contains an injection of *epinephrine,* a synthetic form of adrenaline that stops cells from releasing histamine, the chemical that causes all of the problems in an allergic reaction. It also relaxes the muscles in the throat and airways and tightens the vessels in the nose so you can breathe more freely. This medicine works very quickly, often within ten minutes of being injected. It may make you dizzy for several hours after the injection, so have someone else drive you to the nearest hospital (or call 911) if at all possible.

Drug Allergies

Q. *My mother says I am allergic to amoxicillin because when I was a baby she gave me some and I got a very upset stomach and had diarrhea for several days. I don't think this is really a drug allergy, but I wanted you to clarify this for both of us.*

A. While Mother may know best most of the time, I think you're right on this subject. A true drug allergy is something your mother would not have forgotten. What you experienced as a baby was likely a drug sensitivity or intolerance. In the case of either a drug allergy or a drug sensitivity, your body reacts with varying degrees of violence to something given to make you better. Drug sensitivities aren't as serious a condition as a drug allergy, but rarely is having an upset stomach and diarrhea pleasant. Drug allergies, however, are generally much more of a concern and may quickly turn life threatening if ignored.

What Is a Drug Allergy?

The symptoms of a drug allergy normally start out with a very itchy rash soon after taking the medicine. Other really unpleasant things start happening quickly—like a high fever and flushing, a rapid swelling of the tissues in the throat, difficulty breathing, and a drop in blood pressure. The throat can swell to the point that it is impossible to swallow or breathe. A drug allergy thus elicits the same sort of life-threatening response, **anaphylactic shock,** as a bee sting, although for different reasons.

Drug allergies can be hard to predict. You may have an allergic reaction to a drug you have previously taken with no problems. Any drug can cause an allergic reaction, but typically the *penicillin* family and related drugs (*amoxicillin,* ***Augmentin,*** *ampicillin, oxacillin, dicloxacillin*) are to blame. Other drugs that commonly cause allergies include ***Dilantin*** (*phenytoin*), *insulin,* the *sulfa* class (*sulfasalazine,* ***Bactrim, Septra***). *Iodine* and the contrast dyes used for X rays are also responsible for allergic reactions in many individuals.

How Are Drug Allergies Treated?

Non-drug treatments

The best long-term treatment of drug allergies is to avoid the drugs that cause them. Be certain that both your doctor and your pharmacist are aware of any problems you have had with medicines in the past. This will help prevent your doctor from prescribing and your pharmacist from dispensing a medicine that could cause an allergic reaction.

OTC treatments

For mild drug sensitivities, antihistamines (like *diphenhydramine*) taken by mouth or used in cream form can help the itchy hives. Once the drug causing the allergy or sensitivity has been stopped, these symptoms generally go away on their own within a few days to a week.

Prescription treatments

If you have just taken a drug and feel that you could be having an allergic reaction, don't waste time. Call 911 or have someone take you to the doctor right away. If it is only a mild reaction, the doctor will probably send you on your way with an over-the-counter antihistamine like **Benadryl** (*diphenhydramine*). If it looks to be more serious, they'll bring out the big gun—an *epinephrine* (*adrenaline*) shot. This medicine quickly relaxes the muscles in the airways to allow free breathing. You may also leave the office with a prescription for an **EpiPen** (*epinephrine* or *adrenaline*) for use at home. The doctor may also write a prescription for a corticosteroid (like *prednisone*) to help gradually bring down the swelling in the tissues so you can breathe again.

The Drug Lady Recommends . . .

If you have a history of drug allergies that could be life threatening, wear a *Medic Alert* necklace or bracelet at all times. Sure, they aren't the most attractive pieces of jewelry in the world, but wearing one will let others know that an anaphylactic reaction may be happening if you are unable to communicate. Saving your life is worth it!

Eye Allergies

Q. *My eyes always seem to get very red, itchy, and runny in the spring and fall. Can this be prevented? If not, what can I do to safely treat this annoying and sometimes unsightly condition?*

A. It can be rather embarrassing to have your family and coworkers always ask, "Have you been crying?" or "Was the movie that sad?" When the tissue companies start sending you stock-portfolio information, it may be time to look for a little relief. Eye allergies are as common as the sneezing kind of allergies and are often caused by the very same little flying pollens and allergens. Luckily, they can usually be treated even more successfully than other kinds of allergies.

What Is an Eye Allergy?

An eye allergy is actually a collection of symptoms involving the eyes and different types of allergens or irritants. These irritants can be pollen from trees and plants, cat or dog dander, feathers, makeup (such as eyeliner), or microscopic molds, fungus, or mildew. You may also see this condition referred to as allergic **conjunctivitis,** meaning an allergy of the conjunctiva or membrane surrounding the eye. The symptoms appear as red, itchy swollen eyes that may tear more than usual, which often causes your nose to run. In effect, you're a mess!

The bad news is that if pollen is the culprit, this type of allergy can last up to six weeks or until the plant stops releasing the pollen. Eye allergies blamed on the cat will last as long as the cat is around. However, before you find Kitty a new home, the good news is that eye allergies are easily treated.

How Are Eye Allergies Treated?

Non-drug treatments

One method that is very often overlooked during the pollen season is simply washing the face with a cool washcloth after you've been outside. Washing takes pollen grains away from the face before they can make their way into the eyes. Gently wiping the eyelids, stroking outward and away from the eye, quickly and easily removes the cause of the problem.

OTC treatments

Decongestants. Eyedrops are available that contain a decongestant (for shrinking the blood vessels in the eye). These are called vasoconstrictor drops and they will get rid of the red quickly. The ingredient *oxymetazoline* is one of the longer-acting eyedrop decongestants; *phenylephrine* has a slightly faster response.

Combination Products. When you have any type of allergy, most decongestants work better when combined with an antihistamine. Eye allergies are no different; the decongestant takes care of the redness, while the antihistamine takes care of the itching and watering.

The Drug Lady Recommends...

For fast allergy relief, *Naphcon-A Allergy Relief* eyedrops are a good choice for both a decongestant (*naphazoline*) and an antihistamine (*pheniramine*). This combination was available only by prescription until recently; now you can purchase it over the counter. The active ingredients reduce redness and stop the allergic reaction in its tracks. Because the decongestant constricts blood vessels, anyone with high blood pressure, heart disease, or glaucoma should avoid it. Also, check with your doctor before using in children under the age of six.

Eye Lubricants. An eye lubricant can keep your eyes moisturized when allergies have them prickly- and gritty-feeling. Many people prefer lubricating drops to ointments because ointments can blur your vision. Also, drops are usually easier and less messy to put in the irritated eye.

Irrigation Solutions. When you feel as though the pollen is inches thick and all you want to do is rub your eyes, a saline irrigation solution may be in order. It can be very soothing as it washes out pollen, dust, and other irritants that aren't supposed to be there.

The Drug Lady Recommends...

For those ladies who suffer from allergies caused by mascara and/or who are irritated by contact lenses, *Ocusoft* makes a wonderful mascara just for you. It doesn't promote allergies and is very gentle for already-irritated eyes. Many of my customers find this very effective when mascara is necessary but the allergy season will not cooperate.

Prescription treatments

The prescription drop *Patanol* (*olopatadine*) effectively blocks the action of histamine and stops the itching and redness for up to eight hours with one application.

It is possible for an eye allergy to progress to a full-blown infection very quickly. The constant itching, rubbing, and scratching of the delicate eye membranes can introduce bacteria or even viruses into the eye. If your eye

Putting In Eyedrops and Ointments

Have you ever watched someone try to put in eyedrops? It is difficult to lean back, squeeze the drops, and not blink at the precise moment that huge drop comes hurtling toward your eye. Wasting the drops not only could prolong the condition you're treating, but eyedrops can be *very* expensive, too.

Start by washing your hands. It would amaze you to know how many bacteria are living just on the tip of your finger! Tilt your head backward. Use the back of a chair or sofa to prop your head if necessary. Use that freshly washed index finger to pull the lower eyelid away from the eye. See the nice little pouch that forms? Aim the medicine for that pouch. Don't attempt to put the drops directly on the eyeball. That can be very scary and causes even the best of us to blink before that drop hits; it's an instinctive way to protect the eye, but it wastes a lot of eyedrops. Also, use care not to touch the tip of the dropper to your eyelid.

For ointments: Very carefully, squeeze a ribbon of ointment into the inside margin of the pouch inside your lower eyelid (see above). The doctor will usually tell you how much; a quarter inch is common. Slowly close the eyelids and let the medicine cover the eyeball. You may very, *very* gently massage the eye to assure the ointment spreads evenly. Try to keep your eyes closed for at least sixty seconds for maximum absorption. Use a soft tissue to wipe off the excess. Eye ointments and many drops can cause blurry vision. This can last for some time after applying them, so use care if you must drive or operate machinery. See, that wasn't so bad, was it?

allergy progresses to an infection or even a long-lasting redness, see your doctor. The doctor can prescribe an antibiotic (like *gentamicin* or *erythromycin*) for a bacterial infection, a corticosteroid (like *prednisolone*) for redness and inflammation, or a combination of both an antibiotic and a steroid like **Cortisporin Ophthalmic Suspension** (*polymyxin B, neomycin, hydrocortisone*) to reduce swelling and clear the infection.

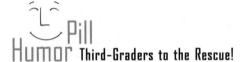 **Third-Graders to the Rescue!**

A group of third-graders was asked to come up with some of their best jokes about allergies. I hope you get a chuckle from their "lighter look" at sniffles and sneezes.

Where is a sneeze usually pointed?
Atchoo!

What happens when corn catches cold?
It gets an ear ache.

What does a pony sound like when it has a cold?
A little horse.

Why did the bee go to the doctor?
It had hives.

What do you get when you cross poison ivy with a four-leaf clover?
A rash of good luck.

What disease does grass get?
Hay fever.

Food Allergies

Q. *My four-year-old daughter has developed a food allergy to milk. She can't tolerate any type of dairy products without having a stomachache and sometimes diarrhea. Does this have anything to do with food we gave her as an infant? Could we have prevented her food allergy?*

A. There could be several ways to trace your daughter's problem. Milk allergies can be inherited from Mom or Dad, or can develop from introduction to cow's milk while a baby's intestine is still porous. In her case, however, it may be that she doesn't have a true food allergy at all. It sounds much more likely that your little girl has a lactose (or dairy-product) intolerance. (See "Lactose Intolerance," chapter 3, page 88.)

What Is a Food Allergy?

Many people think they are allergic to a certain type of food when, in fact, they only have an intolerance to that particular food. Less than one percent of people have genuine food allergies, which result in allergic reactions— where your body sees a particular food as an element to be fought at all costs. This type of reaction includes a rapid swelling of the airways and very itchy hives, and can quickly progress to anaphylactic shock. Severe stomach cramps, diarrhea, and nausea also may accompany a food allergy. Seventy percent of the people who suffer from this type of food allergy are under age thirty, with the majority of those cases occurring in children under the age of six.

Children with food allergies typically begin showing their allergic reaction with a skin rash. Food-allergic children often are allergic in other ways as well; they have many more episodes of hay fever (see "Hay Fever," page 41) and may even be more prone to asthma than others. There are even studies that show a connection between food allergies, attention-deficit disorder, and migraine headaches.

Foods that commonly cause allergies include seafood, peanuts, or spinach. "Extras" put into foods, like certain starches or chemicals, can also

Recommendations from the American Academy of Pediatrics

To help prevent food allergies, the American Academy of Pediatrics' recommendation is that babies stay on breast milk or iron-fortified formula until their first birthday; the reasoning is that the intestine is still porous (has holes in it) and larger protein molecules may travel into the bloodstream and cause an allergic reaction. This also means avoiding the "allergy triggers" of cow's milk, egg whites, peanut butter, and corn and wheat products, especially if others in the family have a history of allergies.

cause violent reactions. Look out for corn starch, food dyes (like Yellow No. 5), and gum arabic. Sometimes our bodies may see these foods or chemicals as being so foreign that they require immediate expulsion. Unfortunately, the body's way of getting rid of this foreign substance may mean nausea, hives, and quick, extreme swelling of the throat.

Food intolerances, in contrast, are not a life-threatening matter. Some people can't eat dairy because it will upset their stomachs terribly; they aren't actually allergic to dairy products, but may lack an enzyme called lactase that is necessary to help digest milk and cheese (commonly known as **lactose intolerance**).

How Are Food Allergies and Intolerances Treated?

Non-drug treatments

Unfortunately, the prognosis for a true food-allergy sufferer is not good. The best treatment of a food allergy is to simply avoid all contact with the offending food. There isn't a shot or a pill you can take that will enable you to eat the foods you are allergic to.

If the problem is a sensitivity to milk (lactose intolerance) and you feel you still need to have some dairy in your diet, yogurt is a good substitute.

The Drug Lady Recommends...

If you are **lactose intolerant**, products like *Lactaid* contain the enzyme *lactase* and can be taken just before dairy products are consumed. Several commercial preparations of lactase are available including a liquid form, to add directly to milk, and capsules that may be swallowed or their contents sprinkled over food. Caplets and chewable tablets are also available and should be taken with the lactose-containing food. Adding lactase to regular milk has been shown to significantly reduce the symptoms of milk intolerance.

The bacteria from live yogurt cultures produce *Lactobacillus acidophilus,* which is very effective in breaking down lactose. Look for yogurt with "live cultures" for your best digestion defense.

OTC treatments

Again, true food-allergy sufferers won't find anything for them on the over-the-counter shelves. The best defense is to stay away from the food that causes the problem. There will always be instances, however, when you might not be aware that a particular food contains what you are allergic to. It is a good idea to have an antihistamine (like *diphenhydramine*) around for emergencies, like for mild hives from "just that tiny bite" you took.

Prescription treatments

If your reaction to a particular food has resulted in swelling and difficulty breathing, see your doctor about an anaphylaxis kit (like **EpiPen,** see page 30) for emergencies. These kits are easy to carry in a pocket or purse and contain a shot of *epinephrine* that just might save your life if you accidentally eat something that your body is extremely allergic to.

Hay Fever

Q. *Does hay fever mean I'm allergic to hay? I have this every year for a couple of months and it makes me miserable. What can I do?*

A. Yes, it is possible that you are allergic to hay if you have hay fever, but it is more likely that you are allergic to lots of things flying around in the air. Hay fever is not usually caused by hay, and it's not really a fever either.

What Is Hay Fever?

Hay fever is really another name for the condition called **allergic rhinitis**—"allergic" for the allergic reaction taking place, and "rhinitis" pertaining to the nose area; however, hay fever affects the nose, eyes, and throat with equal vengeance. *Hay fever* is a term that includes all types of seasonal allergies caused when plants, trees, grasses, weeds, and shrubs release their pollens. When the amount of pollen in the air rises (called "the pollen count"), so do the sniffles and sneezes—add to that itchy, runny noses and eyes, sneezing and swollen sinuses, and sometimes a headache from the sinus pressure, and you've got quite a few unhappy allergy sufferers. Hay fever depends a lot on where you live, too; when the trees and grasses produce pollen for longer periods (as in the Pacific Northwest), you have a longer season for hay fever.

Hay fever can also refer to an allergy to pet hair and dander, dust mites, mold, or feathers. Because these tend to occur year-round instead of just seasonally, these are called "perennial allergies," but they have the same symptoms as seasonal allergies.

How Is Hay Fever Treated?

Non-drug treatments

Many herbalists recommend *stinging nettle* for the stuffiness and congestion of hay fever. Studies show promise that this herb may work well for many sufferers. The dosage used is 300 mg of the nettle leaf (in capsules) two to three times daily during allergy season.

Quercetin helps prevent cells from releasing histamine, which causes an allergic reaction. Taken regularly in a dose of 200 to 400 mg two to three times a day, this antioxidant may slow your body's reaction to allergens.

If pollen is the cause of your allergy symptoms, *bitter gentian root* tea may be used to urge the body to produce extra liquids, like saliva or tears, to flush out the pollen grains.

Avoiding Those Pesky Pollens and Allergens

■ Know the pollen count before you step outdoors. Stay inside on bad days if possible.

■ Use the air conditioner whenever possible.

■ Avoid smoky, stuffy places.

■ Let someone else comb the dog and cat; then stay away for a while after he's done, so the dander will have a chance to settle somewhere other than in your nose.

■ Make your home "dust-mite-unfriendly." Remove old and musty carpets and vacuum often.

■ Don't use feather pillows. Try synthetic hypoallergenic products instead, and read the labels carefully.

OTC treatments

Once your allergen has been pinpointed, you have two choices. You can avoid the allergen altogether or you can take medications to make life more tolerable. Medications are available for both the prevention of hay fever and for treatment once the allergic reaction has started.

For prevention, you might try *cromolyn sodium*. Found in over-the-counter products like **Nasalcrom,** this medication stops an allergy before it begins. However, it is not effective once the allergic reaction has begun, and takes several days to a week of regular use before it will prevent symptoms. Antihistamines, like *chlorpheniramine* or *diphenhydramine,* work well for treatment once an allergy has begun. A word of caution though: antihistamines may make you very sleepy.

The Drug Lady Recommends . . .

For an over-the-counter antihistamine that causes the least amount of drowsiness, try a product that contains *chlorpheniramine*. Products like **Chlor-Trimeton** *(chlorpheniramine)* may still make you tired, but not as much as *diphenhydramine*. Better yet, for daytime use, look for a combination antihistamine-and-decongestant medicine (like **Actifed**). The decongestant will often counter the groggy effects of the antihistamine. Decongestants are commonly found under the name *pseudoephedrine*. Remember, always carefully read the cautions on the package's label.

A Warning About Phenylpropanolamine: *Phenylpropanolamine—PPA*—was an ingredient in dozens of cold and cough remedies for adults and children (including several **Dimetapp,** **Triaminic,** and **Alka-Seltzer** products) as well as many OTC appetite suppressants. A recently released study at Yale found that PPA increased the risk, for women aged 18–49, of hemorrhagic stroke (which is relatively rare among young people). This is a very serious concern—serious enough for the FDA to issue a public health warning about PPA and take steps to remove it from drug products. They are doing this by asking drug companies to discontinue products with PPA or to reformulate them with other ingredients—and I would certainly encourage women in the at-risk age group to use products that don't contain PPA. While most products now available do not contain this ingredient, there may still be some of the PPA products on your shelves at home.

Prescription treatments

First, your allergist needs to know which allergens are causing the problems. Because it is impossible to keep you away from all pollens and allow you to function normally, an allergy skin test may be required. Your doctor may take a blood test to see if your body is producing antibodies—a response that occurs upon exposure to an allergen. If there are large amounts of a specific type of antibody, say the IgE antibody, the test will help determine exactly what's bothering you. Once your doctor knows what is causing the problem, you must learn how to stay away from it; avoidance of the offending allergen is the most effective treatment of hay fever.

Once hay fever has started, your doctor may prescribe a number of treatments. For those who prefer sprays to tablets, there is a prescription antihistamine nasal spray called **Astelin** that is very effective for sneezing, itchy eyes, and runny nose.

Some doctors prescribe antihistamines like **Claritin** first, to prevent the allergy, or nasal sprays with a steroid ingredient (like **Beconase AQ** or **Rhinocort**) to reduce swelling once an attack has started. **Claritin,** like other prescription antihistamines such as **Allegra** or **Zyrtec,** has the advantage of not making you sleepy like their OTC counterparts.

If these treatments aren't enough to make life bearable, your doctor can start giving you allergy shots. When your body is injected with small amounts of the allergen that causes a reaction, it mounts a response by producing antibodies to fight the next exposure. This process starts with tiny amounts of the allergen, and then builds up until the body can be exposed to an allergen without a reaction. This is a most effective treatment for those who are allergic to insect bites, pollen, and pet dander. I hear the shots are really not all that painful, and being able to breathe again is definitely worth it!

Hives

Q. *How can I tell if a rash on my arm is hives or not? Are hives contagious?*

A. Hives are pretty easy to figure out. If you've just eaten something unusual and you break out with red, itchy patches of skin— usually on the chest, arms, or legs—you probably have hives. If you are just in from the sun, taking an unfamiliar medicine, or under a great deal of stress, and your arms, legs, or chest are covered with swollen red areas that itch intensely, you probably have hives. And you don't have to worry about anyone else catching hives—they aren't contagious.

What Are Hives?

Hives are raised, red, and itchy patches of the skin (called wheals) that affect over 20 percent of the population at one time or another; they are the result of an allergic reaction to something with which your body has been in contact. As with other allergic reactions, when the body perceives a threat, it releases histamines. With hives, these histamines cause intense itching, red bumps, and swelling. Our bodies can even perceive environmental factors like illness and emotional stress as an enemy attack, and the result may be hives.

Hives most commonly appear and then disappear within the same day, but if the stress or other agent causing the reaction isn't removed, they can last for several weeks. It is important to be cautious the first time that you get hives because they can be one of the first symptoms of anaphylactic shock. If the hives progress into difficult breathing, call 911 right away.

Finding the Culprit

Most cases of hives can be traced to one (or even more than one) of the factors below:

- NUTS—peanuts, walnuts, or Brazil nuts
- SEAFOOD—shrimp, clams, other shellfish
- MEDICATION—penicillin, flu vaccines, tetanus shots
- FOODS—strawberries, milk, wheat
- INSECT BITES/STINGS—bees, ants, wasps, hornets
- ENVIRONMENTAL PRESSURES—cold, heat, sunshine, latex
- EMOTIONAL/PHYSICAL STRESS—infections, exercise, home and work stress

You may also see hives referred to as **urticaria**. Urticaria usually refers to hives that are limited to a small area, like a patch on your leg. For more involved and swollen areas, like the whole arm or both legs, the scientific term is **angioedema**. What is most important is not the big medical terms, but how to get rid of the hives quickly.

How Are Hives Treated?

Non-drug treatments

First, and most important, you (or your doctor) must identify what is causing the problem and get away from it as quickly as possible. If you've just eaten a particular food or taken a medicine, stop ingesting it immediately and watch carefully for further signs of allergic reaction. If it is a medication causing the problem, call your doctor so that he can advise you on stopping use of that drug. If the sun is a problem, keep covered up or stay in the shade until the bumps subside.

Avoid exposing the hives to heat, or rubbing the itchy areas. I know it's not easy when you're itching like crazy, but the more the area is warmed or rubbed, the more histamine may be released, making the itching worse. For fast relief while you're deciding on the root cause of the hives, apply cold, moistened compresses. You can apply *chickweed* in a poultice directly on the skin (or even added to the bath) to help with the intense itching of hives. A cup of plain oatmeal in the bathwater can also provide soothing relief for itchy skin; the colloid (or gluelike) substance in oatmeal starch acts as a skin protectant, adds moisture, and soothes irritated and itchy skin.

The Drug Lady Recommends . . .

For soothing relief from the itchiness of hives, put your entire body into a tub of cool water with *Aveeno Oatmeal Bath.* The soothing action of the oatmeal acts to cool the skin and ease the itch. Note: Because oatmeal products can make the bathtub slippery, it is a very good idea to put down a tub mat to prevent a fall.

Benadryl for Itching?

One young mother came into the pharmacy and stood a long time by the OTC allergy products. When I asked if I could help her, she explained that her child's pediatrician had recommended *Benadryl* (*diphenhydramine*) for an itchy rash. She was concerned because all of the Benadryl products on the shelf seemed to be for allergies and sinus conditions, not rashes. She thought that perhaps she had misunderstood the doctor's instructions.

The child's mother had indeed heard right. Benadryl (diphenhydramine) is in the class of medicines called antihistamines. An antihistamine stops the allergic reaction in the body whether it comes from an allergy in your nose or from an allergen that causes a rash. Benadryl products are used for itchy rashes (available in liquid form for children), for seasonal and perennial allergies (in tablets or capsules), even directly on skin rashes (in a cream form).

OTC treatments

For milder cases of hives, grab some of the antihistamine **Benadryl** (*diphenhydramine*) for fast itch relief. Available in cream, liquid, capsule, and tablet forms, this medicine helps slow down the allergic reaction that is taking place in your body. *Hydrocortisone* creams are also very effective for controlling the itch.

Prescription treatments

If it is your first case of hives or an unusually severe or long-lasting episode, it is a good idea to visit a doctor as soon as possible. Some cases of hives require corticosteroids (like *prednisone*) or prescription antihistamines (like *hydroxyzine*).

Hives that don't respond to antihistamines or corticosteroids and are hindering your ability to breathe may need to be treated quickly with an *epinephrine* (*adrenaline*) shot. This drug will quickly open the breathing passages and could save your life.

Latex Allergies

Q. *My friend always fills out her medical profile with "latex" as something she's allergic to. I was embarrassed to ask her how she knew she was allergic to latex. Is that really an allergy?*

A. Latex allergies are indeed real allergies. Your friend is suffering from the same condition that plagues nearly 6 percent of the entire population. It may be hard to believe, but latex products (like surgical gloves) have over 200 proteins, which can be potential allergens. Most of the cases of latex allergies occur among health-care providers who must deal with or wear these medical products daily. It is amazing just how much we depend on latex in our daily lives. Products made from latex include condoms, gloves, catheters, tubing for stethoscopes, ports for IVs, envelope glue, carpet backing, and balloons. If you work around these substances, having an allergy to them can mean you will have an adverse reaction to almost everything you touch or use.

What Is a Latex Allergy?

Latex is produced mainly from the sap of the Brazilian rubber tree. This tree has proteins that are foreign to our bodies' own systems. The latex is further processed by adding preservatives and chemicals, which also can cause allergic reactions. Certain fruits, particularly kiwi, avocados, or papayas, may contain these same allergenic proteins.

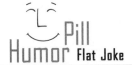

Pill Humor Flat Joke

The doctor tells the patient that he has the new disease called "HEGS."

The patient inquires, "What's HEGS?"

"It's a combination of hives, encephalitis, gonorrhea, and syphilis," the doctor replies.

The patient asks, "What's the cure?"

The doctor responds, "Well, we have to keep you in a hospital room and feed you nothing except pancakes until the disease goes away."

"Pancakes? How can pancakes cure my disease?" asks the patient.

The doctor answers, "Oh, they can't. That's the only food we can slip under the door."

Latex allergies are often referred to as "latex's triple threat," meaning those who are allergic experience a contact dermatitis reaction, an immediate hypersensitivity reaction, and an allergic contact dermatitis. The result is a combination of symptoms that include severe itching and cracking open of the skin, red sores and bumps, swelling of the contact area, runny nose and eyes, difficulty breathing, and in severe cases, anaphylactic shock. A latex allergy can produce an anaphylactic reaction that is just as potentially life threatening as a penicillin allergy. Even more disturbing is that these symptoms don't generally show up the first time you are exposed to latex, but may appear from six to as long as forty-eight hours later. These wonderful symptoms can hang around for up to a week after the latex has been removed.

Causes of Latex Allergy

A latex allergy may begin when one or more of the over 200 proteins found in latex products find their way into the body. This can occur through the skin, from injections, or by breathing in the powder on the inside of balloons or gloves. You may have noticed that gloves have a cornstarch powder inside to help keep hands dry. This powder can hold on to proteins and send them into the air whenever the gloves are taken off.

Latex allergies also can be seen in both men and women who are allergic to condoms. This type of allergy doesn't always occur the first time someone is exposed to latex, but often after the sensitivity builds up over repeated exposure. Allergic reactions to the latex in condoms can result in itching and redness of very sensitive areas.

How Are Latex Allergies Treated?

Non-drug treatments

The most effective way to treat a latex allergy is to prevent it from happening. Unfortunately, this is usually much easier said than done. When your livelihood depends on using latex gloves on a daily basis (as it does for medical personnel) or when your medical condition requires sometimes hourly changes of latex equipment (such as IV bags), avoiding contact with latex is nearly impossible.

The Drug Lady Recommends . . .

If you must wear gloves in your line of work, try wearing non-latex gloves or even cotton gloves under the latex to reduce your exposure to the allergic proteins. For individuals who have experienced a **latex allergy**, it is a good idea to always have an anaphylaxis kit, like *EpiPen*, and to wear a ***Medic-Alert*** emblem, just in case.

In the last few years, the FDA has begun to put more pressure on the companies making latex products to ensure that they are safer for general use. The proteins that cause many allergies are being identified and removed during the manufacturing process.

OTC treatments

Hydrocortisone or antihistamine cream (*diphenhydramine*) applied to the itching area can bring temporary relief. Over-the-counter antihistamines, like **Chlor-Trimeton** (*chlorpheniramine*), are also a short-term solution until the latex problem is removed.

Prescription treatments

Often the latex allergy is so severe that prescription treatment is required. Your doctor may prescribe a steroid, like *prednisone,* to decrease swelling or even a histamine H2-blocker, like **Tagamet** (*cimetidine),* to slow down the allergic response.

THREE

Children's Good Health: "Oh, Baby!"

ADHD ▩ Asthma ▩ Baby Gas ▩ Chicken Pox ▩ Children's Diarrhea ▩

Colds and Coughs ▩ Cradle Cap ▩ Diaper Rash ▩ Earache ▩ Fever ▩

Fluoride Supplements (see Chapter 7) ▩ Head Lice ▩ Impetigo ▩ Jaundice ▩

Lactose Intolerance ▩ Nausea and Vomiting ▩ Pain ▩ Pinworms ▩

Reye's Syndrome ▩ Teething

ALL PARENTS FEEL truly powerless when their children get sick. They depend on us for so much, yet when they look up at us with a fever or in pain, it often makes us realize how much there is to know about their special needs. In many ways we think of our children as small adults, but with medicines this notion can cause them harm. Drugs have different effects on adults than they do on children—sometimes even opposite reactions. Dosage for children is another often-complicated factor a parent must consider. Combine these challenges with actually getting the little one to swallow the medicine, and it really makes you wish they came with instructions! Chicken pox, fevers, earache, and head lice are just some of the common but nevertheless formidable ailments awaiting you and your child. Let's take a look at some of the best ways to tackle them.

ADHD

Q. *I am interested in learning more about what medicines can be taken safely for ADHD. My son was recently diagnosed, and some of the medications scare me.*

A. Your son's diagnosis is shared by as many as 10 percent of all schoolchildren in the United States! In fact, ADD and ADHD are now the most common developmental problems found in childhood. The inability to pay attention is called attention deficit disorder (ADD). If this problem is combined with a high activity level of hyperactivity, the clinical name is attention-deficit/hyperactivity disorder (ADHD).

What Is ADHD?

A child is said to have ADHD when he or she shows a very short attention span, a constant high level of excitement, inability to prioritize and organize, excessive fidgeting and talking, and impulsiveness that isn't quite appropriate for children their age. Most children who suffer from this condition are male, and are on the high side of normal in intelligence. Medical science has many theories for what causes ADHD, but one of the most accepted is that the brain overproduces a chemical so that the child has difficulty processing normal sensory messages.

ADHD may begin to appear around the age of three and continue until the late teens, when it generally disappears. ADHD will generally run in families, too. If the symptoms listed above sound like any normal five-year-old, that simply highlights the importance of making sure you have an accurate diagnosis from your pediatrician (or a specialist) before treating your child with any medications.

Signs and Symptoms of ADHD

Because so many ADHD symptoms are just typical behavior for a growing child, it is important that the doctor have time to make a good diagnosis. It is also appropriate to ask for a second opinion from a doctor who specializes in ADHD. Here are a few common signs of possible ADHD.

- Extreme impulsiveness
- Fidgets excessively
- Difficulty with schoolwork
- Excessive talking and interrupting
- Difficulty following instructions
- Difficulty taking turns
- Not being able to organize tasks
- Easily distracted

How is ADHD treated?

Non-drug treatments

Because so little is known about the cause of ADHD, non-drug treatments are among the most experimental. There is enough support for the role that diet plays that many doctors recommend a high protein, low carbohydrate diet. Since this type of diet is good for children anyway, it's worth a try. There is much more to the treatment of ADD and ADHD than taking medicines. Often the whole family can benefit from support groups and behavioral therapy. This isn't just a condition that affects the child—it affects the entire family. For example, for those children who simply require more structure in their lives, a therapist can work with a family to establish routines that help the child find that structure.

Extra B vitamins, in the form of a *B-complex* supplement, may help restore the delicate chemical balance of the brain.

Evening Primrose Oil (EPO) has been used successfully in some chil-

The Drug Lady Recommends . . .

A complementary natural product showing promise for children with ADD and ADHD is *Efalex*. This product contains a combination of *evening primrose oil, purified tuna oil, vitamin E, omega-3 fatty acids* (DHA,GLA, AA), and *thyme oil*. These oils are thought to be low in children who suffer from ADHD and may play a part in influencing behavior. Ask your doctor about the possibility of adding Efalex to your child's treatment. Also, be aware that it may take up to three months for the child's body to replenish its store of essential fatty acids.

dren who have been determined to have low blood levels of fatty acids. Adding this to some children's diets at a dose of 2–3 grams daily produced remarkable results. Other essential fatty acids include *linoleic, linolenic,* and *arachidonic* forms. These fatty acids are important for proper transmission of nerve impulses. They may act to maintain proper brain and eye function as well as influence behavior.

OTC treatments

ADHD is a condition that shouldn't be left to over-the-counter medicines, although a good daily multivitamin just might help. If you suspect that your child may be suffering from ADHD, call the doctor right away. Help is available for your child and the whole family.

Prescription treatments

Proper diagnosis of ADHD is key. Your child's doctor will make a diagnosis based on a collection of criteria over time. Because of the controversy surrounding indiscriminate ADHD medication prescribing, it is important to share your concerns with the doctor and not to be afraid to ask for a second opinion.

Generally, treatment for ADHD starts with a stimulant like **Ritalin** (*methylphenidate*), long-acting **Concerta** (*methylphenidate*), **Adderall** (*amphetamine salt*), or **Dexedrine** (*dextroamphetamine*). It may seem strange to give these drugs to a child who seems already overstimulated, but they act to calm the hyperactivity in a child's body. Side effects may include a dry mouth, irritability, inability to sleep, or dizziness. These side effects are normal and will generally go away as the child becomes more used to the medicine.

If these stimulants don't give the results hoped for, **Catapres** (*clonidine*) may be added or used alone. Antidepressants, like **Tofranil** (*imipramine*), **Wellbutrin** (*bupropion*), and **Norpramine** (*desipramine*), may also be effective for maintaining a proper brain chemistry balance.

Asthma

Q. *My daughter has been diagnosed with asthma and we have many questions about her condition and especially her medicines and how to use them. Can you help?*

A. Asthma can be a very difficult condition to deal with, both for the child who suffers from it and for the parent who must watch helplessly as the child struggles to take in a breath of air. The wheezing and coughing can be a frightening experience. In the past, having asthma meant skipping and sitting out strenuous activities. Today, however, the prognosis for childhood asthma is good. With proper medication and care, an asthma sufferer doesn't have to miss out on any activities.

What Is Asthma?

Asthma is a lung condition that affects over twelve million Americans. It occurs when the bronchial tubes and/or lungs react to allergens, smoke, cold air, stress, and even exercise and begin to constrict or narrow, very quickly. As the airways become irritated, they swell and begin to secrete sticky mucus in an attempt to fight off what they see as a threat in the form of cold air, exercise, or pollen grains. Allergies and asthma are very closely related. In fact, a large percentage of individuals who suffer from allergies also have asthma.

How Is Asthma Treated?

Non-drug treatments

Because of the seriousness of an asthmatic condition, most health-care providers recommend medical treatment first and the use of non-drug and OTC treatments as a complement to that treatment.

Taking warm, steamy baths with a few drops of *lavender* or *eucalyptus* essential oil does wonders to open and soothe inflamed airways. Use care to avoid getting this oil directly on the skin as it can be irritating to the skin if not properly diluted.

Some asthma sufferers have been shown to have lower-than-normal levels of *magnesium* and certain *B-complex* vitamins. An adult supplement dose of *magnesium* is 200 to 400 mg three times daily; *vitamin B-6,* 25 to 50 mg twice daily; *vitamin B-12,* 1000 mcg per day. Divide the dose in half for children 50 to 100 pounds, and by one-third for children 50 to 25 pounds. For those under 25 pounds, consult the doctor for recommendations. Adjusting the dose and adding these to your older child's daily regimen is a good way to fight asthma more naturally.

Learning to avoid and deemphasize stressful situations is helpful for stress-induced asthma attacks. Identify the triggers that seem to make your child's asthma worse, and keep an ongoing diary. Avoiding irritants in the environment, like cold air or smoky rooms, can thwart an attack before it occurs.

The Drug Lady Recommends . . .

Using a **peak-flow meter** regularly is a way to measure how much the airways are blocked. By having your child exhale into this handheld meter, you can measure how strongly his lungs are able to push air out. Your health-care provider will be able to help you set a range on the meter for your child that shows when everything is clear and when medicine may be needed. By keeping one of these devices at home, you can monitor asthma conditions before they reach a crisis level.

OTC treatments

Those who suffer from asthma attacks should not turn to the OTC shelf for answers. While there are certain products specifically advertised to help with asthma, these may be harmful if not used with appropriate medical care. Products like **Primatene Mist** contain a very small amount of the medication *epinephrine,* advertised as being able to open airways quickly. However, few health-care providers recommend the use of this medicine without proper monitoring. Very often, a first asthma attack will be much milder than progressive ones. Without the right dosage of medicine to help open the airways, your child's life could be in danger.

Prescription treatments

Prescription treatments for asthma are generally one of three types:

- bronchodilators that open the airways quickly
- anti-inflammatory steroids that decrease the swelling in the airways over time
- anti-allergy medicines that work to decrease the allergic reactions that cause some forms of asthma

Bronchodilators like *albuterol* (**Proventil** or **Ventolin**) are used for relief during an asthma attack. They are available in a portable inhaler form and in liquid forms for use in the **nebulizer**. Albuterol is also available in tablet and syrup form.

Anti-inflammatory steroids, like **Azmacort** (*triamcinolone*) or **Flonase** (*fluticasone*), are used to prevent asthma attacks from occurring. These should be used every day and NOT during an actual attack. The medicine in these products acts to prevent allergen exposure–induced swelling in the airways. In emergency situations the doctor may prescribe a stronger steroid like **Prelone** (*prednisolone*) to keep the airways open. This liquid is generally given in a large dose, then decreased or tapered down over the next few days until the asthma is under control. Often this drug is used in combination with one of the bronchodilators for maximum breathing capability.

What Is the Best Way to Use an Asthma Inhaler?

Asthma medicines come in many different forms. One of the most portable ways to carry these medicines everywhere you go is in a metered-dose inhaler (or MDI for short). Asthma medicines taken this way go right into the airways where it will be most effective in the shortest amount of time. Younger children do well with liquid or nebulizer asthma medications, while the MDIs are a better choice for older children who have the dexterity to use them effectively. Practice with your child to be sure the medicine is getting into the airways, where it will be effective.

■ Taking it out of the box is a good first step! Some pharmacies put the prescription label on the outside of an MDI box, so be sure to jot down the prescription number before you throw the box away in case you need to call in for the child's refill.

■ Shake the MDI several times before starting the puffing procedure. Removing the cap from the mouthpiece can prevent injuries from flying caps to friends standing close by.

■ Have the child exhale completely before taking a puff. No "waiting to exhale" here.

■ Hold the mouthpiece about three finger-widths from the mouth.

■ Open mouth. Aim. As your child starts to breathe in, have him press down the top of the container . . . and fire!

■ Keep inhaling until the lungs are full. Take a big breath!

■ Hold this breath for as long as possible. Try counting to five by one-thousands. 1,001 . . . 1,002 . . . 1,003 . . .

■ Exhale.

■ If your child's doctor prescribes more than one puff, have the child wait at least one minute before repeating; longer than a minute is better, but try to hold off at least for sixty seconds.

Anti-allergy prescriptions, like **Claritin** (*loratidine*) or **Zyrtec** (*cetirizine*), block the receptors that react to allergic histamines. Without an allergic reaction, many episodes of asthma can be avoided.

Baby Gas

Q. *A very tired young mother came to my counter with a tiny infant who was bellowing at the top of her little lungs. "We've been up all night and she won't stop screaming. The doctor's office says it's gas, but she just won't burp. What can I do?"*

A. Baby gas—one of the great joys of parenting! Your little angel swallows air or her formula doesn't quite agree with her, and her tummy fills up with gas. Usually burping or other equally pleasant ways of expelling the air will do the trick, but sometimes she just can't get rid of it. She hurts! Poor baby! Gas is very common in babies, so you're not alone. It affects almost half of all newborns within the first two months of life.

What Causes Baby Gas?

The most common cause of gas in your child's tummy is that her new little system must get used to digesting and coping with food. Breast milk or formula contains proteins and milk sugars that must be broken down. Mother's breast milk may even contain traces of gas-producing foods (like cabbage or broccoli) that upset baby's tummy. Moms—watch what you're eating!

Your baby may be allergic to certain ingredients in the milk she drinks or she may suffer **lactose intolerance.** If you are formula-feeding, it may be necessary to switch formulas to find the right match for her system.

Infant gas also can be traced to little screamers who swallow big gulps of air with every yell. This excessive swallowing of air builds up pressure in the tummy, and what goes in must come out. In addition to crying, your baby may show symptoms of gas by pulling her legs up tight against her body or lying in a curled position.

How Is Baby Gas Treated?

Non-drug treatments

For non-drug relief you might try laying your baby on your lap, on her back with her head resting on your knees and her legs toward you. Gently pump her legs up and down in a "bicycling" motion.

As your baby's intestines mature, the gassy stage will pass. Have patience, parents!

OTC treatments

If your baby begins showing symptoms of excess gas—like crying constantly, flatulence, or lying in a fetal position—give the doctor a call before you try the over-the-counter gas remedies. Chances are you'll be directed to the baby-gas department of your local pharmacy, but with little ones, it's best to be absolutely sure first.

The Drug Lady Recommends . . .

As the gas bubbles build up, it is up to you to help the baby get rid of that excess pressure. Products like *Infants' Mylicon Drops,* a brand of *simethecone,* will give rapid relief. Mylicon Drops work gently to break down gas bubbles in minutes and are safe because they are not absorbed into your baby's system. For babies under two years of age, the dosage of Infants' Mylicon Drops is 0.3 ml four times daily, after meals and at bedtime, or as directed by a physician. The drops can also be mixed with one ounce of cool water, infant formula, breast milk, or other suitable liquids to make it easier to get down.

Prescription treatments

Some infants may require something more than the over-the-counter remedies can provide. If discomfort persists, give the doctor a call. Small doses of medicines like **Reglan** (*metoclopramide*) work by emptying the stomach out faster and thereby avoiding the formation of gas. Your pediatrician will have the right answers if the over-the-counter products just aren't quite enough to stop the painful gas.

Humor Pill

Did you hear about the baby born in the new high-tech Seattle delivery room?
It was cordless!

Chicken Pox

Q. *We have the chicken pox! Well, my two children have chicken pox. What can I do to make life around our house more bearable?*

A. Congratulations! It's not often that you get to have chicken pox in a two-for-one deal. Life around your house is going to be lots of fun for the next couple of weeks. Let's see if we can help make things just a little easier.

What Is Chicken Pox?

Most of us remember having the chicken pox in childhood, when we were repeatedly told, "Don't scratch that, you'll leave a scar!" This disease occurs most often in children under the age of nine, but adults have been known to get it a second time, too. Chicken pox is caused by a virus from the herpes family called *varicella*.

The first symptoms usually appear with a low-grade fever and the child feeling grumpier than normal. The rash usually begins on the trunk, but within the next few hours the face and head often will be covered with an itchy mask. The red bumps will develop a liquid-filled blister on top. It's when these blisters break open that the itching becomes the fiercest. There can be up to five hundred of these on one small body at one time! These itchy bumps will continue to appear over the next seven days or so. Hang in there, parents, it will be over soon!

Encourage your children NOT to scratch the pox—they really can leave scars. Your child may not have much of an appetite during this whole ordeal; headache and general fussiness are also the norm. The contagious period starts about twenty-four hours before you ever see a rash and lasts until all the blisters have dried into scabs. Adults can show symptoms up to twenty-one days after being exposed. The chicken-pox vaccine is recommended for children and adults who haven't had the disease.

How Is Chicken Pox Treated?

Non-drug treatments

Baths in cool water with baking soda added can be a wonderful "Ahhh" for itchy skin. Wet compresses of baking soda also can provide quick relief. A cupful of uncooked oatmeal added to the bath may also soothe and cool the blister.

Also, trimming the fingernails short can prevent scratching, keeping those scars to a minimum.

OTC treatments

Oatmeal baths, like **Aveeno,** help soothe hot skin and ease the itch. Aveeno also makes a lotion of colloidal oatmeal that feels wonderful on itchy chicken-pox sores.

For pain relief and fever reduction, **Tylenol** (*acetaminophen*) is a good choice, NOT aspirin—**Reye's syndrome** has been linked to chicken pox (and influenza) and aspirin consumption in children and teens (see "Reye's Syndrome," page 99).

Antihistamines like **Benadryl** (*diphenhydramine*) help stop the itch from the inside. Available in both liquid and chewable forms, antihista-

The Drug Lady Recommends . . .

Those people who think of everything must have come up with *Caladryl* lotion; it does double-duty. This product combines the drying agent of calamine lotion with a topical anti-itch formulation of *Benadryl.* Keeping the bottle cool is also a nice trick to get even more relief. It's important that this product (and many other topical antihistamines) be used only on children over 12 months old. Ask your pediatrician about recommendations for the younger set.

mines are an excellent choice for easing the itchies of many children. Beware that most antihistamines may cause excitability in children, so time the doses accordingly.

Prescription treatments

If your child has a serious medical condition that could weaken his or her immune system, the doctor may prescribe the antiviral medicine *Zovirax* (*acyclovir*). To be effective, it must be given within the first twenty-four hours (that's within twenty-four hours of first seeing the rash). By the time the blisters appear, it's often too late for antiviral medicines to work.

Children's Diarrhea

Q. *My one-year-old son seems to suffer quite a bit from diarrhea. The doctor says that it's normal, but is there anything that I should do?*

A. I imagine the messy diapers are a challenge. It probably isn't terribly comfortable for your son, either. Diarrhea in youngsters is commonly traced to their diet, unlike diarrhea in adults, which is often tied to both diet and stress concerns.

Other types of diarrhea that are of concern in children are caused by viruses, bacteria, or parasites. Diarrhea can also be traced to food poisoning, or a recent sickness that included treatment with antibiotics. It's great that you talked to your child's doctor first, because excessive diarrhea in little bodies can cause problems very quickly.

What Is Children's Diarrhea?

As children's bodies grow, the frequency and uniformity of their bowel movements change. Diarrhea in children is defined medically as a sudden change in bowel habits to include loose, watery stools. Often diarrhea is classified according to how often and how much the child is filling up the diaper. For children who are on solid food, here are some guidelines to follow. (All kids are different, however, so it's a good idea to go by what is "normal" for your own child.)

■ Mild diarrhea: three to four stools in twenty-four hours; these may be loose and somewhat watery, but not particularly large in volume.

■ Moderate diarrhea: five to six stools in twenty-four hours; these may be loose, but not watery enough to leak out of the diaper.

■ Severe diarrhea: seven or more stools in twenty-four hours; these are liquid enough to run down the legs and can require a total clothing change.

How Is Diarrhea in Children Treated?

Diarrhea is one of those childhood conditions that requires vigilance—and possibly quick action. Children can lose a large percentage of their

Signs of Dehydration

Because children have such small bodies, their systems can quickly dehydrate from diarrhea. This is a potentially dangerous condition that can sneak up on even the most observant parent. Here are some signs of dehydration to looked out for when your child is suffering from diarrhea.

For all children:

■ dry mouth

■ no tears when crying

■ inactivity or lethargy

■ sunken eyes

■ cool and blotchy hands and feet

■ fast and weak pulse

■ no urination for several hours

Especially for infants:

■ fewer than six wet diapers per day or if the baby isn't wet for more than 8 hours

■ a soft spot in the top of the head that looks sunken

body fluids VERY quickly, which is the main danger associated with diarrhea in children.

Non-drug treatments

If your child is on solid foods, adding small amounts of bananas, rice (or rice cereal), applesauce, or toast (or crackers) can help give more substance to the stool and still be easy enough on the child's stomach. Clear liquids are also a very good idea.

OTC treatments

When diarrhea strikes your child, a common recommendation from pediatricians is to give him children's electrolyte-replacement drinks like **Pedialyte.** It is very important not to give children any adult diarrhea medicines without consulting a doctor, as they can be damaging to the children's systems. Some OTC diarrhea medications, like **Kaopectate** or **Diasorb,** may be safer for the younger set because they contain the active ingredient *attapulgite,* a claylike substance that binds bacteria and toxins from the colon and acts to absorb water and make the stools firmer.

The Drug Lady Recommends . . .

Keep *Pedialyte* or other types of electrolyte replacements handy, in a favorite form like freezer pops. This way, if a bout of diarrhea comes up in the wee hours of the morning, you'll be prepared. These cool, tasty treats soothe children, as well as providing the necessary salts and sugars that can be lost so quickly with diarrhea.

Prescription treatments

Your child's doctor may prescribe medication to speed up the motion of the digestive system (like *metoclopramide*) or he or she may elect to just wait it out. If it is a bacterium or protozoa causing the problems, an antibiotic may be prescribed.

Colds and Coughs

Q. *What can I use safely for my three-year-old's cold? He's coughing, stuffed up, and miserable, and no one is getting much sleep!*

A. When your little one has a cold and cough, the whole family is miserable. Your child's inability to tell you exactly how he feels leaves many parents playing detective to find the right medicine to fit the symptoms. Parents must also take many factors into consideration when treating cold symptoms—the child's weight and age, past behavior when not feeling well—and then comb through the multitude of children's products lining the pharmacy shelves.

What Causes a Child's Cold and Cough?

New parents typically get a few weeks' reprieve from infant colds and coughs because the baby still has immunities obtained from Mom's antibodies; breast-feeding helps continue this protective action a little longer. Soon, however, the world's relentless attack of viruses and bacteria takes its toll, and your child's system caves in—the sniffles, sneezes, stuffy noses, runny noses, and coughs make their first appearance. Blame rhinovirus, the bug that finds a nice home in the respiratory system and is associated with "the common cold." It is not unusual for babies from six months to two years in age to have six to ten colds every year! That's a lot of "little" colds and coughs.

Children's cold symptoms typically begin with a runny or stuffy nose, low-grade fever (under 101 degrees Fahrenheit), sore or scratchy throat, and cough (either phlegmy or dry and hacking). The good news is that it will typically run its course in about a week to ten days; unfortunately, as of yet, there is no cure for coughs and colds, only symptomatic treatment.

How Are Children's Colds and Coughs Treated?

Non-drug treatments

A cool-mist vaporizer is a must for every home with young children. Colds and coughs can be very drying to the mucus membranes of the nose and throat; adding extra moisture to the air can be a welcome relief.

The Drug Lady Recommends . . .

Giving steamy baths with *Johnson's Soothing Vapor Bath*. This wonderful combination of oils of *eucalyptus, menthol,* and *rosemary* opens stuffy noses and eases coughs by relaxing the child (and parents too). It's safe for babies over three months old.

Administer saline nose drops and use a bulb syringe to gently aspirate nasal mucus to open stuffed noses. To cool a feverish forehead, try the **TheraPatch Fever** cool-gel patch for kids; these cool instantly and last for hours.

Encourage your child to drink plenty of fluids—more fluids generally mean thinner mucus in the nose and chest.

OTC treatments

There are many products on the market designed to treat cold and cough symptoms in children. The best idea is to narrow down your child's symptom list and pick products accordingly.

▨ Fever and aches. For babies up to twenty-three months old or weighing 23 pounds, try **Infants' Tylenol Concentrated Drops;** these work to decrease fever and ease the aches of being sick. The dosage is based on weight for greatest accuracy, so read the directions carefully—and, of course, call your pediatrician before administering any medication to your child. For children twenty-four months old and over 24 pounds, **Children's Tylenol Elixir** or **Soft-Chew Chewables** provide a tasty way to keep fevers at bay.

The Drug Lady Recommends...

Triaminic AM Decongestant Formula (pseudoephedrine) is a popular orange-flavored syrup that children really seem to like, even if it is medicine. The Triaminic products give professional labeling guidelines for younger children based on weight.

■ Stuffed noses. *Afrin Children's Nasal Decongestant Spray* contains the decongestant *phenylephrine* to give quick, short-term relief for children aged six to twelve. Younger stuffed noses may respond well to *Triaminic Infant Oral Decongestant Drops.* Again, always consult your pediatrician before beginning any over-the-counter or prescription medicine.

■ Runny noses. When a runny nose is a symptom, the medication to look for is an antihistamine; these dry the drips quickly. Allergies also respond well to antihistamines like *brompheniramine, diphenhydramine,* or *chlorpheniramine.*

■ Coughs. When your child's cough keeps everyone up at night, a cough suppressant (*dextromethorphan*) with an expectorant (*guaifenesin*) to thin mucus is in order. *Robitussin-DM Syrup* or *Infant Drops* should be a standby in every home.

■ Sore throats. *Dimetapp "Get Better Bear" Freezer Pops* are a great product that can soothe irritated throats. These ice treats contain *pectin* to help stop the sore and scratchy feeling.

Prescription treatments

When a child first begins to show symptoms of a **cold** or cough, many parents run to the doctor for an antibiotic. Unfortunately, this usually isn't the best course to take. Antibiotics aren't effective against a virus. Because a virus usually causes cold symptoms, giving an antibiotic for a simple cold will only increase the resistance of other bacteria his body is fighting.

If the virus weakens your child's system, bacteria may find a home in the ears (see "Earache," page 74), eyes (see "Pinkeye," page 169), or lungs (causing a cough). These are the cases that warrant the use of an antibiotic. Your child's pediatrician will determine which one to write a prescription for based on the child's particular symptoms.

If over-the-counter cough remedies aren't effective for your child, the doctor may prescribe a syrup containing *codeine* to suppress the cough reflex.

Cradle Cap

Q. *Our new baby has a rash on her head that my mother calls "cradle cap." What is this? Should we see the doctor or will it go away on its own? Is there something I can buy over-the-counter?*

A. First, I'd like to offer congratulations on the new addition to your family. Now don't worry—cradle cap is not a serious condition. However, I know that you want her looking her best for those first photos and first visits from her adoring public!

What Is Cradle Cap?

"Cradle cap" is a common name for a specific type of inflammation or rash called **seborrheic dermatitis** (a type of eczema) that sometimes occurs on the heads of newborns. It has nothing to do with a cradle, but the rash does somewhat resemble a crusty, yellow cap. In some infants, seborrheic dermatitis may develop only in the diaper area and the rash will have a thicker, scalier appearance; these scales are also called "plaques." Seborrheic dermatitis appears to run in families. It is not contagious, it is not caused by poor hygiene, it is not an allergy, and it is not dangerous; it is simply a skin condition that your baby has and will probably outgrow. Experts seem to think that it is caused by hormones passed on by Mom before the baby's birth. These hormones stimulate the skin's oil glands and skin cells to go into overdrive, thus causing the rash.

How Is Cradle Cap Treated?

Cradle cap generally disappears completely on its own by the time the child is eight months to a year old. But of course you don't want to wait that long for those adorable pictures. Your baby's pediatrician may have specific recommendations for getting the best results in minimizing the yellow skin rash.

Non-drug treatments

Some doctors find that applying *mineral oil* to the scalp helps dissolve the crusty skin plaques. These can be easily removed from the hair with a soft sponge, a soft toothbrush, or a baby brush. *Baby oil* and *petrolatum jelly* also work well to loosen and remove the scales.

The Drug Lady Recommends . . .

Washing your baby's head every two or three days with a gentle baby shampoo, like *Johnson's Baby Shampoo*, is helpful for moistening and dissolving the scalp plaques. Cradle cap will come back, so continue to wash the affected areas whenever an outbreak occurs. Have patience—your baby WILL grow out of it!

OTC treatments

Your pediatrician may recommend the use of an over-the-counter steroid cream like *hydrocortisone* to decrease the inflammation and spreading of the rash. Sometimes cradle cap is itchy for the little one and this helps decrease the itch.

Prescription treatments

If it looks as though the cradle cap is getting worse or is spreading, call your pediatrician. He or she may prescribe a stronger steroid cream to slow it down. For severe problems, your doctor may prescribe shampoos that contain *coal tar*, or scalp creams that contain *cortisone*. For cradle cap that has open sores, a topical antibiotic like **Bactroban** *(mupirocin)* may be necessary to prevent infection from starting.

Diaper Rash

Q. *What is the best medicine for diaper rash? My baby's behind seems to be bright red no matter what I do. Help!*

A. A bright red baby behind is a condition most parents face. The last thing in the world you want is for your baby to hurt, but unfortunately, at some point in their lives almost all young children will experience the pain and discomfort of a diaper rash. A diaper rash can vary in severity from a mild redness with accompanying soreness to painful, open sores in the diaper area. The good news is that diaper rash can be treated—and children don't stay in diapers forever!

What Causes Diaper Rash?

Most cases of diaper rash occur due to contact of baby's tender skin with the child's urine or stools. Foods eaten by a nursing mom, or baby's formula, may also cause problems. Some other causes of diaper rash may include allergic reactions to soaps, laundry detergents, baby powders, or lotions. If your child is taking antibiotics, they may cause diarrhea, which also increases his chances of developing the rash. With all these possible irritants, it is no wonder that most babies will suffer from diaper rash at some point. Let's take a look at what to do once this happens and how to prevent it as much as possible.

The common factor in all types of diaper rashes is skin wetness. Diaper wetness can increase friction, and makes the skin more pliable and easier to tear. This dampness, in combination with stool enzymes or other irritants, causes redness and painful inflammation. With a diaper rash the skin may appear red, raw, and cracked, and may feel painful or itchy to the baby. Most rashes should clear up within three or four days when treated properly.

How Is Diaper Rash Treated?

Non-drug treatments

The best way to prevent diaper rash is to keep your baby as dry and clean as possible, but we all know that sometimes this is easier said than done. If your baby seems to be predisposed to a sore bottom, you may want to avoid using disposable diapers or rubber pants, and try to stay away from strong detergents and bleaches. Try *Ivory* or those that advertise to be hypoallergenic.

Change diapers frequently and immediately after urination or bowel movements. Wipe the baby's bottom well after changing the diaper. Be sure to dry the area thoroughly before reapplying a clean diaper.

Babies on a high-protein formula may be more susceptible to diaper

Types of Diaper Rashes

The term *diaper rash* is really an umbrella term for many different disorders:

- ▓ Friction rashes—caused by irritating, rubbing contact between the diaper and the baby's skin. It is most commonly found along the inner thighs or where the elastic from diapers tends to gather.
- ▓ Irritant rashes—caused by irritants like laundry detergents, soaps, or lotions. Friction and irritant rashes resemble a Picasso painting of red splotches.
- ▓ Intertrigo rashes—caused by moist heat as when a damp diaper has been left on for too long. A red, thin-looking layer of skin identifies this type of rash.

rashes due to the higher acid content of their urine. This acid produces a type of burn that closely resembles a diaper rash. If this is a problem, changing the baby's formula may be all that's necessary to avoid the red bottom.

The Drug Lady Recommends...

Dry, dry, dry! The drier the bottom, the better the chance the diaper area will stay healthy. Exposing the affected area to air also can aid in the healing process, as can applying the diaper loosely, or allowing your baby to go without a diaper for a while. The more air, the more quickly the rash will heal—and bare baby bottoms are so cute!

OTC treatments

There are several over-the-counter treatments available to help cure diaper rash. As a first step, look to protectants like *zinc oxide* or *petrolatum.* These agents coat and cover the skin, protecting it from contact with urine or stool; names to look for are **Balmex, Desitin,** or **Diaperine.** An *aloe vera* ointment may also help clear up rashes and soothe the burning skin. All of these ointments or creams should be applied in a thick layer with each diaper change or as prescribed by your doctor. Avoid using premoistened towelettes if your child has a rash; they tend to sting.

The Drug Lady Recommends...

Another general-purpose protectant called **A&D Ointment** contains *cod-liver oil* as a source of vitamins A and D. Vitamin A, applied in ointment form, has been shown to play a role in forming and maintaining healthy skin structure. This is an excellent skin protectant not only for diaper rash, but also for other minor skin injuries.

Prescription treatments

If your baby's diaper rash takes the form of a more serious, yeastlike fungal infection (most often from *candida albicans*), prescription treatment is necessary. Your doctor may prescribe *nystatin* powder that is applied directly to the bottom with each diaper change. Some prefer a combination cream, like **Mycolog II,** with both an antifungal (*nystatin*) and a steroid (*triamcinolone*) to help reduce the swelling, redness, and itching.

The baby's rash may also be the signal that something else is going on. It's time to call the doctor if

■ the rash persists for more than four days, or if any of the treatments seem to worsen the rash.

■ the rash stays bright red or raw-looking for several days despite treatment, or if you notice small red dots on the baby's bottom. This might signal a bacterial infection.

■ crusting, large blisters, or pus begin to appear.

■ your baby develops a fever.

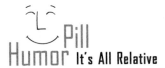

Humor Pill It's All Relative

A man calls the hospital frantically from his cell phone. "My wife is pregnant and her contractions are only two minutes apart! What should we be doing?"

"Is this her first child?" the nurse on the other end asks.

"No, No, No!" the man shouts. "This is her husband!"

Earache

Q. *My child seems to always have an earache. I hate to see her in so much pain. What can we do to make it better?*

A. Seeing your little one in pain with an earache can be a frustrating experience. To add to the frustration, it is sometimes difficult to determine exactly what is the cause of the problem. Because an earache may be due to an infection, too much earwax (see "Earwax," chapter 6, page 162), or even water trapped deep within the ear—the best advice is to see the doctor right away.

What Causes an Earache?

With young children and infants, the earache may quickly appear with symptoms of pain (shown by tugging or rubbing the ears), fever, and more grumpiness than usual. The pain results from a swollen blockage of the eustachian tube (the canal that drains from the ear to the back of the throat). This tube can get plugged when an infection finds a home in the warm, moist environment of the middle ear. Children have narrower tubes than adults do and that, along with their greater susceptibility to colds and respiratory infections, makes them prime targets for ear infections. Babies who are bottle-fed lying down can develop earaches as a result of milk entering the eustachian tubes. Since they can't tell us that they feel bad, infants may show signs of an ear infection by tugging on the ears or shaking their heads from side to side.

With proper medical attention, an earache will usually clear up in ten to fourteen days, but if the fluid in the middle ear gets trapped, there may be lasting problems. Children can sustain long-term hearing loss and delayed communication ability (slow to talk) if the infection goes on too long. It's important to follow up on an earache, because if the inflammation and fluid buildup continue, the eardrum may be damaged.

Earaches in adults and older children may be attributed to accumulated earwax or to water getting into the ear during swimming or showers. If water gets deep into the ear canal and becomes trapped, either by wax buildup or swelling of the eustachian tubes, a condition called **otitis externa** or **swimmer's ear** develops. Frequent swimming or showering can strip the normal lining of the ear canal, which allows bacteria or fungus to grow in the trapped water pockets. Swimmer's ear sufferers complain of a persistent ringing or sloshing in the ear, along with some pain and itching deep within the ear.

How Are Earaches Treated?

Non-drug treatments
Temporary relief from earaches can often be found by applying warm, dry cloths to the painful ear. Moist heat from warmed towels or cloths ap-

Pill Humor Actual stories from the pharmacy

A frazzled young mother came into the pharmacy for a refill on her son's liquid *amoxicillin* for his ear infection. She had just picked up a bottle of the antibiotic medication two days earlier, with the instructions: "*One teaspoonful three times a day for ten days for ear infection.*"

When asked why she needed a refill so soon, she explained, "I don't understand why, but by the time I get a teaspoonful into one of his ears, it spills out of the other one. He gets this sticky pink stuff all over himself and me. Doing this three times a day has been a real battle and we're already out of medicine!"

Her pharmacist quickly changed the bottle's label to read, "*Give one teaspoonful BY MOUTH three times a day for ten days for ear infection.*"

Mother and child both recovered nicely.

---

plied to the ear and neck area can also be soothing to the swollen and painful eustachian tubes. Be careful not to let the cloths or towels get too warm—remember children have very sensitive skin.

OTC treatments

Ear infections should be treated with prescription medications, so it's important to seek medical attention quickly when an earache develops. If you can't get to the doctor right away, try one of the over-the-counter de-

The Drug Lady Recommends . . .

Triaminic AM Decongestant Formula (pseudoephedrine) is a popular orange-flavored syrup that children really seem to like, even if it is medicine. The Triaminic products give professional labeling guidelines for younger children based on weight, but as always, consult your pediatrician.

congestants, like *pseudoephedrine,* to relieve the pressure in the eustachian tubes. Watch children's dosages carefully, however, since many decongestants are not recommended for children under two.

Infants' Tylenol Cold Drops, with *pseudoephedrine* as a decongestant and *acetaminophen* as a fever reducer, are a good choice for the younger ones with an earache. Many children find some temporary relief from **Children's Tylenol** *(acetaminophen)* or **Children's Motrin** *(ibuprofen)* oral suspension in pediatric dosages.

Prescription treatments

When someone in your family has an earache, the best thing to do is to head for the doctor's office. Middle-ear infections are treated with antibiotics, and antibiotics are available by prescription only. The doctor may prescribe the broad-spectrum antibiotic *amoxicillin* for your child (the liquid we call "the pink stuff"). *Amoxicillin* has a bubblegumlike flavor, and most children don't react too violently to taking it. If the dosage is less than a teaspoonful, ask your pharmacist for a special syringe to make sure the medicine is measured correctly.

Antibiotic/corticosteroid eardrops, like *Cortisporin Otic,* penetrate deep into the ear to kill bacteria and relieve inflammation. This is available as both a solution and a suspension. There is also an eardrop specifically for pain relief, called *Auralgan.* It has a numbing agent to ease the discomfort of a swollen ear canal.

How to Put In Eardrops

Getting eardrops into your little person's ears can be a daunting task. Here are some tips for making sure that more medicine gets in the ear than all over your child.

- Have the child lie down or tilt the head so the sore ear is facing up.
- Pull the earlobe down and back to give the medicine best access to the eustachian tube.
- Place the medicine in the ear and allow it to soak into the ear canal for two minutes.
- A small wad of cotton inserted in the ear will help keep the medicine inside where it will do the most good.

The Drug Lady Recommends...

Warm the eardrops first! The eardrops will feel much better going in if you put the CAPPED bottle in a warm cup of water. The warmth also will expand the eustachian tubes a little, allowing the medication to reach its destination faster. Remember—WARM water, not hot.

Fever

Q. *What's the best treatment for my child's fever?*

A. Seeing your little angel with a high fever can be a very frightening experience. Children often become very quiet and lethargic when fighting a fever. Temperatures can rise very quickly and dangerously when a child is sick. Having medicine around the house for those 3:00 A.M. fevers is a good idea for all involved. (See Appendix A, "Family First-Aid Kit," page 343.)

What Causes a Fever?

When a child has a fever, it usually means some type of inflammation or infection has developed. A fever is the body's way of saying, "Hey! Things aren't going so well in here!" The fever is a sign that the body's immune system is attacking the bacteria or virus causing the inflammation or infection.

Sometimes a fever can be difficult to determine because normal body temperature fluctuates all day. Every child is different; but a normal temperature is usually between 97 and 100 degrees Fahrenheit. Your child's temperature usually will be lower in the morning and higher in the evening. Anything higher than 100 degrees is considered a fever.

How Is a Fever Treated?

Non-drug treatments
Some specialists recommend that medicines not be used for a fever until other methods like warm sponge baths are used. Warm water helps

open the blood vessels near the skin and cools the blood. Check with your child's doctor first if you aren't sure how to best treat a fever. If a child has a fever but does not seem to be uncomfortable and is eating well, it is not necessary to treat the fever with either medication or baths.

OTC treatments

Warning: It is important that children not be given aspirin for their fevers. To prevent Reye's syndrome (see "Reye's Syndrome," page 99), never give infants, children, or teenagers aspirin or aspirin-containing drugs for a viral illness. For treatment of fever, use *acetaminophen* (**Tylenol**) or *ibuprofen* (**Motrin**).

Liquid ***Infants' Tylenol Concentrated Drops*** (*acetaminophen*) are a good first choice for fighting fevers. Another popular choice is ***Infants' Motrin Concentrated Drops*** (*ibuprofen*). For older children, both *acetaminophen* and *ibuprofen* products are available as elixirs, suspensions, and chewable tablets. ***Children's Motrin Oral Suspension*** (*ibuprofen*) tastes great, works fast, and lasts longer than ***Children's Tylenol*** (*acetaminophen*).

Ibuprofen is also a great pain reliever because it works as an anti-inflammatory drug as well as a fever reducer. Anti-inflammatory medicines also help bring down swelling from painful conditions like earaches and teething. If hives, facial swelling, or wheezing occur, stop the medication and bring your child to the doctor RIGHT AWAY; an allergic reaction is under way and must be treated quickly. These reactions are rare, but you should always be prepared whenever starting a new medication.

The Drug Lady Recommends . . .

Feverall (*acetaminophen*) in anal-suppository form can be a lifesaver when all else fails and your child can't keep any medicine down. It may not be the most pleasant way to give medicine, but it will get medicine into the body quickly and is usually very effective for reducing fevers.

Types of Thermometers

▪ Glass thermometers. These can be either oral (mouth) or rectal (rectum) types. A rectal thermometer is better for children under five years old, although it can take several minutes for a reading. While accurate and inexpensive, these are not generally recommended due to the chance of breakage.

▪ Digital thermometers. Put in the mouth, these generally work in less than thirty seconds. You get a "beep" when the temperature has been read. These are generally very accurate and cost under $10.

▪ Temperature strips. Placed on the forehead or under the tongue, depending on the brand, these thermometers are easy to use, but not very accurate.

▪ Ear thermometers work in two seconds or less. These are the best for easy use and accuracy, but the high price may put these out of reach of some parents.

Prescription treatments

If a child's fever lasts longer than forty-eight hours or if an infant (three to six months) registers a fever higher than 100.5°F (measured rectally), give the doctor a call. Some children experience mild convulsions or seizures with a fever. If this should occur, it is important to notify the child's pediatrician as soon as possible.

Warning

If you notice your child is experiencing any of the following symptoms with fever, call the doctor IMMEDIATELY: seizures, unusual sleepiness or grogginess, a stiff neck or back, confusion, or a spotted rash. Any one of these may be the first sign of a much more serious condition, and your child requires prompt medical attention.

Fluoride Supplements

(See Chapter 7, page 179.)

Head Lice

Q. *The school sent home a note that said my daughter has head lice! I can't believe it. I wash her hair every day. What can we do?*

A. First, realize that head lice don't visit because you or your children are dirty, unwashed, or not cared for. The little fellas show absolutely no discrimination for social class or wealth. Head lice is the number-two communicable condition among children, after the common cold. More than ten million cases of lice infestation are reported every year. The most common mode of travel for these little bugs is children sharing hats, combs, or scarves.

What Are Head Lice?

Head lice are tiny, whitish insects that live on the scalp and hair shafts. Unfortunately, the lice themselves are not the only problem. The female louse (that's singular for "lice") lays eggs called "nits" and strongly attaches them to the hair shaft; she can lay ten eggs a day for up to forty days. That's a lot of little nits crawling around—it makes me itch just thinking about it! Not only do these creatures crawl around, but they also have to eat to survive, and blood is their favorite meal. As you can imagine, these tiny bites produce a great deal of itching.

How Are Head Lice Treated?

Non-drug treatments
Because the tiny nits attach to the hair shaft with a very sticky, stubborn substance, combing vigorously will not remove them. Neither will the old home remedy of putting **Vaseline** on the hair in hopes of smothering the nits.

Some alternatives for mild cases include the use of a very fine-toothed comb, called a "nit comb," to thoroughly and completely run through every strand of hair. This must be repeated at least every three days. Essential oils of *rosemary* and *lavender* also have had some success in eliminating adult lice, but often are not effective against the nits. Unfortunately, I

The Drug Lady Recommends . . .

The commercial product *Nix* (*permethrin*) is a cream rinse made by the folks at Warner Lambert. It comes highly recommended from health-care providers because one of its ingredients dissolves the sticky coating that holds the nit in place on the hair shaft. It also kills a lousy louse dead in ten to fifteen minutes, with a success rate of 97 to 99 percent when used as directed. The residual effects last up to fourteen days!

haven't found anything in the non-drug category that is 100 percent effective in a case of head lice.

OTC treatments

To start killing the lice, make sure the child's hair is freshly washed, then, while it is still damp, apply a cream rinse with a lice-killing insecticide. Cover the roots and scalp well; leave on the hair for ten minutes, then rinse off completely. That should do it. *Permethrin* even has a residual action—lice are killed for several days after application. But if for some reason your child shares another cap with another "lousy" child, repeat the treatment in seven days. Some minor side effects like burning, stinging, itching, and rash may be experienced. Remember, this is an insecticide, designed to kill bugs—it's powerful stuff!

Other products, like **Rid** by Pfizer and **A-200** by SmithKline Beecham, use *pyrethrins* as an active ingredient. These are available as shampoos, solutions, or gels. Pyrethrins are extracted from the chrysanthemum—yes, really! This insecticide causes the nervous systems of lice to go into overdrive, killing them within ten to twenty minutes, along with 75 percent of their unhatched offspring. Apply and leave on the hair for at least ten minutes, then wash out thoroughly. Watch the eyes and face—it will sting! Redness and itching are side effects, especially for anyone with a ragweed allergy (because this chemical does come from flower extracts).

When you get home from the trip to the drugstore for lice treatment, you'll need to wash all bedding, hats, and scarves thoroughly in hot water. Combs and brushes should be placed in a mild solution of water and bleach to ensure that the nits are completely dead. Check the hair of other family members for several days to be sure the lice haven't spread. It's a time-consuming process, but worth it if you don't have to re-treat the family.

The use of over-the-counter products on the hair and combing the hair out carefully, combined with washing everything after treatment, should produce 100 percent dead lice with no nits left over. Problem solved—and the neighbors never even have to know!

Prescription treatments

Prescription products like *lindane,* in lotion or shampoo form, are also available, but should only be used in severe cases. There have been rare problems associated with lindane, including links to aplastic anemia, leukemia, and other blood diseases. If this is prescribed, discuss the pros and cons with your doctor.

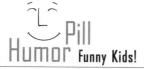

Humor Pill — Funny Kids!

Some school nurses share the smiles from their real notes for "medical excuses."

- ▦ "Mary could not go to school because she was bothered by very close veins."

- ▦ "Please excuse James from P.E. He has loose vowels."

- ▦ "My son has been told by his doctor not to take P.E. Please execute him."

- ▦ "Please excuse John for being. It was his father's fault."

Impetigo

Q. *Our children have various skin conditions from eczema to food allergies. The youngest is always scratching and has now developed impetigo. Could you tell me more about this and what we can do to make it go away? Can the other children catch it?*

A. With your little ones always scratching, picking up an infection like impetigo was almost inevitable. The bacteria that cause impetigo really seem to love areas of the skin that are already broken open by scratching. This makes insect bites, poison ivy, skin rashes, or cuts an especially attractive area for the bacteria to find a home.

What Is Impetigo?

Impetigo is a bacterial skin infection caused by *Staphylococcus aureus* or by Group A strep bacteria. It grows especially well in the areas around the nose and mouth. The rash first appears as small red spots. These spots turn into fluid-filled blisters that leak a golden-colored liquid. This liquid contains very contagious bacteria, so YES—your other children could get impetigo from an infected child. As the blisters open, the skin becomes covered with a crusty layer. Typically the infection takes about a week to run its course, and during this time it may be very itchy. This is also the time when it can spread very easily to other areas already affected by scratches or open sores.

Warning:

It is very important to call the doctor if your child experiences stomach upset, headaches, puffy face, or lower-than-normal urinary output when suffering from impetigo. These may be the signs of **glomerulonephritis,** a kidney disease that may occur as a complication of impetigo.

How Is Impetigo Treated?

Non-drug treatments

The first step to take when the doctor diagnoses a family member with impetigo is to limit your other family members' contact with the impetigo sufferer's personal bedclothes, clothing, or towels. Wash everything thoroughly and make sure everyone in the family uses a clean towel. Also, disinfect areas of the house that the infected child touches frequently, as well as her favorite toys. Toss the washable toys in a bathtub of water with a cup of bleach added. Clothes and bedclothes should be laundered in hot water.

Using a gentle soap like ***Ivory*** or ***Johnson's Baby Wash*** to bathe your child when the spots first appear may clear up mild cases of impetigo.

Tea tree oil has wonderful natural antibacterial properties. A dab of this on a cotton ball applied three times daily may sting a bit, but it will kill many kinds of harmful bacteria on the skin.

Cutting the child's fingernails short can help prevent both spreading the bacteria to other parts of the body and the nails scratching open new areas where the bacteria can thrive.

OTC treatments

For mild cases, the doctor may recommend a triple-antibiotic cream or ointment, like **Neosporin** (*neomycin, polymyxin B,* and *bacitracin),* to keep the bacteria in check. An antihistamine like **Benadryl** (*diphenhydramine*) will help control the itch. Covering the area with a **Band-Aid** is effective for areas your child just can't stop scratching.

The Drug Lady Recommends . . .

While following the doctor's orders for antibiotic treatment, you may continue to wash the areas with warm water and an antibacterial soap like *Dial.* The warm water will help soften the crusted areas, while antibacterial soap will keep bacteria to a minimum.

Prescription treatments

For severe and persistent cases of impetigo, one of the stronger antibiotic creams and ointments available by prescription is called **Bactroban** (*mupirocin*). This works to target certain bacterial skin infections, like those

School and Day-care Rules

While each school or day care has its own rules, typically your child should be kept out of school until he has been on treatment for twenty-four hours with antibiotics taken by mouth, or for forty-eight hours with antibiotic creams alone. For mild impetigo treated with an antibiotic ointment, the child can usually continue to attend day care or school if the sore is covered with a *Band-Aid.*

It is important to make the school or day-care workers aware that your child has this infection to prevent a major outbreak among everyone there.

that cause impetigo. For more serious cases of impetigo, an antibiotic prescription taken by mouth (like *amoxicillin* or *erythromycin*) may be needed in addition to Bactroban. You should notice the infection responding to the antibiotic combinations within three days. If this isn't happening, or if your child begins to run a high fever, give the doctor a call RIGHT AWAY.

Jaundice

Q. *Our newborn baby is yellow! We took him to the doctor, who said it was jaundice. He said we should put him in the sun as much as possible—is this right? What else should we be doing for him? We didn't get any medicine from the doctor.*

A. Just when some of the scariness of having a new baby begins to wear off (for instance, "Does he have all his fingers, . . . toes, . . . etc.?"), he starts turning yellow! This can be a very frightening experience for new parents. Thankfully, it usually isn't serious and is very common among our newest arrivals. Just so you won't worry: 60 percent of full-term infants develop jaundice on the second or third day after birth. It typically disappears after that first week.

What Is Jaundice?

Technically jaundice occurs because of unusually high levels of **bilirubin** in the blood. So, what's bilirubin? This is the yellow pigment in our blood formed from broken-down hemoglobin, an important part of the red blood cells, which carry oxygen. Newborns have a larger amount of hemoglobin than the rest of us. Adults already have bacteria in their bodies that normally break down bilirubin. Because little newborn systems aren't quite used to their "out-of-womb" experience, their bodies can reach a high bilirubin level quickly. There are no bacteria yet to get rid of the bilirubin, so it must be eliminated in bright yellow stools or taken back in by the blood. The skin and the whites of the eyes take on an alarming yellowish appearance, making your newborn's complexion look jaundiced—not at all what you had in mind.

How Is Jaundice Treated?

Non-drug treatments

Sometimes breast-feeding can bring on or prolong jaundice. This is called "breast-milk jaundice." In these cases, the baby is usually taken off the breast for one or two days while Mom continues to pump her milk. This gives the baby's body time to begin producing the compounds necessary to get rid of the bilirubin naturally.

Mild jaundice is usually left to run its course. The baby's body begins to produce the important "bilirubin-digesting" bacteria and the problem soon resolves itself. During that first week, simply feeding the baby frequently will ensure that everything is flowing out before it has an opportunity to be absorbed into the blood.

If your doctor feels that the bilirubin level isn't high enough for the baby to be admitted to the hospital, he may recommend putting the baby near a window for as much filtered sunlight as possible. This triggers the same mechanism in the baby's body as the hospital bilirubin lights (see "Prescription treatments" on page 88).

The Drug Lady Recommends . . .

Here is a firsthand account of the effectiveness of natural sunshine on jaundice. I visited some dear friends just after the birth of their son Ryan. His mother said he was suffering from mild jaundice. I looked all over for the little guy before his mother told me he was "over by the window." There he was in his carrier, sunning himself, the warm Florida sunshine bathing his tiny little legs and chest. The sunshine worked just fine on the jaundice and it looked like he was enjoying himself, too.

OTC treatments

Since newborn jaundice is a condition that generally clears up of its own accord as the baby's system matures, there are no over-the-counter treatments for this condition.

Prescription treatments

If the jaundice becomes severe, the doctor may put the baby under what are called "bilirubin lights" or "bililights." Also called **phototherapy,** this blue spectrum of lights chemically changes the bilirubin into compounds that are much easier for the body to process.

Lactose Intolerance

Q. *The doctor says that my young daughter is lactose-intolerant and that is what is causing her "smelly" diapers. Will this be something she lives with, or is there some formula that I can give to help this?*

A. There are several different types of lactose intolerance, and the type your daughter has will determine whether it is something she'll outgrow or will be around forever. Her pediatrician will be a great help in determining which type she has.

What Is Lactose Intolerance?

Lactose is the sugar found in milk—something we all probably have consumed at one time or another. The body normally produces the enzyme *lactase,* which functions to break down lactose into a more usable form. If you are "lactose-intolerant," this means your body doesn't produce any, or enough, lactase to digest the lactose; when this undigested milk sugar finds its way through the digestive tract, intestinal bacteria take over the job. Unfortunately, this bacterial breakdown of lactose results in hydrogen gas (VERY smelly), diarrhea, and stomach pain.

"Primary lactose intolerance" is a condition that usually begins around the ages of three to thirteen, and will continue through life. If this is what your daughter has, she has a lot of company—over thirty million people, in fact! It seems that within certain populations (Mediterranean, African, Asian, and Native American), 75 to 100 percent of people experience this type of lactose intolerance.

Diagnosis of Lactose Intolerance

Your doctor can perform one of several tests to determine if a true lactose intolerance is present or if something more is going on.

- For infants: A stool acidity test measures the amount of acid in the stool. When lactose makes it to the colon undigested and bacteria take over, high amounts of lactic acid are produced, which show up in this test.

- For older children and adults: The hydrogen breath test records the amount of gas produced when an individual drinks a high-lactose beverage. High levels of hydrogen gas indicate improper lactose digestion.

- Another common test is the lactose intolerance test. With this test, nothing is eaten before the test, and then a high-lactose beverage is consumed. Blood samples are taken over a two-hour period to determine how well the body is digesting the lactose. Low blood-sugar levels mean that not very much of the lactose has been broken down, indicating lactose intolerance.

"Secondary lactose intolerance" occurs when the lining of the intestinal wall where lactase is produced is damaged. Certain antibiotics, and medicines like **non-steroidal anti-inflammatory drugs (NSAIDs**; for example, *naproxen* or *ibuprofen*), or even a severe bout of diarrhea can cause this. This type of lactose intolerance usually takes care of itself as soon as the intestinal lining has had time to heal and begins to produce lactase again.

If your daughter is very young, her condition may be the result of a congenital condition (one present at birth). In "congenital lactose intoler-

The Drug Lady Recommends . . .

If it becomes necessary to give up milk and dairy products, it is important to be sure that the body is getting enough calcium. For adults and children who can chew well, chocolatey calcium supplements like *Viactiv* are a yummy way to get 500 mg of calcium in a tasty treat. Yogurt is also a good alternate source of calcium for those who are lactose-intolerant. Look for active and live cultures, since these help digest the lactose part of the yogurt.

ance," the intestine simply does not make the enzyme lactase. This is a rare condition and is usually diagnosed within the first week after birth. These infants must be fed lactose-free formulas to accommodate their systems.

How Is Lactose Intolerance Treated?

Non-drug treatments

Unfortunately there is no cure for **lactose intolerance.** With primary lactose intolerance, the focus is either on eliminating lactose-containing foods from the diet, or adding the enzyme *lactase* to the system. *Soy* or *rice milk* may provide a tasty substitute for the allergy-causing lactose found in animal-based dairy products. Some are even fortified with extra vitamins and calcium.

For secondary lactose intolerance in infants and young children, changing the formula or milk source often improves the symptoms dramatically. Adults should avoid high-lactose products until the system readjusts.

OTC treatments

If the **lactose intolerance** is mild and your child's desire for milk products is strong, there are over-the-counter products that can make the unpleasant symptoms much more tolerable. Adding the enzyme *lactase* directly to milk products, or taking it before drinking a glass of milk, may be all that's needed to help the body digest and process lactose. This typically decreases the diarrhea and gas experienced with primary lactose intolerance. OTC products to look for are ***Lactaid, Dairy Ease,*** and ***SureLac.***

Prescription treatments

Doctor visits for lactose intolerance will probably be limited to the initial diagnosis. Your pediatrician can provide excellent recommendations for a personal plan to deal with this condition depending on its severity.

Humor Pill

DOCTOR: "How is the little boy who swallowed the four quarters doing?"
NURSE: "No change yet!"

Nausea and Vomiting

Q. *What is the best medicine I can give my child when he is sick to his stomach? We would like to have something around the house because he always seems to get sick in the middle of the night.*

A. I think children have a sixth sense about when all the drugstores are closed for the night. That's precisely the time they decide to start running a fever and get nauseated. . . . Well, not always, but it certainly seems like they do know! Having medicine around the house for such emergencies is always a good idea (see Appendix A, "Family First-Aid Kit," page 343).

What Are Nausea and Vomiting?

Nausea is the very unpleasant, sick feeling in your stomach that you get right before you vomit. Nausea and vomiting go hand in hand. An area of the brain called the "vomiting center" triggers both. (That sounds like such a wonderful place!)

When the body has something inside it that shouldn't be there, then up it comes—quickly. Both the feeling of nausea and the actual vomiting can be caused by an infection (like stomach flu), movement (like car or motion sickness), pain, or irritation of the senses by certain smells and foods.

Vomiting is an automatic response in which the body forcefully expels the contents of the stomach. Your windpipe closes to prevent what's coming up from getting into your lungs, while your abdomen and diaphragm contract forcefully to push everything out quickly. It's an efficient system, but not one we like to use very often.

How Are Nausea and Vomiting Treated?

Non-drug treatments

Nausea and vomiting are usually self-limiting, which means they will stop by themselves. However, if the nausea and vomiting haven't stopped after twelve hours, or seem severe, it is time to give the doctor a call. These become serious conditions when the child cannot keep any fluids down and becomes dehydrated, so fluid intake is important. Try to give small amounts of flat soda (let it sit until the bubbles have dissipated) or clear, non-diet drinks like *Sprite* or *7-Up*. Sugared drinks are better than plain water because they help delay the vomiting reflex. Avoid highly acidic drinks like orange or grapefruit juice, which can cause more stomach discomfort.

Peppermint tea and *gingerroot* tea act as wonderful digestive aids, both in calming the stomach and in soothing the nauseous feeling.

The use of **acupressure,** or applying firm, constant pressure on the lower arm approximately two inches above the wrist crease, often provides natural relief from nausea.

Nux vomica and *arsenicum album* are two commonly used remedies for nausea; these are said to calm nausea by using the ancient principles of **homeopathy.** This practice entails using very, very small doses of ingredients that normally would cause the same symptoms you are trying to treat. While there may not be enough of an active ingredient to heal, it doesn't appear that these homeopathic remedies hurt, either.

OTC treatments

Most over-the-counter antinausea medications are designed to treat nausea and vomiting related to motion sickness by focusing on the middle ear to restore a sense of balance and to reduce the feeling of nausea. Look for names like *Bonine* (*meclizine*) or *Dramamine* (*dimenhydrinate*). The most common side effects are drowsiness and grogginess. Blurred vision and dry mouth also may occur.

The Drug Lady Recommends . . .

Emetrol is recommended for the relief of nausea due to upset stomach from intestinal and stomach flus. This product is safe for children because the active ingredient is not a drug, but a sugar solution of *dextrose*, *levulose (fructose)*, and *phosphoric acid*. It soothes the tummy by decreasing the pressure within the stomach, and the sugars work to delay the vomiting reflex—it tastes pretty good, too. Because of the high sugar content, diabetics should avoid Emetrol.

Prescription treatments

If the nausea doesn't seem to respond to over-the-counter medicines, or lasts more than twelve hours, it's time to call the doctor. For severe nausea, the prescription drug **Phenergan** (*promethazine*) may be given either as a suppository, a liquid, or a shot. For nausea that accompanies surgery or chemotherapy, **Zofran** (*ondansetron*) is very effective.

Pain

Q. *My four-year-old daughter broke her arm in a fall from a swing and she is in quite a bit of pain. I'm a little scared of pain medicines. I don't want her to hurt, but I don't want to give too much, either. The doctor said to give her over-the-counter (OTC) pain medicines during the day and save the prescription medicine for nighttime. What do you recommend as a good OTC pain medicine for children?*

A. Choosing the right pain medicine for a little one can be a difficult decision for all health-care providers—mommies and daddies included. It's especially hard for parents to see their babies hurting.

Because children's bodies are so small and because their little systems metabolize some medicines very differently from adults, it is always wise to use extreme care when giving pain medicines. Some prescription pain medicines, like those containing *codeine,* can slow down a child's breathing and make them very lethargic. These are generally given only at bedtime or when the pain is most severe.

How Is a Child's Pain Level Determined?

Children are usually very honest in their assessment of when something hurts or not, but if they are too young to tell you exactly how badly it hurts, then finding a medication for it is a more complex decision.

An infant's pain is determined by how much or how little he or she cries; a baby's quiet whimpering can be as effective as screaming in determining pain. From ages one to four, children may talk about an "owie," they may favor a particularly painful body area, or they may simply sit very quietly as if this would make the pain go away.

For four-year-olds and up, doctors (and parents) can ask them to rate the pain on a scale of zero to five. Zero means no pain, and five means the worst pain. This also can be modeled using the hands: holding them far apart means a lot of pain and close together means only a little pain.

How Is a Child's Pain Treated?

Non-drug treatments

When the cause of the pain has been identified and the appropriate pain medication prescribed by the doctor, there are things you can do at home to make this experience less unpleasant. Playing a quiet game, watching a funny video, or simply holding and rocking the sick child can go a long way in helping make the pain go away. A warm cloth dabbed with relaxing *lavender* aromatherapy oil and held close to the child can also be a soothing distraction from the pain.

OTC treatments

Aspirin is rarely used in the treatment of pain in children under fifteen years old. This is because of the connection between aspirin and Reye's syndrome, a condition in which children who have a fever in combination with the virus-based illnesses (chicken pox or influenza) can become very ill and possibly die when aspirin is taken (see "Reye's Syndrome," page 99). Parents should NEVER give a child or teenager aspirin, or aspirin-containing drugs, for any illness that causes a fever. It is important to read all OTC product labels VERY carefully. Some common medications that contain aspirin (or *salicylates* related to aspirin) might surprise you; these include **Pepto-Bismol, Excedrin,** and **Alka-Seltzer Plus.**

*Acetaminophen (**Tylenol**)* is commonly seen as a stand-alone OTC product as well as in combination with *codeine* in stronger prescription medicines like **Tylenol No. 3** (*acetaminophen* and *codeine*). Acetaminophen for children comes in several yummy flavors as well as in the favorite forms of liquids, chewable, and junior caplets.

Elixirs, Suspensions, and Drops

It is important to be aware of the different concentrations of products contained in elixirs, suspensions, and drops. For example, acetaminophen suspensions and elixirs have the same strength of 160 mg in one teaspoonful (5 ml), but concentrated infant drops have 160 mg in 1.6 ml. That's a big difference!

Always, ALWAYS follow the package directions and your doctor's instructions. If you ever have a concern about the right dose, call the doctor or ask your pharmacist for a clarification BEFORE you give the medicine.

Ibuprofen (**Children's Motrin** or **Children's Advil**) in suspension, chewable, or junior tablet form is another excellent choice for children's pain relief. This medication is classified as an anti-inflammatory and works by decreasing inflammation as well as blunting the body's perception of pain.

The side effects of acetaminophen or ibuprofen are generally very mild. There may be some upset tummies, but this is unusual. While

The Drug Lady Recommends . . .

Ibuprofen (**Motrin**) is an anti-inflammatory pain reliever that works especially well for "boo-boos" that involve swelling. Broken arms, toothaches, even joint and muscle pain can be relieved with ibuprofen. Ibuprofen comes in a suspension liquid, and in chewable and junior tablet forms, with berry, orange, bubblegum, and grape flavors. Names to look for are **In-fants' Motrin Concentrated Drops** (ages 6 months to 23 months), **Children's Motrin Suspension** (ages 24 months to 11 years old), and **Children's Motrin Ibuprofen Chewable Tablets** (ages 4 to 11 years old).

ibuprofen doesn't contain aspirin, sometimes it can cause an "aspirin allergy" type of reaction; this can show up as wheezing, itchy hives, a fast, irregular pulse or heartbeat, a change in color of the skin (indicating shock), shortness of breath, and swelling of the face. It doesn't happen often, so you shouldn't worry needlessly, but this is something to keep in mind anytime someone in the family takes ibuprofen. These medicines typically don't cause drowsiness or grogginess, but if your child is sick, you may notice more of this type of behavior.

Prescription treatments

Prescription pain medicines for children can be a simple combination of products, like **Tylenol No. 3** (*acetaminophen* and *codeine*), for mild to moderate pain—or the medicine may be as strong as *morphine* for severe pain. Your child's doctor is the best judge to determine the correct doses and time to give the medicines. Often children's doses are very precisely calculated based on your child's size, so it is very important to give the medicines exactly as directed.

Most of the stronger prescription pain medicines cause quite a bit of drowsiness and may produce stomach upset too. Narcotics, like codeine, can slow a child's breathing and make it shallow as it takes effect. For the first few doses of a prescription pain medicine, it is a good idea to keep a close watch on your child for possible side effects or reactions to the medicine, like those listed above.

Pinworms

Q. *The day-care center called and said that pinworms may be going around among the children. What do I look for? If we get them, what is the most effective way to get rid of them FAST?*

A. If pinworms do come to visit, your family has a lot of company. In the United States, it is estimated that at least 25 percent of all kids will have (or already have) pinworms. If it's any comfort, the tiny pinworm is considered the most common intestinal parasite in the U.S. Don't panic if your family does see the little guys—they aren't dangerous and can be very quickly and effectively taken care of!

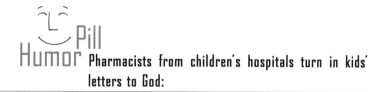

Humor Pill Pharmacists from children's hospitals turn in kids' letters to God:

Dear God:

I didn't think orange went with purple until I saw the sunset you made on Tuesday. That was cool!

Eugene

Dear God:

Did you mean for the giraffe to look like that, or was it an accident?

Norma

Dear God:

Instead of letting people die and having to make new ones, why don't you just keep the ones you have now?

Jane

Dear God:

Who draws the lines around the countries?

Nancy

Dear God:

Thank you for my baby brother, but what I prayed for was a puppy.

Boyce

Dear God:

Please send me a pony. I never asked for anything before. You can look it up.

Bruce

Dear God:

I want to be just like my daddy when I get big, but not with so much hair all over.

Sam

What Are Pinworms?

Pinworms are white, wriggly worms that thrive in your child's lower intestinal tract (the colon). Adult worms are only about a half-inch long when fully grown. They spread from one person to another through the thousands of tiny eggs they lay. When it is time for the female pinworm to reproduce, she moves out of the colon through the child's anus and onto the surrounding skin, which causes intense itching. Some of the eggs she lays may float in the air to land on other objects in the room, but most stay close. They grow to maturity in just six hours. Some crawl back into the anus, where they will continue the cycle. Other eggs may be transferred from child to child, from objects on which the eggs have landed, as well as from eggs traveling under small fingernails from scratching around the anal area. You should be aware that little girls can easily transfer the eggs to their vaginal areas, too, and may experience pain when urinating.

The first sign of pinworm infestation is itching in the rectal area, particularly at night. If your child is complaining, or if you suspect pinworms, check his or her anal area a few hours after bedtime while she's asleep. That's when the adult worms can be seen moving around. Sometimes you may see them wriggling around in the child's stool. (This is definitely not the most pleasant of parental duties, but it is a reliable way to determine whether pinworms are present.)

For a more accurate diagnosis, take a small piece of adhesive tape and touch it (gently) to the child's anal area; the adult worms will stick to it and your pediatrician can confirm that these are pinworms.

How Are Pinworms Treated?

Non-drug treatments

There is no direct non-drug treatment for pinworms, but there are a number of things you can do to prevent their recurrence. Make sure to wash all bedclothes, towels, and underwear in hot water. Toilet seats and bathtubs should also be disinfected with a diluted bleach solution. It is a good idea to use a disinfectant on favorite toys, as they could be a home for the eggs. Teaching your children to wash their hands regularly is a good way to help prevent the spread of pinworms to other people.

OTC treatments

Because pinworms are so common, they are one of the few parasites that can be treated effectively with an over-the-counter product.

The Drug Lady Recommends . . .

Pin-X, a onetime treatment for pinworms, is made from a base of the powerful "pinworm eliminator" called *pyrantel pamoate.* It has a nice caramel taste and should be taken only once, at any time of day, either alone or with milk or fruit juice. There is even a convenient weight dosage chart on the package.

Prescription treatments

The doctor may prescribe **Vermox** (*mebendazole*) for family pinworm treatment when OTC products haven't been effective. It's a chewable tablet that each family member can take, and it is very effective against the worms. It doesn't kill the eggs, however, so washing all bed linens and items the child has come into contact with is very important. Treatment again in two weeks is recommended—just to be sure the pesky little fellas have been taken care of.

Reye's Syndrome

Q. *What is "Reye's syndrome?" I know that aspirin can cause it, but I took lots of baby aspirin when I was child and no one had ever heard of this. Is it new? What should I look out for with my child?*

A. Reye's syndrome was actually discovered in 1963. This condition just wasn't as well publicized (or well known) as it is today; doctors aren't even absolutely positive that aspirin causes the syndrome, but there are too many incidences of aspirin use and Reye's to take any chances. It is a rare condition, affecting fewer than twenty children each year in the United States. However, the seriousness of this condition and the fact that warnings about it are on every bottle of aspirin are enough reason to learn about it in detail.

What Is Reye's Syndrome?

Aspirin packages warn parents not to give aspirin to anyone under the age of fifteen who is experiencing any type of illness that is accompanied by a fever. The reasoning for this seems to be that a viral particle (typically from the chicken pox or influenza virus) can react with aspirin to produce a compound the body perceives as deadly. The brain becomes inflamed and swells, and the liver, which typically filters toxins out of the body, becomes overwhelmed and can't get rid of normal ammonia and other harmful chemicals, which build up rapidly and eventually affect brain function. Once the reaction starts, it can progress very quickly.

The symptoms usually appear four to seven days after the original illness begins. The child feels sick, has episodes of vomiting, and shows changes in mental function, including grogginess, disorientation, or confusion. Eventually the child can become delirious and even slip into a coma.

How Is Reye's Syndrome Treated?

Non-drug treatments

Call your doctor right away if your child is recovering from a viral illness and suddenly develops severe nausea, vomiting, or behavioral changes.

The Drug Lady Recommends . . .

As with many illnesses, the very best treatment for **Reye's syndrome** is prevention. Use pediatric forms of *Tylenol* (*acetaminophen*) or *Motrin* (*ibuprofen*) for children's pain and fever relief. Be alert to the fact that *aspirin* can sneak into your medicine chest. Some medicines that contain aspirin (or *salicylates* related to aspirin), which you might not be aware of, are *Pepto-Bismol*, *Excedrin*, and *Alka-Seltzer*.

There are many other causes of these symptoms, but it is best to talk to your doctor so that Reye's syndrome can be ruled out. This is NOT a condition for self-treatment.

OTC treatments

There is no over-the-counter treatment for Reye's, and it is important to get medical help quickly if any of the symptoms described above appear after a viral infection.

Prescription treatments

Often when a child is brought in with symptoms of Reye's syndrome, a liver biopsy and a spinal tap are done to confirm the diagnosis. Treatment consists of supporting the child's heart, lung, and brain functions while keeping levels of ammonia in the blood low until the symptoms of Reye's syndrome disappear. Steroids may be given to reduce swelling in the brain.

Teething

Q. *Our baby is getting her first tooth! She's drooling more than usual and seems unhappy. What can we do to help? What medicines are safe to put in her mouth?*

A. A first tooth is indeed a momentous occasion—for the parents and the baby! Now it's time to pull out the "drool bucket" because your little one will be rapidly producing large amounts of saliva. Her disposition may also shift toward the fussy side, and anything within six feet of her mouth is fair game to chew on.

What Is Teething?

A baby's first teeth start to appear anywhere from six months of age to one year. The lower front teeth (central incisors) are generally the first to show, with the upper front central incisors following closely behind. The other teeth are still forming under the gum, so dentists recommend starting fluoride treatments at around six months of age in areas where fluoride is not added to the drinking water. (See "Fluoride Supplements," chapter 7, page 179.)

Symptoms of teething may include heavy drooling, fussiness (especially at night), swollen gums, refusing to eat, or gumming any object within reach. Contrary to what our parents thought, teething should not cause a fever.

What Can You Do for a Teething Child?

Non-drug treatments

First, always consult your child's pediatrician before putting anything into your child's mouth to relieve teething pain. Here are some items to ask about:

Teething rings and soft cloths kept in the refrigerator (NOT the freezer—they will be too hard) are often a welcome surface for your baby to gum heartily. Cleaning the new teeth and gums with a soft cloth or a soft-bristled toothbrush may ease pain as well as arm the child with good oral hygiene habits.

Homeopathic remedies for teething include *mercurius sol* 6C, *chamomilla* 6C, or *calcarea carbonica* 6C. A trusted brand to look for is **Hyland's Teething Tablets** or **Teething Gel.**

OTC treatments

Keeping baby comfortable is the top priority. **Baby Orajel** contains a numbing agent, *benzocaine,* at a concentration of 7.5 percent. It is to be applied directly to the sore area of the emerging tooth, not more than four

The Drug Lady Recommends . . .

Pain-relieving medications like *Infants' Motrin Concentrated Drops* (*ibuprofen*) are anti-inflammatory pain relievers that work especially well for the swelling and inflammation of teething. The eight-hour dose is 50 mg (1.25 ml dropperful) for babies 12–17 pounds, and 75 mg (1 and ½ dropperful) for 18–23 pounds.

times a day, and only for babies over four months of age unless directed by your pediatrician. There is also a stronger product called **Baby Orajel NightTime** with 10 percent benzocaine to help relieve the baby's discomfort so the whole family can rest.

Infants' Tylenol Concentrated Drops work to decrease the aches and pains of teething. The dosage is based on weight for greatest accuracy. Weight-based dosage for a four-hour dose of 160 mg/1.6 ml of *acetaminophen* are: 40 mg (0.4 ml) for children 6–11 pounds; 80 mg, (0.8) ml for 12–17 pounds; and 120 mg (1.2 ml) for 18–23 pounds. It is important to use only the dropper specifically designed for the medicine you have purchased. Many products have different dose measurements as well as different concentrations of medication. Don't assume that the dose for one brand is the same as for all others.

Prescription treatments

Teething is a condition that generally does not require a doctor's visit. However, if your child is experiencing a great deal of discomfort, is running a fever over 101 degrees Fahrenheit, or shows signs of infection, bring him in to see the doctor right away.

Coughs, Colds, Flu, and Sore Throats: That Favorite Time of Year

Bronchitis ▓ Common Cold ▓ Coughs ▓ Flu ▓ Sinusitis ▓ Sore Throat

MANY OF US carry a certain dread when we hear mention of "cold and flu season." It's that time of year when we feel helpless against the ravages of a microscopic virus that can make us feel miserable. Often it's when we're at our sickest that we must scour the aisles in our local drugstores searching for the drug that will make us feel better. Standing groggily bewildered in front of the over-the-counter cough, cold, fever, pain, sore throat, flu, and sinus medications while running a fever and coughing is not the best way to treat your symptoms. In this chapter I'll try to save you both time and misery by simplifying your choices, based on the symptoms you're experiencing, so you can face this cold and flu season secure in the knowledge that you have the tools to make yourself and your family as comfortable as possible.

Bronchitis

Q. *Almost every year I develop a case of bronchitis that often lasts for weeks and sometimes even turns into pneumonia. What causes this and what can I do to avoid it next time?*

A. When your coworkers start putting up quarantine signs around your desk and your family runs away when you start coughing, it may be time to get some help. Bronchitis is definitely a condition to take seriously. If left untreated, it can very rapidly progress to pneumonia and land you in the hospital. While this may sound like a good way to get some rest, just keep thinking about what a wreck the house will be by the time you're well!

What Is Bronchitis?

Bronchitis is the inflammation of the bronchial tubes leading to the lungs. The cause can be bacterial or viral, but until you see the doctor for a culture, there is no way to know for sure. If it's bacterial, an antibiotic usually does the trick. Viruses are trickier because our antibiotic arsenal won't work on them; typically a viral infection is just left to run its course.

Bronchitis starts when bacteria or a virus irritates the bronchial tubes, causing them to swell. Your body produces mucus to help fight the irritation, and soon the coughing starts. Other symptoms of bronchitis include pain in the middle of your chest, a flulike weakness, fever, muscle soreness, headache, and wheezing.

A person can develop either "acute" or "chronic" forms of bronchitis. "Acute bronchitis" typically comes on like a cold, with symptoms of fever and coughing that produces a great deal of mucus. Young children and the elderly are especially susceptible. The good news is that acute bacterial bronchitis usually goes away within two to four days with antibiotic treatment. If the bronchitis is viral in origin, you'll have to be happy with simply taking it easy and concentrating on making yourself as comfortable as possible until the virus runs its course. Treatment for the aches, pains, and coughing (see below) will make this time much more bearable.

In "chronic bronchitis," the same symptoms occur year after year, for weeks to months at a time, and are usually much worse in the winter. The cough starts out dry, then progresses to wheezing and shortness of breath after each cough attack. Most cases (over 80 percent) of chronic bronchitis can be traced to smoking. Chronic bronchitis can quickly progress to a life-threatening lung disease called **chronic obstructive pulmonary disease (COPD)**, the fourth-leading cause of death in the United States. Antibiotics, in combination with medications that open the airways (bronchodilators), are often a first resort. Oxygen may be required if the condition doesn't respond quickly. Because of the seriousness of this condition, your doctor should closely monitor the course of treatment.

How Is Bronchitis Treated?

Non-drug treatments

Because bronchitis can be serious, a doctor should look at it before any self-treatment is tried at home. The measures below are great for helping the prescription medicines work, but they should never be used instead of a doctor's care.

Tips on How to Avoid Bronchitis

You can lower your chances of getting bronchitis if you

- don't smoke
- eat healthy foods
- exercise regularly
- wash your hands often

- Drinking plenty of liquids will help thin the mucus in the bronchial tubes.

- Use a vaporizer, humidifier, or steam from hot water to help open up your chest. Adding *sage* and *eucalyptus* to the steaming water is also helpful. Get plenty of rest and try to give your body every opportunity to get well by eating healthy foods. Fruits and vegetables, high in antioxidants, help protect the body against infections.

Since the treatment of chronic bronchitis is primarily aimed at reducing irritation in the bronchial tubes, try to keep away from smog or particles in the air that irritate your lungs, or smoke that can irritate bronchial tubes and lungs. Stay away from those smoky card games and bundle those fall leaves instead of burning them.

OTC treatments

A pain reliever like **Tylenol** (*acetaminophen*) or **Advil** (*ibuprofen*) may help the headache, body aches, and muscle pain associated with bronchitis. A cough syrup with *guaifenesin* (an expectorant) may be helpful. Expectorants are thought to reduce the thickness of the mucus lining in the bronchial tubes.

The Drug Lady Recommends . . .

An excellent expectorant-only product is called simply *Robitussin Cough Syrup*. Please, PLEASE take this (or any other over-the-counter cough syrup) ONLY if your doctor gives the go-ahead. It is not recommended for cases of chronic bronchitis. Bronchitis can be very serious and very damaging to the lungs. We want you around and breathing well for a long, long time!

Prescription treatments

For bacterial infections, an antibiotic (like *amoxicillin* or **Septra**) may be ordered by the doctor. A potent cough suppressant, *codeine,* is often given for short-term cough control and to allow necessary rest.

In addition to antibiotics and cough syrups, bronchodilator drugs (like *albuterol*) may be prescribed to help relax and open up air passages in the bronchial tubes. Steroid inhalers like **Beconase** (*beclomethasone*) must be used regularly to provide relief from chronic bronchitis. These work by decreasing tissue swelling to allow freer breathing.

Common Cold

Q. *I'm so confused! I have a cold—just a cold. I feel lousy and I can't breathe. What's the difference between an antihistamine and a decongestant? What do I need to take to breathe again? Please just point me to the right product!*

A. They call it a common cold. Sorry, but when it happens to most of us, having a cold is anything but common; the sneezing, coughing, and stuffiness are enough to make us feel miserable. We want to get rid of it quickly so we can resume feeling normal again. Let's see what works.

What Causes the Common Cold?

A cold is usually caused by a bug in the very large and nasty *rhino* (from the Latin word for *nose*) family of viruses. This rhinovirus makes a home in the respiratory tract and begins with a sore throat, stuffy or runny nose, and sneezing and coughing. So many people suffer from these symptoms that they are referred to as "the common cold." A cold typically lasts one to two weeks whether it's treated or not, so the key to finding relief is to make the symptoms as bearable as possible. Antibiotics are not effective against the cold virus, and as of this writing no one has developed a good vaccine to prevent us from getting colds.

How Is the Common Cold Treated?

Non-drug treatments
Sometimes it is hard to get the real story regarding natural and alternative cold products. One hears many claims of miracle cures, especially for colds. Well, there isn't really a miracle. Your body is exposed to a cold

virus and you "catch" it. Congratulations! But there are some herbals, like *echinacea,* that will stimulate your immune system and help you fight the infection faster.

Several studies have shown the beneficial effects of echinacea in increasing the body's production of white blood cells. These cells act to fight off infections by killing bacteria and viruses and moving them out of the system faster.

Echinacea doesn't prevent the cold from coming on, but it does help get rid of it faster. In fact, it can decrease cold symptoms by a day or more if taken at the first sign of a cold. Common dosage is 325 to 650 mg of the freeze-dried plant taken in capsule form, three times daily at the first sign of a cold and on through the duration of the cold. Liquid extracts in tincture forms may also be effective for fighting the cold virus. It's important that you take echinacea only when you start to feel sick, not every day. In fact, one study showed that taking echinacea every day to prevent the common cold actually increased the length of time the person stayed sick!

Zinc lozenges, in brands like **Cold Eeze,** make the cellular surface less inviting for viruses to find a home. If the virus can't find a home, it can't cause cold symptoms. Echinacea should also be avoided by those with autoimmune conditions, like Rheumatoid Arthritis or Multiple Sclerosis, as it may overstimulate the immune system and make these conditions worse.

The Drug Lady Recommends . . .

 Avoid that morning glass of milk when you have a head or chest cold. Dairy products can actually increase the body's production of thick, sticky mucus.

OTC treatments

As if having a cold weren't bad enough, to try and treat yourself you have to browse through a dizzying array of products in search of the elusive cure. There are virtually hundreds of different medications—antihistamines, decongestants, pain relievers, and combination products—with

Decongestant or Antihistamine?

In a nutshell, an **antihistamine** dries up what's dripping and stops the itchy, watery eyes. When your head is all blocked up and breathing seems like a lost art, the key is to unstuff it as quickly as possible with a **decongestant.** An easy way to remember this is

▦ A decongestant will decongest you, leaving you unstuffed but drippy, with a "keeping you awake" side effect.

▦ An antihistamine will dry you up, but you still may be stuffed up, with a "sleepy" side effect.

huge, medical-sounding names like *pseudo*something or *chlorbromo*something. What's effective? What's safe? Where do you even begin?

First let's decide what you need. A symptoms checker, if you will. Let's see . . . stuffed nose, stuffed head, and sinus pressure. You need a **decongestant**—fast. For sneezes, sniffles, and itchy eyes, an **antihistamine** is in order. Let's find out a little more about both of these.

Decongestants

A decongestant is a medicine that constricts or tightens swollen blood vessels in the nose. This decreases the inflammation in the nose and sinus area and allows you to breathe again, but it doesn't dry you up. When you take a decongestant, you should be prepared, with lots of tissues handy, as the drips will appear full-force.

One of the most popular tablet forms of decongestant goes by the name of **Sudafed** (*pseudoephedrine*). If breathing normally again quickly is high on your list of priorities, then a decongestant spray used directly in the nose may be what you need. Here again, you have to make choices. There are well over thirty different strengths, brands, and formulations. Stick with a long-acting active ingredient like *oxymetazoline.* You'll see this in products like **Afrin, Neo-Synephrine, Vicks,** and **4-Way** nasal sprays.

With decongestants you don't have to worry about the drowsiness found with antihistamines, but they do tend to make your heart beat faster (a type of stimulant effect). That is not a good thing if you're taking med-

>
> ## The Drug Lady Recommends . . .
>
> Nasal decongestant sprays work very well—sometimes too well. Watch out for a common problem seen with over-the-counter decongestant sprays, called **rhinitis medicamentosa**, and translated into plain English, it means DON'T USE THESE PRODUCTS OVER THREE DAYS IN A ROW. With this condition, you'll first notice a decreased effectiveness of the decongestant, then the congestion comes back with a vengeance. This "rebound congestion" can be twice as bad as that you initially experienced.

icine to control your blood pressure, or if you're trying to get some sleep. Because of the way decongestants affect the body, individuals with heart disease, prostate enlargement, thyroid disease, and diabetes should also avoid decongestants unless specifically given the okay by their doctor.

Antihistamines

We often think of antihistamines as a treatment for allergic reactions to pollen, molds, spores, and microscopic animal hair that find a home in the moist areas of the nose and throat. When this occurs, the body tries desperately to get rid of the offending substance (called an **allergen**) by sneezing, or flooding it out and releasing a chemical called **histamine.** Within a few minutes you've got watery, itchy eyes. Within hours, your sinuses become inflamed and swollen. You can't breathe and your head feels like it's filled with soggy cotton, sort of like how you feel when you have a cold— and that's why antihistamines can be helpful for this ailment as well.

Antihistamines block the action of histamine during an allergic response and prevent the drippy nose and stop the itchy eyes. Some names you see on the shelves are **Benadryl** (*diphenhydramine*), **Chlor-Trimeton** (*chlorpheniramine*), and **Tavist** (*clemastine fumarate*). (With generic or chemical names like these, aren't you glad their brand names are a little easier to pronounce?) All of them work equally well to relieve drippy cold symptoms, but they can make you very sleepy. So use caution (or avoid these altogether) if you are driving or operating heavy machinery. If you

The Drug Lady Recommends...

If you're looking for an antihistamine that will cause the least sleepiness of those available over-the-counter, try the *Chlor-Trimeton* (*chlorpheniramine*) brand. If this brand still doesn't allow you to function without snoozing, ask your doctor about non-sedating prescription antihistamines like *Claritin* (*loratidine*) or *Zyrtec* (*cetirizine*).

have emphysema, chronic bronchitis, glaucoma, or an enlarged prostate, antihistamines are also NOT advised.

Coughs

Q. *What is the best over-the-counter treatment for a nagging cough?*

A. The first step in treating a cough is to determine exactly what type of cough you have. I know you're thinking, "A cough is a cough"—but there are different kinds! And different types of coughs require different treatments. I have a warning for the faint of heart: We're going to be talking a great deal about one of my favorite topics—mucus. You can't talk about coughs without mentioning mucus, so for the overly fastidious, we'll be talking about it a lot.

What Is a Cough?

A cough is not actually an illness in itself, but part of a reflexive action that is so common, we do it almost every day. Coughing keeps the airways clear so we can breathe freely. Many times we aren't even aware we've coughed if it's just a couple of little hacks. However, when bacteria, viruses, and even allergens attack the body, it fights back by producing large amounts of mucus. This mucus protects the respiratory tract and makes it harder for these offenders to find a good foothold—they get stuck in the goo before they can make their way farther into your body. A productive cough is the body's way of getting this mucus out before the bacteria or viruses get

What's the Difference Between a Cold, Flu, and Allergy?

Let's start with the easiest one. An **allergy** is the body's attempt to fight off an offending allergen, which can be anything from animal dander to ragweed. Allergies are not contagious and usually come around seasonally if they are pollen-related, and year-round if they are related to pets or dust. There are many different classes of allergies, including skin, eye, respiratory, food, drug, latex, and insects. (See Chapter 2, "Allergic Reactions.")

A **cold** is most commonly caused by a virus in the *rhino*-family that makes itself at home in the respiratory tract and may begin with a sore throat, nasal symptoms (stuffy or runny nose), sneezing, or a cough. A typical cold lasts one to two weeks whether it's treated or not, although if the symptoms get too miserable, they can be addressed individually. (See "Common Cold," page 108.)

The **flu** (short for "influenza") is characterized by a sudden onset of fever along with head or muscle aches; sore throat, weakness, and a feeling of exhaustion are also common. (See "Flu," page 115.) The virus responsible is *H. Flu.* and may be one of several strains that are further divided into types A, B, and C. Type A is the one that changes most often, so medical science always struggles to keep up with a vaccine to prevent it. You actually begin to show symptoms of the flu from one to four days after exposure to the virus. Usual duration of the flu is one week, but the weakness may linger for another week or more. Many cases of the flu can be prevented with a vaccine.

down into the lungs. A dry cough (sometimes called "non-productive") exists when the body reacts to an irritant.

Warning: If you begin a new medication for high blood pressure (like **Prinivil** or **Zestril**) and notice a cough soon afterward, call your doctor right away. This is a common side effect of drugs called ACE inhibitors (angiotensin-converting enzyme inhibitors). ACE inhibitors control blood pressure by decreasing the substance that allows the body to retain salt and water. Other commonly prescribed drugs in this category are **Capoten** (*captopril*) and **Vasotec** (*enalapril*).

Coughs and Cough Syrups

Coughing is our body's way of getting rid of something irritating. We classify coughs according to how well they get rid of those offenders (productive or non-productive) and cough remedies as to how they treat the cough (suppressants or expectorants). A **productive cough** is one which brings up lots of sticky mucus from the far reaches of your respiratory tract. This type of cough can usually be traced to some type of infection. Productive coughs are generally treated with an **expectorant** (like *guaifenesin*) to thin the mucus and make it easier to move up and out before the bacteria or virus has an opportunity to find a new home.

A **non-productive** (or dry) **cough** occurs when you feel an irritating tickle in the back of your throat and there is no excess mucus produced. Non-productive coughs may be caused by sinus drainage, smoke, exposure to irritants in the air, and even certain types of medications. This type of cough is most effectively treated with a **cough suppressant** (like *dextromethorphan*), which acts to calm and quiet the cough.

How Are Coughs Treated?

Non-drug treatments

Drinking a big (8-ounce) glass of water is often as effective as an over-the-counter **expectorant** for thinning mucus. Drinking lots of water can be one of the fastest (and least expensive) ways of getting rid of a productive cough. Water also keeps your throat soothed when you have a non-productive cough.

For nighttime coughs, try sleeping with your head elevated six to eight inches. This will help keep the mucus from pooling in the back of your throat and triggering an annoying cough all night long.

OTC treatments

Coughs are treated with either a **cough suppressant** (like *dextromethorphan*) for a **non-productive cough** (to stop the cough) and an **expectorant** (like *guaifenesin*) for a productive cough (to thin the mucus in your respiratory tract, making it easier to expel).

Plain ***Robitussin*** (without any DM's, PE's, or CF's after the name) with the expectorant *guaifenesin* as its active ingredient is a great choice for

The Drug Lady Recommends . . .

One of the standards in the pharmacist's medicine chest for many years has been the *Robitussin* brand. This entire line of products covers almost every type of cough known to man (or woman). *Robitussin DM* (*guaifenesin* and *dextromethorphan*) is a great cough suppressant/expectorant combination to have around the house. This cough syrup thins the mucus and slows down the cough reflex and will hold you over until a doctor can determine what type of cough you have.

those rattling coughs. For long-term cough suppression (at least for a good night's sleep), a favorite of many is the twelve-hour dosing of **Delsym** (*dextromethorphan*).

An **antihistamine** can help if drippy sinuses at the back of your throat cause a cough-provoking "tickle." These drugs will dry up the sinus drainage. Also, keeping a cough drop and a bottle of water close by can keep your throat moist and stop the irritating tickle.

Prescription treatments

If any cough lingers for over ten days, it is a good idea to give the doctor a call. You could have a more serious bacterial infection that would benefit from an antibiotic. If over-the-counter **cough suppressants** aren't doing the job and your body needs the rest, your doctor may prescribe *codeine* to stop the cough. It works very well and very quickly and puts you to sleep fast. This is not a drug to use during the day when you need to function coherently.

Flu

Q. *I think I have the flu. How can I tell if it's the flu and not just a bad cold? What can I do to feel better?*

A. It's often difficult when you are sick to tell exactly what you have. You feel generally rotten. Your symptoms may look like a bad cold, with a runny nose, sore throat, cough, body aches, and fever. The only

Humor Pill

A young boy with a bad cold was taken to the doctor by his mother. After examining him, the doctor said, "There is not much I can do. He has a virus. It just has to run its course."

After they left the doctor's office, the boy said to his mother, shaking his head, "Boy, Mom, that doctor sure is dumb. He thinks that I'm a computer."

difference between a bad cold and a flu is the severity of symptoms. Fortunately, there are now ways to decrease the severity of the flu or at least make the miserable symptoms more bearable.

What Is the Flu?

The word **flu** is a shortened form of "influenza." Influenza is a viral infection that attacks the respiratory system. Currently, there are three different types of flu: A, B, and C. Type A is the form that changes or mutates from year to year. Because of these mutations, it is impossible to become permanently immune to the influenza virus.

Doctors usually make the diagnosis of flu based on how bad your symptoms become. Fever above 101 degrees Fahrenheit, chills, and severe body aches are often the determining factors. You begin to show symptoms of the flu from one to four days after exposure to the virus, and it usually lasts a week, even though a feeling of weakness may linger for another week or more. The flu is spread by direct contact with the virus and is highly contagious. When an infected person sneezes or touches an object, the virus is left behind.

How Is the Flu Treated?

Non-drug treatments

Because the flu is so highly contagious, it is important to wash your hands frequently during the flu season. Drinking plenty of water helps keep the airways moist and also helps flush viruses out of the system before they have time to find a home.

Vitamin C has been shown to have a protective effect against some forms of influenza. Taking just 500–1000 mg daily may decrease both your chance of getting the flu and the length of time it lasts.

Echinacea, with its immune-system boost, is an herbal that is showing promise for decreasing the severity of flu symptoms. Capsules or tablets of dosages of 325 to 650 mg three times daily seem to work best. Echinacea should be taken at the first sign of illness, and not on an everyday basis. It is also not recommended for individuals who have autoimmune conditions, like Rheumatoid Arthritis or Multiple Sclerosis, as this extra immune boost may actually make these conditions worse.

OTC treatments

With the flu, sometimes the best remedy is to just make yourself as comfortable as possible until the symptoms subside—in other words, address the symptoms and get plenty of rest. **Tylenol** (*acetaminophen*) or **Motrin** (*ibuprofen*) can ease the body aches, pains, and fever. **Decongestants** (like *pseudoephedrine*) will help the stuffy nose, and an **antihistamine** (like *diphenhydramine*) helps dry up the runny nose and watery eyes.

If nausea is a problem, be sure to keep your body fluid levels up. Drinking high-electrolyte beverages like **Pedialyte** will ensure that your body is able to give its best to fight the virus. While this is generally thought of as a children's product, it works well for sick adults, too.

The Drug Lady Recommends . . .

A soothing hot liquid is a way to deal with most flu symptoms. One of my customers' favorites is *Thera-Flu Flu, Cold, and Cough Relief.* This medicine has *acetaminophen* for headache, body ache, and fever; *dextromethorphan* for cough; *pseudoephedrine* as a **decongestant**; and *chlorpheniramine* as an **antihistamine**. Many people also find that the lemon flavor helps ease the pain of their sore throats.

Just add hot water to the medicine from the packet and sip it down. Ahh . . . It may make you *very* sleepy, so take this one only at night or when you're safely at home to rest.

Prescription treatments

Some of the latest prescription medicines on the market are promising in their ability to decrease the severity of flu symptoms. There are a few rules, however: Antiviral medicines like **Tamiflu** (*oseltamivir*) and **Relenza** (*zanamivir*) must be taken within the first two days of symptoms appearing. This can be difficult, especially when it is so hard to determine whether you have the flu or a bad cold. Studies have shown that if these medicines are taken soon enough after your symptoms start, they can decrease your "flulike" feelings by a day to a day and a half.

Flu Shots and Flu Sprays

For those at higher risk for contracting the flu, a flu shot gives them a fighting chance. In fact, according to one study done between 1992 and 1994, only 1.7 percent of those who got the flu shot came down with flu, while 13.4 percent of those who didn't have the shot got the flu—that's over a 90 percent effectiveness rate! Flu shots are recommended for high-risk youngsters who have weakened immune systems (like those with AIDS or diabetes); the elderly; pregnant women (AFTER the first trimester); and health-care workers who are exposed to others who may be carrying the flu virus.

Flu sprays are a new drug form for protecting against the flu. Schoolchildren all over the world are cheering that the needles might finally be put away! An intranasal flu vaccine (this means it is inhaled through the nose) is being tested with excellent results: The nasal spray demonstrated a 93-percent protection rate among schoolchildren. Pretty impressive!

Sinusitis

Q. *My nose and head are so stuffed I can barely breathe. Is this a cold or sinusitis? What is the best medicine I can take for this head congestion?*

A. Having difficulty breathing is never a pleasant feeling. Chronic head congestion is often referred to as sinusitis. Sinusitis is frequently associated with the common cold, but is actually an inflammation of the sinus membranes that can be caused by allergies, or by a bacterial or viral infection. This constant congestion can make you feel as though your head is stuffed with soggy cotton and like your brain works that way, too.

What Causes Sinusitis?

Sinus head congestion can be caused by many factors, including a cold, flu, sinus infection, or allergy. The mucus membranes in spaces behind the eyes and nose (sinuses) become irritated and inflamed; soon they swell and block the airway. A headache, runny nose, and severe head stuffiness with pressure develop. Fever, bad breath, weakness, and an inability to smell are often other unpleasant attractions of this condition.

Sinus Infections

It can be difficult to tell the difference between symptoms of a sinus infection versus other types of respiratory problems. Common symptoms of a sinus infection may include a runny nose, nasal and head congestion, facial pain in the sinus areas (forehead and below and in between the eyes), toothache, and fever. A nasal discharge that appears greenish usually signals an infection. To determine the extent of your sinus inflammation, the doctor may use magnetic resonance imaging (MRI) to look at the sinus cavities. Many symptoms of a viral or an allergy-induced sinus infection disappear within forty-eight hours, even without treatment. However, if you have a bacterial sinus infection, you may need to be treated with antibiotics. Most bacterial sinus infections can be quickly treated with a course of antibiotics like *Bactrim (trimethoprim/sulfamethoxazole)*, which your doctor can prescribe.

How Is Sinusitis Treated?

Non-drug treatments

Adding a few drops of *eucalyptus oil* to a steam vaporizer can be wonderful for opening up congested noses and heads. Taking hot showers or baths that produce large amounts of steam is also very effective for opening up the nose. *Chamomile, yarrow,* and *stinging nettle* teas have also been shown to be successful in both decreasing mucus production in the nose and bringing down inflammation in the sinus passages.

OTC treatments

Nasal decongestants such as **Sudafed** (*pseudoephedrine*) may help relieve some of the sinus pressure and increase sinus drainage. You can also try some **Tylenol** (*acetaminophen*) or **Motrin** (*ibuprofen*) for the headache and fever. If you suspect you have a sinus infection, or your symptoms continue to worsen, you should contact your doctor. Combination products with both a pain reliever and decongestant are excellent for a one-stop pill pop—**Advil Cold and Sinus** (*ibuprofen/pseudoephedrine*) is a good choice.

The Drug Lady Recommends . . .

Decongestant rubs are great. I remember the soothing feeling of **Vicks VapoRub** whenever I was congested as a child. A wonderful way to "unstuff" is to rub these ointments containing *menthol, camphor,* or *eucalyptus oil* directly on the throat and chest. This combination of warming and congestion-clearing medicine has eased many stuffed noses and rattling chests over the years. **Mentholatum** has a wonderful cherry-smelling chest rub for children and Vicks provides the same combination of ingredients for adult use without the cherry smell.

Prescription treatments

If your head is stuffed from a sinus infection, the doctor may prescribe a course of antibiotics to clear it quickly. Prescription **antihistamines** may also be effective in treating head congestion, especially if this stuffiness is caused by an **allergy.** There are combination prescription medicines, like **Claritin D,** that contain **antihistamine** (*loratidine*) and **decongestant** (*pseudoephedrine*) in one pill. The decongestant helps the antihistamine by relieving symptoms of stuffy nose and congestion.

Nasal sprays like **Beconase AQ** (*beclomethasone*) or **Flonase** (*fluticasone*) are steroids that can help with the congestion and postnasal drip that often come with allergies.

Sore Throat

Q. *What is the best treatment for a sore, scratchy throat? It hurts to eat and swallow.*

A. Ouch! It feels like someone has used sandpaper on your poor irritated throat. You never realized before just how many times a minute you swallow until it hurt this much. You need relief and you need it fast. Sometimes sore throats come right along with the whole basket of cold or flu symptoms, or they may appear on their own.

What Causes a Sore Throat?

There are actually many causes of sore throats. Bacteria or viruses can cause an infectious sore throat. Postnasal drip from an allergy can bring a miserable irritation to the back of the throat. Shouting all afternoon at the football game or being exposed to excessive smoke also may bring throat pain. You can even have a dry sore throat from breathing in cold air through your mouth.

Because so many different things can cause a sore throat, it's a good idea to get your throat checked by the doctor at the first sign of trouble. If you're not a fan of the doctor's office, at least promise me that you'll definitely go in if you also have a fever higher than 101 degrees Fahrenheit, okay? Your doctor will take a look and might take a throat culture, which usually can be read in the office. The doctor is looking for the presence of bacteria, usually from the *strep* family. A sore throat and fever without any other cold symptoms can mean **strep throat.** Strep can be fought with a course of antibiotics. Remember to take every single pill that the doctor prescribed even if the sore throat feels better. Your body is still fighting the bacteria—give it all the help you can.

How Are Sore Throats Treated?

Non-drug treatments
If your doctor has ruled out a bacterial infection, the best "at-home" treatment is to keep your throat moist. Drinking plenty of water is good. Gargling with warm salt water can be soothing as well. Orange juice may be high in *vitamin C,* but it may also sting. For adding extra C with a sore throat, a 500 mg supplement in tablet form may be the best course.

Here are a few other ways to fight sore throats at home:

▓ Warm towels or cloths placed directly on the neck can feel great.

▓ Little ones can benefit from a steam-mist vaporizer, to keep throat tissues moist while they're sleeping.

▓ Changing the family's toothbrushes every month can also toss out harmful bacteria and prevent sore throats from recurring.

The Drug Lady Recommends...

Some practitioners have noticed that individuals who get frequent sore throats have lower-than-normal levels of *zinc*. One theory for the mechanism of its action seems to be that zinc coats a cell's outer membrane and prevents bacteria or viruses from sticking to it. Zinc lozenges with 15 to 25 mg of zinc per lozenge should be started at the first tickle of a sore throat. These can be taken every two hours for several days until the sore throat eases. Studies show this helps shorten duration of sore throats by at least two days. *Nature's Answer* makes a lozenge in two pleasant flavors, cherry and lemon.

OTC treatments

Lozenges (cough drops or hard candy) and sprays that contain numbing agents (like *phenol*) can help reduce the pain short-term. **Cepastat** lozenges (with *phenol, menthol,* and *eucalyptus oil*) can be used to relieve the pain of swallowing with a sore throat. If you need additional pain relief, over-the-counter pain medications like *acetaminophen* (**Tylenol**) or *ibuprofen* (**Motrin, Advil**) may be helpful.

The Drug Lady Recommends...

When quick sore-throat relief is a priority, try **Cepacol Maximum Strength Sore Throat Spray.** You spray this directly into your mouth, aiming toward your aching throat. Swallow, and within seconds, no more pain! It uses the numbing agent *dyclonine hydrochloride* to provide temporary relief for sore-throat and mouth pain. It's not the best-tasting medicine around, but the makers of this product are trying to overcome this with both cherry and "cool menthol" flavors.

Prescription treatments

If the doctor has done a throat culture and determined the cause of the sore throat, you'll receive an antibiotic for a bacterial infection or orders to make yourself comfortable until the virus runs its course. Be sure that your doctor knows of any antibiotic allergies that you might have before he or she writes the prescription.

Warning

Take a sore throat seriously! Left untreated, a sore throat can progress to **rheumatic fever,** a more serious condition that can cause heart-valve damage. Another worry is that a bacterial infection that begins in the throat may also find a home in the kidneys, where even more damage can be done. This condition is called **glomerulonephritis**. Sore throats with chronic hoarseness also can be a warning sign of throat cancer. If it hurts for over a week, no matter how busy you are, go in to see a doctor. If it's nothing, you can fuss at me for worrying.

Embarrassing Questions: "Could You, Er, Tell Me, Um, What to Do About...?"

Bad Breath ▓ Constipation ▓ Crab Lice ▓ Dandruff ▓ Diarrhea ▓ Excessive

Hair Growth ▓ Gas ▓ Hemorrhoids ▓ Scabies ▓ Sweating ▓

Urinary Incontinence

OFTEN THERE ARE things that you just don't want to discuss with a clerk at the local pharmacy or grocery store. Gas, excessive sweating, hemorrhoids, even constipation can make even the most confident individual blush a little when confessing them to a stranger. When our bodies begin to do strange things, it's often hard to find someone to ask for this personal type of advice. Now with your very own pharmacist-in-a-book, you can tackle those totally natural, but embarrassing, bodily functions with ease and aplomb.

Bad Breath

Q. *I have a problem—my breath smells bad. My wife noticed this and has said something about it on several occasions. What can I do to control this? It makes me very self-conscious when I'm close to other people.*

A. It's understandable that you feel self-conscious when it feels like every time you speak, heavy waves of unpleasant smells emerge from your mouth. Bad breath is common, but thankfully there are very effective ways of dealing with it. Let's find out what causes it and get your breath smelling fresh ASAP!

What Causes Bad Breath?

Bad breath, also called **halitosis,** can be either a symptom of a deeper problem or simply the body's way of dealing with the foods we eat. The first place to look for the offensive odor of bad breath is in your diet. When we eat foods that are high in smelly oil content (like onions or garlic), these oils are absorbed into the lungs and breathed out. Small food particles are left in the mouth and the normal bacteria do their job and start breaking it down for digestion. Unfortunately, this breakdown often produces a very unpleasant smell. "Coffee breath" and "smoker's breath" also come from substances we ingest.

If your mouth is dry, an abundance of bacteria may be breaking down food particles, but nothing is flushing out the results from your mouth. Also, specific medical conditions, like acid reflux, diabetes, or lung problems, can be a source of foul-smelling breath. For example, sweet, fruity-smelling breath may be one of the first signs of diabetes.

How Is Bad Breath Treated?

Non-drug treatments
For the majority of bad-breath cases, brushing and flossing your teeth will do the job. For best results, brush and floss after each meal to remove food particles before the bacteria have a chance to turn them into an odor problem.

After brushing, a tongue scraper also can be used to remove the sticky concoction of bacteria and food particles from the surface of the tongue, and will leave your mouth feeling and smelling amazingly clean. Sipping a *peppermint* tea or chewing on a fresh *spearmint* or *parsley* leaf are other ways to freshen the breath.

OTC treatments

The OTC mouthwash aisle contains a confusing array of products with many different formulations and all kinds of promises. OTC mouthwashes work best by covering up and destroying the source of odors in the mouth. The high alcohol content helps to kill bacteria already present and works to digest food particles. Fewer bacteria equal less sticky plaque attached to the teeth and less odor in the mouth.

The combination of *sunflower oil* and *parsley oil* in **Breath Assure** works well for many bad-breath sufferers.

Mints containing the volatile oils of *peppermint, spearmint,* or *wintergreen* mask other odors already present, but don't cure the root of the problem.

For bad breath made worse by a dry mouth, try a saliva substitute, like **Salivart.** Artificial saliva helps to flush out the mouth and also has the benefit of soothing gum tissue irritated from prolonged dryness.

Prescription treatments

The American Dental Association (ADA) recommends that "if marked breath odor persists after proper toothbrushing, the cause should be fur-

---

The Drug Lady Recommends . . .

For double-duty in removing sticky plaque and freshening the breath, try *Plax* mouthwash. The *tetrasodium pyrophosphate* formula helps to make the plaque, bacteria, and food particles less likely to hang around in the mouth. This unique solution helps loosen and detach sticky plaque before it has a chance to harden on the teeth. The instructions call for rinsing the mouth for thirty seconds BEFORE brushing for best results.

ther investigated." Give your dentist or doctor a call pronto. He or she can rule out any other mouth problems and advise you on what other medical conditions could be responsible for this continuing odor.

Constipation

Q. *I'm tired of spending so much time in the bathroom! What causes constipation? What is "normal"? What can I do to make it go away? I'd really like to avoid it completely.*

A. It seems like every third TV commercial touts the importance of being "regular" or offers remedies for those who aren't—but what exactly is "regular"? Americans greatly vary in their bowel habits, from three times a day to three times a week. What works for you is considered regular.

What Causes Constipation?

Constipation is normally caused by diet, a sedentary lifestyle, or a medication's side effects. More often than not, constipation can be traced to diet and not taking in enough fiber or fluid. It is very important to drink enough water; if you don't, your insides can get tied up for days.

Have you ever eaten that triple-cheese pizza and wondered why you couldn't go to the bathroom for a week? Some processed foods like cheese can actually harden in the colon and put a stop to the whole elimination process.

Lack of exercise will let everything you eat sit right where it is digested—in your colon. Sitting for hours at a desk, or in front of the TV, also does nothing to help move everything down and out. Get up and exercise— your colon will thank you.

It's ironic, but overuse of laxatives to relieve constipation can actually cause more constipation. The drugs in stimulant laxatives, like *senna, cascara,* or *phenolphthalein,* actually irritate the colon in order to produce a bowel movement. When the colon is sufficiently irritated, it simply stops responding to the laxative. Then you take more laxative to get results, and the cycle begins again.

Other medications, such as *codeine* (for pain) or *amitriptyline* (for depression), may also cause occasional constipation. Read the side-effect profile carefully on any drugs you are taking; they may be the culprits for your constipation problem.

How Is Constipation Treated?

Non-drug treatments

Fiber, fiber, fiber! To avoid constipation, you must eat your veggies. Unprocessed grains and the good fiber from fruits can keep your intestines squeaky-clean. Be careful, though, and remember to drink water. Too much fiber without adequate water will quickly lead to that plugged-up feeling.

Another hint: If you feel like you have to go, then by all means, go! Holding in a bowel movement can compound constipation. If you feel like it—do it!

The Drug Lady Recommends . . .

There are three things you should do before you ever buy that first laxative: drink lots of water, get up and exercise, and add some fiber to your diet. Fiber makes you regular by adding bulk to the stool. Drinking at least 64 ounces of water each day, and walking instead of sitting, often will move things right along.

OTC treatments

The safest medication form for over-the-counter relief is the stool softener. These are found in drugstore aisles as **Colace** or *docusate sodium*. Stool softeners work by increasing the amount of liquid in formed stools. This makes the bowel movement easier to pass. Take stool softeners with lots and lots of water. Stool softeners are often the best choice for children because they do not cause cramping and work without harsh medicine.

The old standby **Phillips Milk of Magnesia** has unplugged many individuals over the years. The active ingredient, *magnesium hydroxide*, helps to pull water from the intestines, making bowel movements easier to pass.

The Drug Lady Recommends . . .

Stimulant laxatives should be used VERY occasionally, if at all. Stimulant laxatives contain irritating substances that force the colon to move the stool. Using these more than occasionally can damage the large intestine.

Stimulant laxatives work very quickly, but also sometimes very violently. These products get rid of everything quickly and often produce stomach cramping and pain. Brand names are **Correctol, Ex-Lax,** and **Dulcolax.** Their active ingredients are *senna, anthraquinones, cascara sagrada, bisacodyl,* or *phenolphthalein.*

Fiber laxatives like **Metamucil** and **Citrucel** are wonderful for chronic constipation (although if you would just eat your veggies, you might not need the laxative). Be aware that you MUST drink at least eight glasses of water a day while you are taking this laxative or the fiber can form a lump in your gastrointestinal tract. Fiber laxatives can also absorb some medications, such as vitamin supplements, so use caution before combining them with your other medicines.

When constipation has become severe or impacted, a laxative enema, like **Fleets,** may be advised. Enemas are also used to prep patients for certain surgeries or colon exams, or before the birth of a baby.

Prescription remedies

When strong painkillers (like *morphine*) that constipate are used in surgery, laxative suppositories (inserted into the rectum) are often prescribed.

Constipation also can be caused by more serious problems like a low-thyroid condition (hypothyroidism) or lesions in the colon. Symptoms to look for before calling the doctor include: dull headaches, loss of appetite, low back pain, or a stomach that sticks out or is bloated. If you are using laxatives more frequently but getting worse results each time, call your physician.

Humor Pill
True Story from the Pharmacy Files

A customer comes in several days after filling a prescription for laxative suppositories.

The pharmacist inquires about her condition: "So how are you feeling? Did the medicine help?"

"Well, yes and no," the customer answered. "Yes, I feel better, but I don't think my medicine helped."

"Why not?" the pharmacist asked.

She leaned close and whispered, "Because it tasted so bad that I only was able to swallow one!"

Crab Lice

Q. *I think I have crabs! I'm itching like crazy in embarrassing places. How can I tell if it's crabs or just an itch? What can I use for a quick treatment?*

A. Just the idea that little creepy-crawly creatures could be moving around on your body is enough to make anyone itch. And that's just what crab lice do—very well. These insects look just like tiny crabs when you look at them up close. Crab lice can also lay tiny eggs called "nits," which attach to the pubic hair. These nits will look very much like a white fleck of skin, but are difficult to remove from the hair. The good news is that there is treatment and it can be started quickly. Good-bye, crabs!

What Are Crab Lice?

Crab lice ("crabs," for short) are lice, approximately two millimeters long, that prefer the pubic-hair area but can also be found in chest hair or in the underarms. They received their name because when you look at them closely, they have claws similar to those of ocean crabs. These claws allow them to hold on tightly to a hair shaft, where the crabs do what they do best—reproduce. The female lays three to four eggs each day, which she attaches firmly to the hair. When the nits hatch eight to ten days later, a new colony takes over.

The itching is a result of the inevitable feeding cycle of the crabs. They eat by sucking your blood. Each tiny bite causes an irritation that you want to scratch, so itching is usually the first symptom.

Crabs are spread by close physical contact, most often through sexual contact, although a few cases have been traced to shared towels or toilet seats. Of all the things you can share with someone you care for, crabs are not the most pleasant. Also keep in mind that you can actually have crabs for several days to a week before you notice any symptoms.

How Are Crab Lice Treated?

Non-drug treatments

Because the key to eliminating lice is to completely and totally kill each individual louse and the nits that are cemented onto the hair, I have found no proven natural remedies that will be 100-percent effective. It's time for the really strong stuff. These little fellas are tough.

However, while you are busy taking care of the lice on your body, this is also a great time to wash your clothes, bedding, or towels that could have come into contact with the crabs. Hot water, soap, and using the HOT setting on the dryer are a must because lice can live up to twenty-four hours after they have left your body.

OTC treatments

Thankfully, there are some very effective medications that you can find right on your drugstore shelf. Keep in mind that these medicines are pesticides, and should be used with great care. Pesticides interfere with the nervous system of the bugs in order to kill them. Overuse, or inappropriate use, of these lice treatments could do the same to your nervous system—so be careful!

Nix Lice Shampoo contains *permethrin*, thought by many to be the most pleasant of the pesticide products to use. I prefer this one because it can be applied as a cream, lotion, or shampoo and seems to be the most effective way to get rid of the little bugs in the fewest applications. Nix also reports the fewest side effects.

Rid Lice Shampoo is another bestseller. It contains *pyrethrin,* an effective crab-lice killer. Because pyrethrin is made from chrysanthemum extracts, those with ragweed allergies should avoid this product. And here is the tough part: To work most effectively, Rid Lice Shampoo should stay on for at least ten minutes, but no longer than ten minutes. So set a clock; when the ten minutes are up, rinse quickly. Remember, this is VERY powerful stuff: Follow the package directions carefully.

When you have rinsed the shampoo out thoroughly, a fine-toothed comb or a special lice/nit-removing comb may be used to help remove dead lice or their eggs (nits) from the hair. Most kits come with a nifty little comb inside. Often one treatment will be enough, but you should expect to repeat this treatment after seven to ten days, for up to three weeks, if all the lice and nits have not been eliminated.

Prescription treatments

If your crabs have gotten out-of-hand, and the over-the-counter medicines just aren't working, you may want to see a doctor. First, he can rule out the possibility that something else besides crab lice might be going on. Second, he can prescribe a very strong anti-lice medication called *lindane* that is available in lotion and shampoos. Lindane is not recommended for infants or pregnant or breast-feeding women; there have also been reports of rare neurologic problems occurring in children after use of lindane. If you must use this product, do so VERY carefully!

Dandruff

Q. *I can't seem to shake the flakes—I have incurable dandruff! It is so bad that my entire wardrobe is made up of light-colored clothes, even in the winter. Help!*

A. Hiding in summer clothes all through winter isn't fun. Just think of all of the great winter fashions you're missing, too! Dandruff is a problem shared by over sixty-three million Americans, but that isn't much consolation when you're constantly brushing flakes from your shoulders. The good news is that dandruff is curable—even yours! It just takes a little time and patience.

What Causes Dandruff?

Believe it or not, dandruff is not always caused by a dry scalp or not washing your hair often enough. A tiny fungus called *Pitysporum ovale* (*P. ovale* for short) can be blamed for most cases of dandruff. This friendly fungus finds a great home in the cells of your scalp. When it irritates the cells and causes them to reproduce much faster than normal, the dead white skin cells are discarded onto your shoulders.

Seborrheic dermatitis, an inherited inflammation of the upper layers of the skin, is another common cause of dandruff. When the skin is dry and inflamed, it causes flaking of the skin on the scalp, on the face, and behind the ears.

How Is Dandruff Treated?

Non-drug treatments

For the dry-scalp problems, adding *flaxseeds, flax oil,* or *fish oils* to your diet may help the flaking.

The Drug Lady Recommends . . .

If your goal is to kill the fungus in a more natural fashion, then a powerful natural antifungal like *tea tree oil* might be in order. You may add several drops directly to your favorite shampoo or look for tea tree shampoos in your local health-food or natural-products store. Watch for the tingle—you'll know its working. It may take a week or so, but tea tree oil is very effective in the treatment of dandruff.

OTC treatments

Because dandruff is such a common condition, over-the-counter treatment for it is big business. The key to the complete elimination of dandruff is simple: patience. Any of the shampoos you use must remain on your hair for a minimum of one minute each time you shampoo. Some should remain on for as long as five minutes. Sing a song, count sheep, or do whatever it takes. If you follow the package instructions, dandruff relief is within sight.

One of the active ingredients you will see in dandruff shampoos is *coal tar* (like the product **Ionil T**). Coal tar is a multipurpose element; it is antiseptic (kills germs), antifungal (kills *P. ovale*), and anti-itch (stops the itch).

Another important active ingredient is *selenium sulfide*. Products like **Selsun Blue** decrease the rate at which the cells on the scalp reproduce. Fewer cells forming equal fewer flakes on the head.

A common dandruff-fighter that has been around awhile is **Head & Shoulders,** with *pyrithione zinc* as its active ingredient. Pyrithione zinc works much like selenium sulfide to slow down the rampant cell growth on your scalp.

The Drug Lady Recommends . . .

The newest kid on the dandruff front is *ketoconazole,* known in over-the-counter circles as *Nizoral AD 1% Shampoo,* but the prescription people know it well as the number-one prescribed dandruff shampoo (*Nizoral 2%*). Ketoconazole specifically targets and kills the *P. ovale* fungus.

Prescription treatments

For severe cases of dandruff, or those that simply don't seem to be responding to over-the-counter medicines, it may be time to call in the big guns for a full dermatological workup. If the over-the-counter *selenium sulfide* doesn't do the job, there is prescription strength available in 2.5 percent. Ditto for the *ketoconazole*. Prescription strength is 2 percent (**Nizoral 2% Shampoo**), while non-prescription strength is 1 percent (**Nizoral AD**).

When the itching becomes severe or causes redness, lotions with mild corticosteroids may be prescribed. These are very effective for non-fungal forms of dandruff. You see these lotions as prescriptions for **Hytone** (*hydrocortisone*) or **Kenalog** (*triamcinolone*). These should be used only under a doctor's supervision and for only two weeks at a time. Steroids can cause damage to your skin and increase suceptibility to infection if used for long periods of time.

Diarrhea

Q. *I seem to have diarrhea at least once a week. My diet is okay (most of the time), but my job is pretty stressful. Could stress be causing this? What can I do to get rid of this annoying diarrhea permanently?*

A. Okay, let's see if I've got this straight. You eat okay sometimes, you're stressed at work, and you have diarrhea—any connection? Probably. You know the symptoms: loose watery stools, stomach cramps, and an urgent need to "go."

Stress and diet are big contributors to occasional diarrhea. If it's a weekly bout of diarrhea that you're trying to avoid, take a look at what's going on around you when it happens. Your stomach could be trying to tell you to ease up on the hot, spicy stuff just a bit, or to watch how you're feeling during those high-pressure sales meetings.

What Causes Diarrhea?

Thankfully, most types of diarrhea run their course (no pun intended) within a few hours to a few days. The causes can be varied. Common causes include bacterial and viral diarrhea, food poisoning, inflammatory diseases of the colon, and certain antibiotics. Diarrhea is how our body says, "Get this nasty stuff out of me right now." It is very important to let diarrhea have its way—at least for a short while.

How Is Diarrhea Treated?

Non-drug treatments
Clear liquids are often the very best first choice for diarrhea treatment. Replacing fluids lost through diarrhea is very important. If you are able to

eat something, foods that thicken the stool, like rice, yogurt, bananas, or cheese are also a good choice.

Herbal remedies can be helpful for occasional diarrhea. If you are suffering from stomach cramps, *chamomile* tea can ease the irritation. Herbs high in tannins, like *blackberry, blueberry,* or *raspberry* leaves, have been used historically to relieve diarrhea. If your problem is caused by a bacterial infection, the herb *goldenseal* is known for its antibacterial properties.

OTC treatments

There are very effective over-the-counter anti-diarrheals now on the market. Of course, there is the old standby **Pepto-Bismol,** but avoid this one if your doctor has said no to taking *aspirin* or *salicylates.* Its active ingredient is *bismuth subsalicylate,* an aspirin family member. Just one word of warning— Pepto-Bismol can cause your tongue or stool to turn black for the entire time you take it. This is normal, nothing serious, so don't worry.

Kaopectate contains *attapulgite,* a form of clay that acts to absorb extra water and changes your stool consistency to a firmer state. This is a safe choice for the younger set, too.

If the diarrhea causes dehydration, it may be necessary to supplement with high-electrolyte drinks like **Pedialyte.** This is commonly used for children with diarrhea, but is effective for fluid-deficient adults, too. In a pinch you may also try commercial sports drinks, like **Gatorade.** However, these may be very high in sodium and are not recommended for those on a sodium-restricted diet.

The Drug Lady Recommends . . .

Look for *loperamide* in anti-diarrheal medications. One such product is *Imodium-AD.* This is the most effective and fastest over-the-counter treatment for diarrhea and cramping. Loperamide works by slowing down the motion (peristalsis) of the intestine and allowing stools to form normally. This is often effective in just one dose, in both adults and children six years and older. It may make you a little sleepy, so use caution if you are driving or operating machinery (like the lawn mower).

Prescription treatments

The prescription drug **Lomotil** (a combination product, with the generic names *diphenoxylate* and *atropine*) acts by slowing down the motion of the digestive system, known as peristalsis. This can interact with other medications, so be sure your doctor is aware of any other medicines you are taking.

You also may need to have lab tests to determine whether bacteria or protozoa are causing your illness. If the diarrhea is persistent, your doctor may prescribe an antibiotic to eliminate the bacteria.

If your little one is suffering from diarrhea, look for signs of dehydration after the first symptoms appear. Check the skin often for dryness or loss of elasticity (it sinks in when a finger is pressed on it but doesn't spring back)—a "bread dough" type of feeling. Infants can have a sunken soft spot on the top of their head if they are losing water too rapidly. (See "Children's Diarrhea," chapter 3, page 63.)

If the diarrhea won't quite go away after forty-eight hours, or if you notice that your stools look black or bloody, call your physician right away. Ditto if there are large amounts of mucus with the bowel movement, or you experience severe stomach pain or high fever. These conditions could signal that something much more serious, like gastritis or a bleeding ulcer, is happening inside of your body. Take care of this pronto!

Excessive Hair Growth

Q. *What is the best way to get rid of excessive hair? I am a woman and have hair growing on my upper lip and my chin. Is there something abnormal going on with me? Can I safely remove it?*

A. Sprouting a mustache or a beard when you're a woman can be a very unsettling experience. From birth we've been taught that men shave their faces and women shave their legs and underarms. Now you find you're shaving everywhere. Please don't feel as though you are alone. In fact, 10 percent of the female population suffers from excess hair growth (called hirsutism in scientific circles).

What Causes Excessive Hair Growth?

Hirsutism can be a result of many factors. It may just be that your body is going through a hormonal change; puberty, pregnancy, and menopause can trigger excessive hair growth. Sometimes you just can't escape your genes. Heredity is the main cause of excessive hair growth, especially if you are Caucasian or of Mediterranean descent. The hair follicles get larger and the hair itself turns dark and coarse. Certain medications, like steroids, birth-control pills, or *minoxidil* (a blood-pressure medicine and the active ingredient in **Rogaine**), can also produce excessive hair growth. Another cause is a possible ovarian tumor. These can cause the body to produce too-high levels of testosterone.

Warning:

If your excessive hair growth comes on suddenly (within a period of four or five months) and is accompanied by unexplained weight gain, a deepening voice, and menstrual changes, call your personal physician right away. It may be nothing serious, but tumors of the ovary, thyroid, or adrenal glands can cause these particular symptoms. Polycystic ovary syndrome, or the condition when the ovaries become enlarged with fluid-filled cysts, is also the cause of up to 10 percent of all hirsutism cases. This disorder causes an increase in male hormones (androgens) and a corresponding increase in body hair and other male characteristics (like a deepening voice). Your doctor can make a diagnosis based on certain hormone levels in the body. Treatment will depend on the symptoms and severity of the problem.

How Is Excessive Hair Growth Treated?

Non-drug treatments

The herbal supplement *saw palmetto,* due to its anti-testosterone properties, has been used for treatment of excessive hair growth in women. Does it work? European studies have shown that an extract from the saw palmetto berries taken twice daily in a dose of 160 mg can decrease the effects of testosterone in the hair follicle. It may take up to three months to see diminished hair growth. Your results will also depend on the cause of your excessive hair growth. It will work best if the hair growth is caused by greater-than-normal levels of testosterone.

OTC treatments

The good news is, there are lots of over-the-counter options for hair removal. The bad news is that many of these hair-removal methods hurt! Waxing pulls the hair out by the roots. Electrolysis electrocutes the root of the hair. Bleaches lighten darker, more noticeable hair. Harsh depilatory chemicals effectively melt the hair away. Smoothness comes only at a great price. Side effects of these products are redness, rashes, burning, and tenderness. The hair may be gone, but now you have a rash mustache!

When there are only a few hairs to deal with, tweezers or shaving can do the trick. Be aware that once hair is shaved or plucked, it will grow back much coarser than before.

There are only two permanent ways to remove hair: electrolysis and laser-light treatments. Both of these kill the hair follicle at the root—electrolysis does so by electrocution, and laser by using strong beams of light. It may take several treatments to completely clear an area due to the different life cycles and different speeds of growth of hair follicles.

The Drug Lady Recommends . . .

■ For waxing, try *Nair 15-Second Microwave Wax Hair Removal Kit.* (Yes, it hurts a bit, but at least it's quick!)

■ For a depilatory, try *Nair 3-in-1 Lotion Hair Remover.* (It smells good and keeps the skin moisturized to help prevent rashes.)

■ For bleaches, try *Jolen Crème Bleach.* (Follow package directions carefully, as it can burn sensitive skin.)

Prescription treatments

The prescription drug **Aldactone** (*spironolactone*) is commonly given to women who experience excessive hair growth when other physical problems, such as ovarian tumors, have been ruled out. Generally doctors prescribe this for cases of excessive testosterone production or hormonal changes associated with menopause. It has few side effects (increased urine production or low blood pressure are the most common) and has been shown to be effective within two to five months after treatment starts.

Vaniqa *(eflornithine)* is the first topical treatment for decreasing facial hair in women. It works by stopping the enzyme *ornithine decarboxylase,* which stimulates hair growth. Unfortunately, it doesn't remove the hair, it only slows its growth, so traditional forms of hair removal are still necessary. Darn!

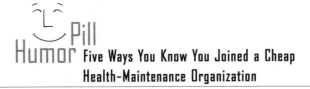

Pill Humor — Five Ways You Know You Joined a Cheap Health-Maintenance Organization

1. Tongue depressors taste faintly of Fudgsicle.

2. The kidney dialysis machines are pedal-powered.

3. Annual breast exams are conducted at the local Hooters restaurant.

4. You swear you saw a crab fork and salad tongs on the instrument tray just before you went under for surgery.

5. You ask for a prescription for Viagra. You get a Fudgsicle stick and some duct tape.

Gas

Q. *I have this terrible problem with gas after I eat. It has gotten so bad that I'm afraid to eat anything at work for fear of an embarrassing "explosion" in my cubical.*

A. It's like living with a live volcano in your stomach every day. You know the signs—the rumblings and gurglings that are a sure signal of an imminent eruption that would put the Mount St. Helens volcano to shame. Unfortunately, this eruption usually manages to time itself exactly when you've stepped into the crowded elevator on the way to the forty-third floor.

What Causes Gas?

When it becomes a choice between eating your meals at home and avoiding your coworkers at every turn, it's time to do something about the gas problem. Gas (flatulence) can be a result of many factors, including improper digestion, dietary changes, or even stress. When you feel anxiety, there is a tendency to swallow air rapidly. This air fills up the stomach and intestine and must go somewhere fast—it exits either as a burp or as gas.

While fiber is a great thing for our bodies, it is not quite so friendly to those around us. Those healthy foods like cabbage, beans, corn, or broccoli can produce an unhealthy atmosphere very quickly when they are added to your diet unexpectedly. The key is to gradually increase your fiber intake until your system is used to the change.

Sugar-free candy or gum that contains *sorbitol* can also cause excess gas. Many people don't have the enzyme that effectively breaks down sorbitol, so the intestinal bacteria change it directly into gas.

Lactose intolerance, or the inability to effectively digest milk products, also can cause many digestive problems, including gas and stomach cramps. In these cases, the *lactase* enzyme can be helpful when taken before eating or drinking dairy products.

How Is Gas Treated?

Non-drug treatments
If you've ruled out dietary changes or stress, you might try to eat and drink more slowly so you swallow less air with your food. Calming your stomach with a warm *peppermint* tea can help digestion. After eating, try going for a short walk around the building instead of immediately camping out in your cubicle. This can relieve the pressure on your stomach and allow you to digest better.

OTC treatments

It may look as though there are more anti-gas products on the OTC shelf than anyone could ever use, but there are definitely differences. The key is finding the one that works best for you.

If you aren't sure exactly which foods cause your gas problem, or if you simply need relief right now, *simethicone* will be your best choice. Simethicone works by decreasing the tension of gas bubbles already in your gastrointestinal (GI) tract. This allows the bubbles to pop very easily, so the passing gas is not quite as explosive. Products to look for are **Gas-X** or **Tempo Chewables**. Be sure to double-check the amount of simethicone in the products you buy; even though it may say "extra strength," one particular brand may have less simethicone per dose than another.

If your gas can be narrowed down to the times you consume dairy products, but you love to eat cheese, you can take **Lactaid,** which has a special enzyme (*lactase*) that breaks down milk sugars quickly, before they have time to produce gas or stomach distress.

The Drug Lady Recommends . . .

To prevent gas from forming, try **Beano.** This works especially well for high-fiber-diet gas. Beano contains the enzyme *alpha-galactosase,* which breaks down these kinds of foods before they are turned into smelly gas. So, when you know that you're going out for a chili lunch, pop a little bottle of Beano in your pocket. It just takes three to eight drops added to the first bite of food to do the job. Be sure to let the food cool a bit, because temperatures over 137 degrees Fahrenheit can deactivate the enzyme.

Prescription treatments

If your gas continues to be a problem despite over-the-counter treatments, it is time to call your doctor for a look. If your diagnosis is acid-reflux disease (an indigestion-related condition), then an acid proton pump inhibitor (which decreases the amount of acid your stomach produces) may be needed. **Prilosec** (*omeprazole*) is commonly prescribed for this situation.

If it is determined that you have an ulcer, your doctor may prescribe an H$_2$ acid blocker like **Zantac** (*ranitidine*) or **Pepcid** (*famotidine*).

The Drug Lady Recommends . . .

Before getting that very expensive acid-blocker prescription filled, you might want to try them in their over-the-counter (OTC) forms to be sure they work well for you. The OTC products are typically one-half the strength of their prescription counterparts, but have the same ingredients (and cautions) as the prescription medicines. OTC products to look for are *Zantac 75*, *Tagamet HB*, or *Pepcid AC*.

Hemorrhoids

Q. *I can't believe I have hemorrhoids! What can I do to get rid of them? How can I be sure that it isn't something more serious?*

A. Ouch! Hemorrhoids are definitely a painful problem. They may start innocently enough, with a slight tenderness or discomfort, then rapidly progress to bleeding and itching. It is hard enough to be suffering with the problem; you don't need the embarrassment of having to ask the clerk what is the fastest and best product. You need relief and you need it fast—no questions asked. Here is what you need to know about hemorrhoids.

What Are Hemorrhoids?

Hemorrhoids are swollen veins in the lower rectum and anus (the opening at the end of the rectum where the bowel movement passes). The veins in the anus tend to stretch out under pressure. This pressure can be in the form of straining during a bowel movement, or during pregnancy when the uterus presses on the hemorrhoidal veins. People who have a diet low in fiber and those who spend lots of time "reading" in the bathroom more commonly suffer from hemorrhoids.

The most common symptoms with hemorrhoids are burning, pain, itching, and bright red blood on the toilet paper. If you notice an unusual discharge from the anus, blood in the bowel movement, or severe pain, call your physician right away. These symptoms can be a signal that something more serious is going on and should be looked at by someone familiar with that area of the body.

Remember that certain lifestyle factors tip the scales in favor of developing hemorrhoids. If you sit or stand for long periods of time at work, eat donuts and other wonderful low-fiber foods for most meals, and don't drink enough water for your system to flush itself out normally, hemorrhoids could be an unpleasant little surprise.

You may also see hemorrhoids referred to as "piles," although why someone came up with that awful term, I can't imagine. Hemorrhoids come in two distinct styles. Those most often seen are the internal variety. These are painless, but can cause quite a bit of bleeding. Swollen internal veins can stretch over time. These are called hemorrhoidal prolapses and are identified when the vein moves through the anus to outside the body. The other form of hemorrhoid is the external kind. These show up as a swollen area around the anus that can be readily seen or felt. External hemorrhoids are easily torn when wiping, so be gentle!

How Are Hemorrhoids Treated?

Non-drug treatments

Treatment of hemorrhoids should begin with using soft, unscented toilet tissue. It's worth the few extra pennies to get the softest tissue possible for that delicate area. Don't rub! Pat gently when wiping.

Sitting in a **sitz bath** of warm water for fifteen minutes can also relieve the symptoms of hemorrhoids. You can use the inexpensive plastic sitz baths that fit over the toilet seat for even more convenience.

OTC treatments

To get a thorough but gentle cleaning, try baby wipes. These are soft and lightly lubricated. If they're gentle enough for a baby's tushie, they should be great for yours. Some of these even have *aloe vera* added to help relieve the burning and irritation.

The Drug Lady Recommends . . .

When your anal area is irritated, burning, or itching, there is very little that feels better than applying a cool, soothing pad liberally soaked with a medicine designed specifically to relieve those symptoms. Soft, hemorrhoidal pads such as *Tucks Hemorrhoidal Pads* contain *witch hazel,* a common **astringent** that dries and cools the itch and burn of hemorrhoidal irritation.

Most hemorrhoidal preparations have an ingredient that protects the anal area from irritation by fecal matter. These protectant barriers, like *petrolatum, zinc oxide,* or *lanolin,* give the skin underneath a chance to heal. For hemorrhoids that are swollen, vasoconstrictives (such as *ephedrine, epinephrine,* or *phenylephrine*) are commonly used to tighten the veins. Because they have an effect on shrinking blood vessels, these should be used with caution if you have diabetes, high blood pressure, enlarged prostate, or high thyroid levels. *Preparation H* is the most common brand of product that has both protectant and vasoconstrictive agents.

If your hemorrhoids are painful, the "*-caine*" products (*benzocaine, dibucaine, tetracaine,* or *lidocaine*) might be just what you need; these are local anesthetics, which means they numb the area where the hemorrhoids are causing the problems. *Pramoxine* is another anesthetic that can be effective, though not related to the "*-caine*" family. *Americaine* and *Anusol Hemorrhoidal Ointments* are wonderful products for their numbing effects.

Prescription treatments

When your hemorrhoids simply won't go away or they have become so bothersome that you just can't take it any longer, it may be time to see the doc. He or she may prescribe an added medicine called a corticosteroid to be used as a part of your hemorrhoidal treatment. Typically it is *hydrocortisone 2.5%* that is used in these preparations. Hydrocortisone is very effective in reducing inflammation from hemorrhoids. Some prescription products go by the names of *Anusol HC* or *Proctofoam HC.*

Scabies

Q. *The day care said that scabies was going around. What is (are?) scabies? How can I tell if my family has it (or them)? I would be so embarrassed! What can we do to prevent scabies?*

A. Believe it or not, scabies are a fairly common skin infection caused by a tiny little mite. This little bug finds a nice home in the top layer of skin. Most often, scabies outbreaks are seen in places where there are lots of people, like nursing homes or day-care centers. If someone in the family has it, you'll know—they'll be scratching like crazy. You also can usually tell if someone has scabies by the short, dark, wavy lines on the skin's surface. Since close personal contact spreads scabies, it is impossible to prevent them; the only way to avoid them is to avoid the exposure.

What Are Scabies?

Is it a "scabi" or scabies? The official word is *scabies*, plural. Scabies are small (0.4 mm) mites with four pairs of legs. Their sole purpose in life is to tunnel under your skin and lay their eggs, which hatch within two weeks. (Yuck!) Sometimes the whole family can be infected before you are aware that anyone has it. The mites prefer the webs of the fingers, wrists, elbows, armpits, and groin area. If this is the first exposure, your family may not show symptoms until two to six weeks after the mites have found a home. Then the itching begins. Small, very itchy blisters may appear after a bath or when your child scratches the skin.

A secondary infection sometimes can occur when the itching becomes severe. Bacteria can find a home along with the scabies mites, and a prescription antibiotic may be necessary. If itching is still present once treatment has begun, antihistamines can relieve the discomfort.

How Are Scabies Treated?

Non-drug treatments

Because the scabies mites must be completely annihilated to stop the itching and interrupt their reproductive cycle, there are no effective non-drug treatments of which I am aware.

Limiting contact with and thorough washing of the affected individual's clothing, toys, towels, and bedding should help prevent the spread to other family members. Often the source of the mite can be traced to an area of the yard or even a favorite swimming hole, as this is where the little fellas live. Once identified, these areas must be avoided.

OTC treatments

Unfortunately, this is one of the few skin conditions where over-the-counter medicines will not be effective. This is strictly a prescription-only endeavor.

Prescription treatments

To determine if the infection is scabies, your doctor may take a skin scraping and look for mites under the microscope. If scabies are diagnosed, you'll take home a prescription for **Elimite** (*permethrin*). Follow the directions to the letter or the medicine may not be effective.

The Drug Lady Recommends . . .

I checked with the Center for Disease Control (CDC) and was told that the only approved treatment of scabies was the prescription drug *Elimite* (*permethrin*). This medicine is applied from the neck down over the whole body. That's the WHOLE body—from the neck to the soles of the feet! It should be left on for at least eight hours (overnight is good), then washed off thoroughly.

This should kill the mites. Itching may continue, but should go away within a day or so. Sometimes a second application is necessary. These guys are tough, but thankfully, they are not invincible.

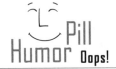

Pill Humor Oops!

We've all had the experience of not being recognized by our patients if we meet them outside of the pharmacy. It must be the white coat. One pharmacist tells of an evening at a very trendy Seattle restaurant with his family when a female customer and her husband sat beside them at the bar. She looked at him quizzically for a moment when he said hi, then loudly blurted out, "Oh, hi! How are you? I just didn't recognize you with your clothes on."

Sweating

Q. *I have a problem with excessive sweating. It usually just happens when I'm nervous, but it is very bad. What can I do?*

A. Excessive sweating can be caused by a lot of things, including nerves, stress, or even a more serious medical condition like diabetes or a thyroid imbalance. The body sweats to lower its internal temperature, but it is possible for our inner thermostats to get a little wacky. When that happens, it is called hyperhidrosis, or excessive sweating.

What Causes Excessive Sweating?

Certain medical problems, like high thyroid levels or high blood sugar, may make you sweat profusely. If your excessive sweating comes on suddenly, it's a good idea to have your doctor do a checkup just to rule out any serious problems.

Hyperhidrosis can make your underarms feel as though you have a fountain installed. *Drip. Drip. Drip.* It can also affect the palms of the hands, the feet, and the groin. This condition is caused by an overstimulation of the nerves that control sweating. With these areas staying wet most of the time, it is only a matter of time before bacteria or yeast begin to grow, leading to body odor (**bromhidrosis**). (See "Body Odor," chapter 12, page 301.)

How Can You Treat Excessive Sweating?

Non-drug treatments

Walnut leaf compresses applied to the palms of the hands and the soles of the feet for several minutes each day will help dry the areas. The recommended amount for a compress or soak is 2 to 3 grams in 3 ounces of water. Unfortunately, walnut leaf doesn't have a long-term effect.

Dried *sage* in a dosage of 5 grams (1 teaspoonful) taken daily in a glass of water may actually slow down perspiration temporarily. However, sage isn't safe for pregnant women or those with a history of seizures.

OTC treatments

Over-the-counter **antiperspirants** can help control sweaty underarms. These come in a variety of forms such as roll-ons, sticks, pads, creams, sprays, and gels. The antiperspirant part of the product has *aluminum* in it. The aluminum works by actually shrinking the sweat glands, decreasing the amount that you perspire, and bacteria don't have as much to feast on. Antiperspirants are also important when you're wearing a dark shirt and don't want everyone to know that you're stressing out. Damp underarms just aren't cool.

Deodorants are often combined with antiperspirants to help hide the odor by killing bacteria as it grows in the warm, moist areas under your arms. Deodorants alone don't decrease the amount that you sweat, they only cover up what's there.

The Drug Lady Recommends . . .

Look for the active ingredient *aluminum zirconium trichlorohydrex glycine* in your deodorant/antiperspirant combinations. I know that's quite a mouthful, but you'll see this in brands like *Ban Ultra-Dry* and *Secret Platinum Protection*. Also, according to tests from the Food and Drug Administration (FDA), the roll-on is the most effective application form.

Prescription treatments

When over-the-counter methods have failed, your doctor might try the prescription medicine called **Drysol** (*aluminum chloride hexahydrate*). Drysol is reported to work in 80 percent of the people who use it for excessive sweating.

The Drug Lady Recommends . . .

Follow the directions on the *Drysol* bottle carefully. It should be applied at bedtime when the skin is dry. Cover the treated area with a protective plastic wrap, like *Saran-Wrap,* to allow the medicine to soak in. It should be washed off the next morning and no other antiperspirant should be applied. This procedure should be repeated nightly until the sweating is under control. Fortunately, according to the product information, many people respond in just two treatments. Excessive sweating from the palms of the hands and soles of the feet may take longer to respond, due to the thicker skin of these areas.

If Drysol isn't effective, there is a type of surgery that cuts the "overstimulated" nerve. It's not for everyone, but at least there is an option for a total cure.

Urinary Incontinence

Q. *My mom has a question that she's embarrassed to ask about. She occasionally has times when she accidentally wets herself. It usually happens when she's laughing or hurrying to get somewhere. What can she do to avoid this?*

A. Please tell your mom that "The Drug Lady" says she has absolutely nothing to be embarrassed about. Urinary incontinence is a common problem. In fact, it occurs in as many as one in three Americans aged sixty or over and is twice as likely to affect women as men. The good news is that with the proper treatment, over 80 percent of those who suffer from incontinence can be helped.

What Is Urinary Incontinence?

Urinary incontinence is the inability to hold your urine, whether the urge to urinate is present or not. There are several different types of incontinence. The most common is **stress incontinence.** This sounds like what your mother has. She may notice that her pelvic muscles are weaker and that urine can leak at the most inappropriate times. Laughing, coughing, sneezing, or any sudden body movement can allow that little dribble to escape.

There is also **urge incontinence,** or the sudden, urgent need to go to the bathroom. Often there isn't time to make it to the toilet before it's too late. This is more common when there is some nerve damage along the spinal cord at the brain-bladder pathway. **Overflow incontinence** happens when our bodies produce more urine than the bladder can hold.

Overuse of *diuretics* (water pills), bladder stones, bladder infections, or simply the inevitable loss of muscle tone in the vaginal tissue can also cause incontinence over time.

How Is Urinary Incontinence Treated?

Non-drug treatments

Caffeinated products like coffee and tea can irritate the bladder and cause leakage. Stay away from these as much as possible and you should see some improvement. Highly acidic foods like tomatoes and citrus also should be avoided because they can irritate the bladder. While changing a diet may not solve the problem entirely, it could improve urine control.

For women, exercises combined with biofeedback can also sometimes completely eliminate the need for more drastic measures like surgery. **Kegel exercises** (developed by Dr. Arnold Kegel, MD) strengthen the vagina, bladder, and urethra so the urine flow can be more easily controlled. You can practice Kegel exercises by trying to hold your urine flow when you're on the toilet. Partially empty your bladder, and then try to slow and then stop the flow. According to Kegel, you should try this several times a week to see how your bladder control is improving.

To strengthen the bladder even more: Tighten and hold these same muscles for a count of four seconds, rest for ten seconds, then repeat ten times (this should be done when you're NOT in the process of urinating). Be patient—it can take up to three months before you notice an improvement. An unexpected positive feature of this exercise is the increased sexual responsiveness you may notice with your newly strengthened vaginal muscles.

OTC treatments

For those occasional accidents, or to be covered "just in case," there are excellent incontinence pads that absorb both urine and odor. ***Depends Undergarments,*** for example, are available in many convenient sizes and different degrees of absorbency.

The Drug Lady Recommends . . .

Many of my customers prefer the *Serenity* brand of incontinence protection guards. These have a special layer that forms a gel when wet. This layer also has an odor-control ingredient inside that traps urine smells very well. No one ever needs to know there is a problem.

Prescription treatments

During menopause, the muscular lining of the vaginal walls begins to shrink due to a decrease in estrogen levels. Often an estrogen cream like **Premarin** is used in combination with the **Kegel exercises** to strengthen muscle tone of the vagina. In more severe cases, your doctor may recommend a **pessary,** which is a small ring inserted near the cervix to support and hold up the pelvic muscles and to prevent urine from escaping.

Many times, urinary incontinence occurs because the bladder or other urinary organs have moved out of their normal positions, as in the case of hysterectomies or pregnancy or with the process of aging. Surgery to resuspend the bladder and restore the urethra to its normal position may be necessary when all other methods have been exhausted. Many new techniques are being tried, such as an implant of collagen around the urethra that can help close the bladder sphincter and prevent leakage.

Taking Care of Your Eyes and Ears: "The Better to See and Hear You With, My Dear"

Allergic Conjunctivitis ▮ Cataracts ▮ Dry Eyes ▮ Ear Infections ▮ Earwax ▮
Eyesight Correction ▮ Flying and Ear Discomfort ▮ Pinkeye ▮
Swimmer's Ear ▮ Tinnitus or Ringing in the Ears

WE USE THEM to see the colors of the world and to hear the music of the sounds around us. The eyes and ears give us a portal through which to experience many of life's exciting events. So it's very important that when these wonderful organs begin to act up, we take care of the problem the right way. Whether it's an age-related condition that we can possibly prevent, or just an annoying itch, taking care of the eyes and the ears is an important job.

Allergic Conjunctivitis

Q. *What is allergic conjunctivitis? My doctor says I have this, but I thought it was an eye infection.*

A. An eye infection certainly can develop from allergic conjunctivitis, but that's not the original cause of the problem. "Allergic" in the name should give it away. Conjunctivitis is an inflammation of the eye that can be caused by many things, but in this case it's caused by an allergy to some substance in your environment—pollen, smoke, air pollution, etc. If this condition is left untreated, there is a good chance that you might develop an eye infection. There are other types of conjunctivitis as well—both bacterial and viral.

What Is Allergic Conjunctivitis?

Allergic conjunctivitis is an inflammation of the delicate membrane (the conjunctiva) that lines the eyeball and the inner eyelid. It is caused by allergies—usually the same seasonal allergies that cause all the sniffling and sneezing. The symptoms of this condition are redness, swelling, fierce itching, and lots of tears. Your nose may run as well. (See "Eye Allergies," chapter 2, page 34.)

There are several other causes of conjunctivitis, including a bacterial or viral invasion of your eyes. Bacterial conjunctivitis, also called **pinkeye,** is diagnosed when the eyes have a heavy, sticky, yellowish discharge in addition to burning and redness. Pinkeye must be treated with prescription antibiotic drops. (See "Pinkeye," page 169.)

Viral conjunctivitis—caused by a virus, of course—causes lots of tears and a thinner mucus discharge that is usually confined to one eye. Unfortunately, antibiotics aren't effective for viruses and this type of conjunctivitis must run its course. Both bacterial and viral conjunctivitis are highly contagious and can be spread easily from eye to eye or from person to person. It is important to wash your hands regularly, to keep your hands away from your itching eye(s), as hard as that may be, and to not share eye cosmetics with others.

How Is Allergic Conjunctivitis Treated?

Non-drug treatments

Warm, damp washcloths may be used to gently wipe the eye. Change the washcloths after each use, and wash them well. Bathing the eye with gentle over-the-counter eyewashes, like *normal saline,* can be effective in removing the foreign **allergens** that are causing the itching and redness.

Staying away from the allergens that cause allergic conjunctivitis, like smoke, cat hair, or high pollen counts, is the best prevention, but not always the most convenient or realistic.

OTC treatments

Antihistamines are often the first lines of OTC therapy for allergic conjunctivitis. You can take them by mouth, like **Benadryl** (*diphenhydramine*), or put them directly into the eye as drops like **OcuHist** (*pheniramine*).

Eyedrops like **Visine-A Eye Allergy Relief Antihistamine/Decongestant Drops** and **Naphcon-A** have both an antihistamine for the itching (*pheniramine maleate*) and a decongestant for the redness (*naphazoline*). For really irritated eyes, expect it to sting a bit, but this is good stuff!

The Drug Lady Recommends...

Because it seems that I always get something in my eye right in the middle of an important deadline, I keep *Lavoptik Sterile Isotonic Buffer Eyewash* around the house. It is an excellent way to flush the eyes when the pollen counts are high. It even comes with an eyecup to make flushing the eye easier.

Prescription treatments

It is possible for an eye allergy to progress to a full-blown infection very quickly. The constant itching, rubbing, and scratching of the delicate eye membranes can introduce bacteria or even viruses into the eye. If your eye allergy progresses to an infection or even a long-lasting redness, a visit to the doctor is in order.

If your hands are constantly in and around your eyes, you may bring in bacteria that will need to be treated with an antibiotic eyedrop, like **Garamycin Ophthalmic** (*gentamicin*). For more serious cases of allergic conjunctivitis, the doctor may prescribe an antibiotic/steroid combination, like **Cortisporin Ophthalmic** (*polymyxin B, neomycin,* and *hydrocortisone*), both to fight infection and to reduce redness and inflammation. The corticosteroid eyedrop, **Pred Forte** (*prednisolone acetate*), is effective in bringing down swelling and relieving itching, redness, and irritation in the eye.

Cataracts

Q. *I have a family history of cataracts and I would like to do everything I can to not have them develop. Is there something I can do to prevent cataracts?*

A. It's nice to see people being proactive about their health! While surgery is the only way to correct a cataract, there are some things you may be able to do to decrease your chances of developing cataracts.

What Causes Cataracts?

Cataracts appear to be caused by changes in the proteins that are part of the lens of the eye. The lens is usually completely clear, but with age and damage, it can become cloudy. This produces a gradual, painless loss of vision.

Simple aging causes cataracts in about 75 percent of cases. Other causes are exposure to damaging ultraviolet light of the UVB spectrum (from direct sunlight), steroid drugs, and complications of diabetes.

How Are Cataracts Treated (and Prevented)?

Non-drug treatments
Adding **antioxidants** to your diet in the form of fresh fruits and vegetables may give some protection at the cellular level. Free radicals (highly destructive oxygen molecules) constantly bombard and damage delicate

eye cells. Antioxidants extinguish these free radicals and offer defense against this damage. You'll also see antioxidants available in tablet or capsule form. Look to *vitamin E, vitamin C, beta-carotene, coenzyme Q-10,* and *grapeseed extract* as powerful antioxidants. One study showed that a simple multivitamin supplement, taken daily, could reduce your chances of developing cataracts by 67 percent!

OTC treatments

Something as simple as wearing sunglasses to filter bright sunlight and damaging UVB rays can greatly decrease the risk of cataracts. It is important to check the sunglasses' rating to be sure that they filter at least 99 percent of the UVB rays. Many styles are available, and the complete wraparound variety offers the best protection. Read the labels on the glasses carefully and don't be afraid to ask your pharmacist if you're unsure.

The Drug Lady Recommends . . .

If you're outside and don't want the hassle of holding on to both your reading glasses and your sunglasses, the folks at Optx 20/20 have the answer. Now it's not necessary to remove your sunglasses and have your eyes exposed to bright (and damaging) sunlight. The *Optix 20/20 Reading Lenses for Sunglasses* stick with water to the inside of your sunglasses. These neat plastic pieces are reusable, too.

Prescription treatments

The only treatment for cataracts is surgery to remove the cloudy lens and replace it with a new, clear one. Unfortunately, cataracts come back in about 30 percent of cases. The best option is prevention. See your eye doctor regularly, and protect those delicate eyes.

Dry Eyes

Q. *What can I do for dry eyes? It feels as though I'm blinking my eyes on sandpaper!*

A. Dry eyes are a common problem for people working in front of computer screens for many hours each day, or for those who wear contact lenses. Dry eyes are also common for individuals who work around wind, smoke, or chemicals. The burning, gritty feeling seems to get worse as the day goes on.

What Causes Dry Eyes?

There are many causes of dry eyes. Inadequate blinking, contact-lens irritation, smoke, or pollutants can result in dry eyes. Even a medical condition called **keratoconjunctivitis sicca** (dehydration of the eye from a lack of tears) is responsible for this annoying state. Dry eyes may be one of the first symptoms of a more serious medical condition, including rheumatoid arthritis (RA) or systemic lupus erythematosus (SLE). Women are more susceptible to dry eyes than men, possibly due to hormonal changes. Low levels of *vitamin A* can cause an eye-surface dryness called **xerophthalmia.**

How Are Dry Eyes Treated?

Non-drug treatments

Eye compresses with the herbs *eyebright* and/or *fennel* cool the redness and tiredness from dry eyes, and using a humidifier in the home will keep moisture around longer.

Give your eyes a break from the monotony of a computer screen for a few minutes each hour. Close your eyes and allow your natural tears to bathe the eyeball. Count to one hundred. Ahh . . . doesn't that feel better already?

OTC treatments

Artificial Tears and other brand names have ingredients that are similar to the eyes' natural tears. That's a good thing when your eyeball feels rough as a cat's tongue. They also contain demulcents, or ingredients that lubricate, protect, and coat the eye membranes. Lubricant ingredients (like *propylene glycol, glycerin,* and *cellulose ether*) help the eyelid slide more easily over the eyeball. Products to look for are **Refresh Plus, Ocurest,** and **Comfort Tears.**

The Drug Lady Recommends . . .

Celluvisc Lubricant Eye Drops' individual single-use containers restore the moisture your eyes crave with a gentle protecting and lubricating formula that has some of the same healthy qualities as natural tears. Due to the thicker formula, Celluvisc is an ideal eyedrop for those stubborn dry eye conditions.

Prescription treatments

If OTC remedies aren't working, or if the dry eyes came on suddenly, see your doctor for a medical checkup to rule out other medical conditions that have dry eyes as a symptom. For severe cases of dry eyes, surgery may be needed. Tear ducts may be opened, or the eyelids may have to be closed a bit to decrease tear evaporation.

Pill Humor Things You Don't Want to Hear During Surgery

- "Oops!"
- "Has anyone seen my watch?"
- "Okay, now take a picture from this angle. This is truly a freak of nature."
- "Come back with that! Bad dog!"
- "Everybody stand back! I lost my contact lens!"
- "I wish I hadn't forgotten my glasses."
- "What do you mean he wasn't in for a sex change?!"
- "Don't worry, I think it's sharp enough."

Ear Infections

Q. *What is the best treatment for an ear infection? My family seems to get them quite often.*

A. Otitis media or infection of the middle ear is a common problem. It typically follows a bout of a cold, flu, or sinus infection, but may also be related to allergies. Because the middle ear uses the eustachian tubes to drain fluid to the throat, a swelling or infection here can produce pain and prevent the fluid from escaping. Middle-ear infections are more commonly found in children under the age of six because their eustachian tubes are shorter, but adults are susceptible, too. The best advice for an ear infection is to get to the doctor right away. The sooner the cause is determined and the proper medication prescribed, the quicker everyone will be hearing well and smiling again.

Otitis externa, or infection of the outer ear, in adults and older children may be attributed to improper use of materials to clean the ears, to earwax (see "Earwax," page 162), or to water accumulating in the ear during swimming or showers (see "Swimmer's Ear," page 170).

What Causes Ear Infections?

Symptoms of a middle-ear infection generally come on quickly with the closure or blockage of the eustachian tube. Pain (either sharp or dull and throbbing), fever, head congestion, a feeling of fullness in the ear, and a slight loss of hearing are common adult symptoms. With children, especially the younger set, you may notice that they tug or rub the ears or shake the head from side to side. This is one way to let you know they hurt. You may also notice a decrease in appetite or difficulty eating for children with ear infections. Irritability, crying, and fever are also signals that all is not right with the little one.

There are other causes of ear infections your doctor may look for, too. For those who are frequently in a pool or the shower, an infection may develop from water that gets trapped deep within the ear canal. Bacteria find a nice home there and a condition called "swimmer's ear" develops. (See "Swimmer's Ear," page 170.) Sufferers describe symptoms of persistent ringing or sloshing, accompanied by some pain and itching deep within the ear canal. Earwax accumulation can harden in the outer ear canal, effectively blocking the eardrum. This type of ear infection generally clears up quickly once the earwax is removed. (See "Earwax," page 162.)

How Are Ear Infections Treated?

Non-drug treatments

While the first line of treatment for an ear infection should be to head to the doctor, warm (damp or dry) washcloths applied to the neck area can be both soothing and help to expand the eustachian tubes. Aromatherapy with *eucalyptus oil* can open clogged airways and make the patient feel more comfortable. Simply add a few drops to a warm towel and inhale deeply. Ahhh . . .

OTC treatments

If you can't get to the doctor right away, try an OTC **decongestant** to relieve pressure in the eustachian tubes. *Pseudoephedrine* is a common decongestant that you should have around for earache emergencies. *Tylenol* (*acetaminophen*) or **Motrin** (*ibuprofen*) can provide temporary pain relief.

Prescription treatments

When someone in your family has an earache, the best thing to do is head for the doctor's office. Middle-ear infections may be treated with antibiotics, which are available by prescription only. A doctor may prescribe

The Drug Lady Recommends . . .

Warm the eardrops first. The eardrops will feel much better going in if you put the CAPPED bottle in a warm cup or sink full of water. The warmth will also expand the eustachian tubes a little, allowing the medicine to reach its destination faster. Use care to not warm the drops too much; the inside of the ear is a delicate area.

an antibiotic (like *amoxicillin* or **Augmentin**) either alone or in combination with an eardrop. Antibiotic/corticosteroid eardrops, like **Cortisporin Otic** (*neomycin, polymyxin B,* and *hydrocortisone*), penetrate deep into the ear to kill bacteria and relieve inflammation. This is available as both a solution and a suspension.

How to Put In Eardrops

Getting eardrops into your own or your family members' ears can be a daunting task. Here are some tips for making sure that more medicine gets in the ear than all over your clothes.

- Lie down or tilt the head so the sore ear is facing up.

- Pull the earlobe up and back to give the medicine best access to the eustachian tubes.

- Place the medicine in the ear and allow it to soak in for five minutes. For children, two minutes is fine.

- A small wad of cotton inserted in the ear will help keep the medicine inside where it will do the most good.

There is also an eardrop specifically for pain relief called **Auralgan** (*antipyrine, benzocaine,* and *glycerin*). It has *benzocaine* as a numbing agent to ease the discomfort of a swollen ear canal.

Earwax

Q. *Is there an over-the-counter way to safely clear my ears of extra earwax?*

A. Earwax isn't a topic that most of us like talking about very much. However, earaches in adults and older children may be attributed to accumulated earwax (also called cerumen). Earwax serves an important function, but it may also cause painful problems.

What Causes Earwax?

Earwax is actually a sticky, brownish secretion that the body produces naturally in the outer ear canal. It functions to trap small debris and prevent their entry into the inner ear canal. Earwax is one of the body's natural protective measures. However, this wax can build up and even trap water deep inside the ear canal, where bacteria and fungi find a home.

How Is Earwax Treated?

Non-drug treatments

It is very important that you DO NOT try to remove earwax with cotton swabs. This will only push the wax deeper into the ears, and possibly plug up the ear canal faster.

Olive oil (also called "sweet oil") may be put into waxy ears for a softening effect. Place just a few drops directly in the ear canal, then gently wipe the excess from the ear. Use a bulb syringe with warm water to gently flush out the now-softened wax. This may be repeated daily for three days until the wax is removed.

OTC treatments

There are several good over-the-counter products for the removal of earwax. These focus on softening the wax so it can be more easily removed. Some earwax softeners are *carbamide peroxide, propylene glycol, glycerin,* and dilute *hydrogen peroxide.*

The Drug Lady Recommends...

The *Bausch and Lomb Ear Wax Removal System* contains the active ingredients *carbamide peroxide* and *anhydrous glycerin*. The glycerin softens the wax, while the bubbles released from the carbamide peroxide gently loosen the buildup. The customer uses the bulb syringe provided to gently flush the ear canal with warm water. Presto! Clean ears.

Debrox also makes a carbamide peroxide drop to place in the ear to soften, loosen, and remove earwax. It foams in contact with earwax, so don't be alarmed at the sudden crackling and popping sound you may hear. (This product should be used only in children over the age of twelve unless the doctor says it's okay. Also, the FDA has given these products approval as "occasional use" agents, so twice daily for up to four days should do the job nicely.)

Prescription treatments

If your ears are ever painful, please see your doctor; there may be hardened or impacted earwax that has to be removed by the doctor. Many ear infections also mimic the feeling of fullness that impacted earwax may bring.

Eyesight Correction

Q. *My eyesight just isn't what it used to be, and the over-the-counter reading glasses are confusing! Could you tell me how to pick the best pair for me?*

A. First, before buying OTC reading glasses, I would recommend seeing your eye doctor for a complete eye exam. Scheduling an exam every two years could actually save your sight (as well as prevent headaches from an improper strength in glasses).

What Causes Eyesight Difficulties?

There are various eyesight conditions that may prevent us from seeing clearly. Farsightedness (**hyperopia**), **nearsightedness** (myopia), and **astigmatism** are called refractive disorders, and are conditions created by the shape of the eyeball. These all should be treated by an eye doctor (optometrist or ophthalmologist) and usually can be corrected with prescription lenses or contacts. Today, laser surgery is another option for correcting these disorders.

Presbyopia, blurred vision at normal reading distance, is common as we age, and is due to the natural stiffening of the lens in the eye. Our eyes cannot focus on close objects. While we still can see distant objects clearly,

Types of Eye Specialists

There are several different types of health-care professionals that we think of as "eye doctors." Here are the differences.

- An optometrist is trained to test the eyes. This is who you visit when you need a prescription for glasses or contact lenses. The medical title is "O.D.," or doctor of optometry.

- An ophthalmologist is a physician who specializes in treatment of diseases and disorders of the eye, such as cataracts or glaucoma. This type of doctor will have an "M.D.," or medical doctor, after his or her name.

- An optician has extensive training in making the glasses and contacts that we rely on to see. This specialization does not carry a title after the name.

we cannot refocus on near objects (like the newspaper). If your condition is mild presbyopia, reading glasses may be all that are needed.

How Are Eyesight Difficulties Treated?

Non-drug treatments

A great deal of attention has been placed on the value of vitamin supplements in preserving the integrity of our eyes. *Vitamins A, C,* and *B-2* (*riboflavin*) and *zinc* are important antioxidants in protecting the delicate cells from damaging free radicals. *Lutein,* found in dark green leafy veggies like spinach or collard greens, is a free-radical fighter shown to have special affinity for the damaging free radicals in the eye. Free radicals are constantly bombarding and breaking down our bodies on the cellular level; unfortunately, it is almost impossible to avoid them. Free radicals abound in smoke, pollution, pesticides, and in much of the very air we breathe.

The Drug Lady Recommends . . .

The vitamin supplement called *Ocuvite* is a wonderful combination of antioxidant vitamins and minerals. It contains 200 percent or more of the adult RDA of the important antioxidants *zinc* and *vitamin E.* It also contains *vitamin C, beta-carotene, selenium,* and *copper.*

OTC treatments

For **presbyopia,** over-the-counter reading glasses may be all that you need, but finding the right strength can be confusing. Often you'll see tags attached to each pair of glasses with a number on them. The level of magnification in the lenses of reading glasses is called "diopter strength."

A very weak magnification would be found in reading glasses with a diopter strength of 1.00. Reading glasses often start with a diopter strength of 1.25, and stronger lenses are offered in diopter strengths that increase by a factor of 0.25 (e.g.: 1.50; 1.75; 2.00; 2.25; 2.50; etc.). Presbyopia may get worse over the years, and the strength of magnification in your reading glasses may have to be increased every year or two. Having your eyes checked every two years will ensure that you don't need more extensive correction than OTC reading glasses can provide.

The best way to determine which pair of reading glasses is right for you is to try them. Hold newsprint at a typical distance (about 14 inches) from your eyes and see if the glasses make it easier to read. Try the diopter strengths on either side of the one you choose, just to be sure that this makes the words crystal-clear!

Prescription treatments

As we age, it may be necessary to give up on the over-the-counter reading glasses and go in to the eye doctor for a prescription. Don't wait. If your vision is blurry or you have any difficulty reading with non-prescription lenses, see the optometrist right away. Your eyesight is much too precious to lose!

Flying and Ear Discomfort

Q. *My ears hurt terribly whenever I fly in an airplane. What can I do to prevent this from happening?*

A. Airplane flights aren't always pleasant, and when you must deal with pain in your body, they are twice as hard. Thankfully, there are very effective ways of dealing with ear pain. Now, if the child in the seat next to you could just equalize HIS ears, the flight would be wonderful!

What Causes Ear Discomfort While Flying?

When you fly, pain in the ears can occur because of a blockage in the **eustachian tubes** (the tubes that connect the middle ear and the throat, and equalize air pressure in the head). On takeoff and landing, the pressure inside the middle-ear canal and that outside the body become unequal because the air pressure in the airplane cabin is changing. Normally the eustachian tubes quickly adjust and allow this equalization, and no pain occurs. But if the tubes are blocked by congestion, a vacuum will form, and fluid presses painfully against the eardrums. Ouch!

How Is In-Flight Ear Discomfort Treated?

Non-drug treatments

Drinking water, chewing gum, or yawning can open eustachian tubes briefly enough to allow the pressure inside to equalize. Bring along a pack of gum or a bottle of water for painful takeoffs and landings.

Feeding a bottle to infants and young children during the flight can be a great way to help them cope with this strange pain in their ears.

The Drug Lady Recommends . . .

When I was learning to scuba-dive, our instructor taught us a great way to equalize pressure in the head. Gently pinch your nostrils closed and very carefully hold your breath, exhale SLIGHTLY against your pinched nose. This blows air into the ear tubes and can be effective in opening the tubes and relieving pain. This looks a little funny when you're sitting on a plane, but if it works, don't worry about that!

OTC treatments

To prevent in-flight ear pain when you have a cold, you should take a **decongestant** (like *pseudoephedrine*) at least an hour before flying. Parents can prepare for a plane trip by giving the children a dose of a decongestant specially designed for them. Decongestant drops are a "must-have" for frequent little travelers because they can relieve the painful pressure from takeoffs and landings, especially if there is some head congestion already present. Look for **Infants' Tylenol Cold** concentrated decongestant drops for babies (use the dose based on their weight) and **Dimetapp Children's Decongestant** pediatric drops for those over the age of two.

Using a decongestant spray like **4-WAY**, which contains the decongestant *oxymetazoline*, can be effective for use just before you take off. However, those who have heart disease, high blood pressure, thyroid disease, diabetes, or difficulty in urination due to an enlarged prostate should not use decongestants unless specifically advised to do so by their doctor.

Prescription treatments

If over-the-counter **decongestants** just aren't strong enough to help, you might ask your doctor for a product like **Entex PSE**, a combination of three ingredients: *phenylpropanolamine* and *pseudoephedrine* (decongestants) and *guaifenesin* (an expectorant to break up mucus). It packs a powerful punch to open those plugged ears.

WARNING: PPA Cautions

Phenylpropanolamine—PPA—was an ingredient in dozens of cold and cough remedies (both prescription and non-prescription) for adults and children, as well as many OTC appetite suppressants. A recently released study at Yale found that PPA increased the risk, for women aged eighteen to forty-nine, of hemorrhagic stroke (which is relatively rare among young people). This is a very serious concern—serious enough for the FDA to issue a public health warning about PPA and take steps to remove it from drug products. They are doing this by asking drug companies to discontinue products with PPA or to reformulate them with other ingredients—and I would certainly encourage women in this age group to use products that don't contain PPA. While most products now available do not contain this ingredient, there may still be some of the PPA products on your shelves at home.

Pinkeye

Q. *My mother says it looks like my baby has pinkeye. What is pinkeye? How do we get rid of it?*

A. Not to diminish your mother's diagnostic abilities (mothers are often the very best), but I would suggest that you take the baby in to a doctor just to be sure. The baby may have any one of several eye conditions called conjunctivitis. Conjunctivitis may be bacterial (like pinkeye), viral, or simply an allergy (allergic conjunctivitis); each type has its own method of treatment and should be diagnosed by the doctor. DON'T take a chance with that baby's precious eyes!

What Is Pinkeye?

Pinkeye, or bacterial conjunctivitis, is an inflammation of the membrane (the conjunctiva) that lines the eyelid and eyeball. It occurs when bacteria make their way into the eye and find a home in this warm, moist environment. The inner eyelid may look red and bloodshot. The "whites of the eye," or sclera, have a bright red appearance due to the inflammation of the conjunctiva. Pinkeye causes pain, itching, and redness, so it's not hard to see how it got its name. If your child wakes up with her eyelids stuck together, and a thick, greenish/yellowish discharge is coming from the eye, it is probably caused by a bacterium.

Bacterial conjunctivitis needs to be treated with antibiotics prescribed by the doctor, and typically runs its course in ten to fourteen days. During that time it is contagious, so day care or schools may ask that the child be kept at home until the symptoms disappear. Check with your child's day care or school for their policies.

How Is Pinkeye Treated?

Non-drug treatments

Gently wiping the outside of the eyes with a warm, damp washcloth can be soothing, and helps the eye flush out the invading bacteria. Using mild baby soap on the outside of the lids can help decrease the amount of bacteria introduced by little hands, but be very careful not to get it into the child's eyes.

Frequent hand-washing and replacing washcloths with each use will decrease the chance of bringing in more bacteria to an already-irritated eye.

OTC treatments

Over-the-counter eyedrops are generally not recommended for treating pinkeye, but may be helpful when an **allergy** is involved (**allergic conjunctivitis**). (See "Eye Allergies," chapter 2, page 34.)

The Drug Lady Recommends . . .

An over-the-counter eyewash of dilute *boric acid* or *normal saline* can be helpful to gently flush the eye. An eyewash serves to both clear the eye of bacteria and to soothe the irritation. (Use an eyecup to place the liquid into a child's eye.) However, this treatment will not kill the bacteria, so a prescription antibiotic may be in order if the symptoms don't clear up within twenty-four hours.

Prescription treatments

Eyedrops by prescription, like *Cortisporin Ophthalmic Suspension,* contain the antibiotics *neomycin* and *polymyxin B* to kill the bacteria responsible for pinkeye, along with a steroid (*hydrocortisone*) to reduce inflammation and redness.

Swimmer's Ear

Q. *In the summer when I swim laps, I always feel like I have water trapped in my ears. Sometimes it sloshes terribly and hurts, but that usually goes away. Is this "swimmer's ear"?*

A. Having a pool sloshing around inside your head can be very annoying, especially if this water is providing a cozy home for bacteria or fungi. While having water in the ear isn't specifically called "swimmer's ear," it may lead to swimmer's ear. Let's see what works for getting this water out fast.

What Causes Swimmer's Ear?

If water gets deep into the ear canal and becomes trapped, either by wax accumulation or swelling of the eustachian tubes, a condition called **otitis externa** or "swimmer's ear" develops. Frequent swimming or showering can strip the normal lining of the ear canal and allow bacteria or fungi to grow in the trapped water pockets. Sufferers complain of persistent ringing or sloshing, along with some pain and itching deep within the ear.

How Is Swimmer's Ear Treated?

Non-drug treatments

Home remedies for water in the ear have been used effectively by many moms over the years. Pour a half-and-half mixture of *isopropyl alcohol* and *white vinegar* into a small dropper bottle. Use one to three drops of this after swimming or showering to evaporate the excess water. The vinegar also sticks around to lower the pH (making it more acidic) in the ear canal; bacteria and fungi don't like to live in acidic areas. Non-drug measures are great for prevention, but the actual treatment of swimmer's ear may require a trip to the doctor for antibiotics.

OTC treatments

Once an infection has been ruled out, your best course of action is to take steps that prevent swimmer's ear from coming back, or simply to remove the extra water sloshing around. Solutions like ***Auro-Dri*** and ***Swim-Ear*** get into the ear canal with the active ingredient *isopropyl alcohol*. This mixes with the water, stops the growth of bacteria and fungus, as well as allowing the water to evaporate much more quickly.

The Drug Lady Recommends . . .

Star-Otic uses *acetic acid, boric acid,* and *Burow's solution* (*aluminum acetate*) to keep the ear canal highly acidic to stop these organisms from returning. *Propylene glycol* is also an important ingredient that acts as a drying agent. Just put three to five drops into the ear canal before and after swimming or bathing, and stop use if any irritation occurs.

Prescription treatments

If pain is present, call the doctor. You may be prescribed an antibiotic to take by mouth, or in an eardrop form. For pain relief, you may need a medication like **Auralgan** (*antipyrine* and *benzocaine*) to ease the discomfort. If there is no pain or infection, OTC products usually do the job.

Tinnitus or Ringing in the Ears

Q. *What causes ringing in the ears? What can I do to treat it?*

A. Persistent sounds like humming, ringing, or buzzing that only you can hear can be very distracting. This condition is called tinnitus. You may notice that these sounds can vary from being something you notice only on occasion, to a condition that makes ordinary concentration difficult.

What Is Tinnitus?

Tinnitus is defined as a noise in the ear that only you can hear. It may be a buzzing, ringing, chirping, roaring, whistling, or even a hissing sound, and can vary from being mildly annoying to driving you to the point of severe depression.

Tinnitus may be caused by a blockage in the ear canal, overexposure to loud noises, or by a reaction to certain medicines (like *aspirin, quinidine,* and *quinine*). Tinnitus may also be one of the first signs of a more serious medical condition (like high blood pressure or low thyroid levels), so it's important to let your doctor take a look before you try treating this yourself.

How Is Tinnitus Treated?

Non-drug treatments

Keeping a "white noise" machine close by the bed may help you sleep better. Background music played softly often masks the annoying sounds of tinnitus.

Certain substances like *caffeine, aspirin,* tobacco, and alcohol may make tinnitus worse. Try avoiding them for a few weeks to see if you notice a positive effect.

The Drug Lady Recommends . . .

The herb *ginkgo biloba* is showing great promise as a natural tinnitus remedy. This herb seems to work within the circulatory system to increase blood flow. The dosage is 40 to 60 mg of the standardized extract (24-percent *flavone glycosides*/6-percent *terpenes*) taken three times daily. Have patience; it may take up to six weeks before you notice an effect.

OTC treatments

There are no over-the-counter treatments available for tinnitus.

Prescription treatments

If tinnitus is interfering with your life, your doctor may fit you with a special hearing aid that masks the sounds of tinnitus and makes your hearing clearer. Another therapy is "auditory habituation." Here, a small device inserted into the ear constantly plays a white noise that is lower in volume than the tinnitus noise, so the brain learns to ignore the tinnitus. This has been shown to be very effective as a permanent treatment.

Pill Humor

What do you get if a philosopher has both insomnia and dyslexia?
Someone who stays up all night contemplating whether or not there is a Dog.

Lips, Gums, and Teeth:
"Smile Pretty!"

Canker Sores ■ Cold Sores and Fever Blisters ■ Fluoride Supplements ■

Gingivitis ■ Lip-Balm Addiction ■ Toothache ■ Tooth Whiteners

MANY PEOPLE SAY that the first thing they notice about a person is his or her smile; for, as small as the mouth is in proportion to the rest of the body, there are an amazing number of things that can happen inside. Your mouth is a very sensitive area and anyone who has ever suffered a toothache or a canker sore can tell you how difficult it can be to eat, drink, or even talk. Let's look at some of the most common conditions associated with the mouth, lips, gums, and teeth.

Canker Sores

Q. *I routinely get small, very painful ulcers in my mouth. What are these? What can I do for relief?*

A. Those mouth ulcers are commonly known as canker sores, and they can be very painful! Chewing can be difficult and acidic foods cause agony. However, there are effective ways of easing the pain while the canker sore runs its course.

What Is a Canker Sore?

You know you have a canker sore (also called an **aphthous ulcer**) if the mouth wound is small, shallow, and covered by a grayish-white membrane. The edges of the canker may be bright red. Sometimes you will know one is coming by a tingling or burning sensation twenty-four hours or so before it appears. Many people may develop these ulcers after accidentally biting the inner cheek or lips. The medical cause is unknown; it may be due to a virus, stress, anxiety, a lack of vitamins, food allergies, or even a symptom of premenstrual syndrome (PMS).

To prevent canker sores from forming, avoid traumatizing the lining of the mouth. That means don't chew on your lips and take it easy with that toothbrush. You could be holding a weapon! Brush at least twice daily to keep the mouth as clean as possible. Check your toothpaste ingredients, as some studies have shown that the ingredient *sodium lauryl sulfate* may worsen or even cause the ulcers.

How Are Canker Sores Treated?

Non-drug treatments

Home remedies for canker sores include moistened tea bags. You can apply the moistened tea bag (regular black tea is sufficient) directly to the sore area. The tannic acid in the tea acts as an astringent and provides some pain relief. Herbal remedies for canker sores include *slippery elm* or *zinc* lozenges for pain relief.

A distinct correlation has been seen between low levels of certain vitamins and amino acids (like *vitamin B-12* and *lysine*) and more-frequent canker sores. Often, simply adding a multivitamin or lysine supplement to your diet will decrease or even eliminate the canker-sore outbreaks.

OTC treatments

For pain relief and a cleaner mouth, rinse with *2% hydrogen peroxide;* this is helpful for killing mouth bacteria that may irritate the ulcer. Dilute with an equal amount of water, swish in the mouth for at least one minute, then spit out. **Gly-oxide** is a product containing *carbamide peroxide* as its active ingredient. It works by foaming around the sore and cleaning the area. Small sips of **Maalox** or **Phillips Milk of Magnesia** can coat and protect the sores.

Most canker sores heal within two weeks, but when you're in pain, those two weeks can seem like an eternity. There are some over-the-counter remedies available that contain a local anesthetic (like *benzocaine*) to relieve pain instantly. Look for names like **Americaine** or **Orajel** for a numbing effect.

The Drug Lady Recommends . . .

Zilactin Canker Sore, Cold Sore, Fever Blister Reliever has *benzyl alcohol* as an active ingredient to relieve pain. It advertises a patent-protected, bioadhesive film that forms within sixty seconds and holds the medication in place for up to six hours. This special coating reduces the irritation caused by normal eating and drinking.

Prescription treatments

If you have many ulcers, or the pain interferes with eating or speaking, you may want to see a doctor. He may prescribe a topical steroid cream especially formulated for the mouth, like **Kenalog in Orabase** (*triamcinolone 0.1%*). This sticky paste covers the ulcer and protects the area while it heals. It has to be applied rather often, but does offer healing relief.

There is also a prescription product called **Aphthasol Paste** (*amlexanox*), which studies have shown decreases the length of time these ulcers hang around by a day to a day-and-a-half. For children over the age of eight years, the doctor may want to try a liquid antibiotic, like *tetracycline;* if held in the mouth for several minutes, the antibiotic will cover the ulcer and speed healing.

Cold Sores and Fever Blisters

Q. *What is the difference between a cold sore and a fever blister? I can never tell which one I have. How do I get rid of them?*

A. Because we often hear cold sores and fever blisters referred to as two separate conditions, it can be confusing. However, cold sores and fever blisters are the same condition. Because they are often uncomfortable and unsightly, let's see what to do to get them to go away fast.

What Causes a Cold Sore/Fever Blister?

Herpes simplex virus Type 1 is the culprit of cold sores and fever blisters, not a fever or cold as the names suggest. However, a fever, a cold, stress, sunburn on the face, or even a mouth trauma brought on by a trip to the dentist may be a trigger to stimulate the viral outbreak. Cold sores are very contagious by any direct contact with the virus (like kissing or drinking out of the same cup) and it is estimated that the virus at one time or another has infected nearly half of the population.

Fever blisters and cold sores typically occur outside or around the corners of the mouth. They resemble blisters with a dry, crusty top, and although they may be unsightly, these sores aren't typically very painful. If you do develop cold sores, be prepared to live with them forever; the virus never goes away but stays dormant until triggered again.

How Are Cold Sores/Fever Blisters Treated?

Non-drug treatments

Natural products like *zinc*, a trace mineral, may get rid of the sore faster. Taken orally (by mouth), a dosage of 50 mg daily may reduce the severity and the frequency of cold sores.

If you feel the tingling sensation, put an ice cube on the sore for about five minutes every two to three hours. Studies have shown that the virus can't thrive in a cold environment and you may be able avoid the outbreak entirely.

The amino acid *lysine* is important for repairing damaged tissue. Lysine is found naturally in certain foods including red meat, milk, lima beans, and soy products. It is often used as a natural treatment for cold sores and fever blisters. For those who never manage to eat right, the supplement dose is 500 mg in tablet or capsule form, taken three times a day at the first twinge of a cold sore.

OTC treatments

Benzocaine, benzyl alcohol, dibucaine, and *camphor* are common ingredients used to dry up the sore, numb the area, and promote faster healing. *Cocoa butter* is also used to soften surrounding skin. This helps decrease cracking and splitting around the mouth.

Lemon balm cream, under the brand name **Herpilyn,** contains a powerful concentrate of the highly tannic leaves of the lemon balm plant, which seems to deactivate the herpes virus.

The Drug Lady Recommends...

A new product in the cold sore arsenal is **Abreva** by SmithKline Beecham. Its active ingredient *docosanol 10%* is thought to provide protection for the healthy cells surrounding an active cold sore. By preventing the virus from entering the cells, it may shorten healing time and the length of time the cold sore produces unpleasant symptoms. For best results, apply at the first "tingle" and use five times daily until the cold sore improves.

Prescription treatments

Prescription antiviral creams, like **Zovirax** (*acyclovir*) or **Denavir** (*penciclovir*), produce a rapid healing of the sore if used early enough in the outbreak cycle. (Remember this if you notice that "tingle" a few days before your wedding!)

Fluoride Supplements

Q. *Are fluoride supplements necessary? My children are not crazy about the taste and I'm not sure they need them.*

A. To help you decide, here a few facts about fluoride that you might want to share with the kids. First, fluoride is proven to be the most effective factor in preventing tooth decay. Even if they think they don't care about tooth decay, remind them how rotten teeth look—yucky. They'll also be spending less time in that dentist chair. The National Institutes of Health recommend fluoride supplementation as safe, inexpensive, and effective for tooth-decay prevention. Fluoride protects teeth that have emerged from the gum, as well as those still below the gumline.

What Are Fluoride Supplements?

The decision of whether or not to give children fluoride supplements is usually based on where you live. In areas where the water is fluoridated (or has fluoride added), pediatricians may not always recommend supplements to protect children's teeth. If the water in your area has one part fluoride per one million parts water (1 ppm), this will prevent tooth decay in 60 percent of children. A glass of 1 ppm fluoridated water equates to 0.25 mg fluoride.

How Are Low Fluoride Levels Treated?

Non-drug treatments
Natural sources of food high in fluoride are apples, canned sardines and salmon, eggs, and calf liver. The amount of fluoride in these foods may depend on the level of fluoride in the soil or water where they are grown or produced.

OTC treatments
Fluoride is found in commercial toothpaste and mouthwash as *sodium fluoride*. It is the most common ingredient added to toothpaste because

of its cavity-fighting capabilities. High-fluoride toothpastes and mouth-washes include *Aquafresh Extra Fresh Fluoride* toothpaste and *ACT Anticavity Fluoride Treatment Rinse* by Johnson & Johnson.

Prescription treatments

In areas that don't have fluoride in the water, the doctor may give you several choices. The general recommendation is to prescribe fluoride supplements in areas with less than 0.3 ppm fluoride in the water supply.

For children, from six months old to the age when they can chew tablets, liquid fluoride supplements can be given. Your doctor may give a prescription for a liquid fluoride supplement alone (*Luride*) or a combination with a liquid multivitamin (*Poly-Vi-Flor*). The active ingredient in both of these is *sodium fluoride.* For ages six months to three years, the dose is 0.25 mg (or half a dropperful) daily. Children ages three to six can graduate to the "big kid" tablets. This gets a little confusing because sodium fluoride tablets come in doses of 1.1 mg and 2.2 mg. The dose for three- to six-year-olds is 0.5 mg fluoride or a 1.1 mg sodium fluoride tablet. Children from age six to their teens should be given 1 mg fluoride or a 2.2 mg sodium fluoride tablet. These come in several flavors and are given once a day. It may require a little trial and error to find your kids' favorites. Don't mix these with milk or dairy products, as doing so may greatly decrease the absorption of fluoride. For best availability of fluoride, give these supplements at least two hours before or after having that glass of milk.

In areas where the fluoride content in water is 0.3 to 0.6 ppm, the dosages given above should be half as much. Ask your dentist or the water company about local water fluoride levels.

The Drug Lady Recommends . . .

There are some dangers associated with too much fluoride, as you may already know. Too much fluoride while the teeth are developing can cause a condition called **dental fluorosis**. This shows up as white spots on the teeth. You should monitor children under age six when they are using a fluoride toothpaste. They should use only a pea-sized dab of toothpaste on their toothbrushes.

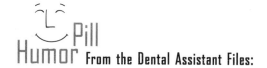

Humor Pill From the Dental Assistant Files:

Mary S. reports one of her first week's blunders while working for a dentist in Florida who was located in the same building as a proctologist. She brought in a patient from the waiting room named Smith for an exam and began prepping him for a cleaning. He looked slightly puzzled, but let her begin. After about ten minutes, he leaned over and whispered to her, "This is nice, but I think you might be working on the wrong end of me." Oops! It turned out that *HER* Mr. Smith was still patiently sitting out in the waiting room.

Gingivitis

Q. *My friend had gingivitis and lost a tooth as a result. I've read that gingivitis can be helped by vitamin supplements. Are there other ways to prevent this? I really want to avoid it!*

A. Take advice from your friend and do everything you can to avoid the inflamed gum condition known as gingivitis—it can lead to serious mouth problems if left unchecked. Gingivitis is treated with a variety of medications in the antibacterial arsenal, but dietary supplements may not be the best first choice. Gingivitis can be a serious condition and should be taken care of by a dentist first—then you may consider adding the vitamins.

What Is Gingivitis?

Gingivitis is an inflammation of the gums—also called gingiva—in which accumulated plaque (the sticky, bacteria-filled film that builds up on the tooth enamel) causes them to look red and swollen, and to bleed very easily. It can be dangerous because this inflammation can spread from the gums to the teeth and deeper into the bone. Teeth can be loosened and even lost if gingivitis is not treated effectively. That's why getting rid of plaque is the key to preventing gingivitis.

Only in rare cases does a vitamin deficiency cause gingivitis. Some factors, such as pregnancy, puberty, menopause, and some drugs (like birth-control pills or **Dilantin**), can make gingivitis worse. Once the condition is diagnosed, it may take several weeks before it can be completely eliminated.

How Is Gingivitis Treated?

Non-drug treatments

The best policy with gingivitis—as in so many areas of health—is prevention. In this case, brushing and flossing will keep it from occurring in the first place.

For those rare cases when a vitamin deficiency is the cause of gingivitis, adding extra *vitamin C* or *niacin* to the diet may be enough. *Folic acid* also has been shown to have beneficial effects for some individuals. Don't buy all of these supplements separately, though. Save your money and just focus on a good multivitamin/mineral combination.

The Drug Lady Recommends . . .

One of my favorites (and the favorite of most pharmacists asked) is the multivitamin/mineral combination in the **Centrum** brand. They advertise having everything—"From A to Zinc"—and they aren't joking. This is an excellent comprehensive multivitamin for supplementing a diet that may not be quite as good as you'd like, or simply to give your body a better shot at fighting disease.

OTC treatments

Tartar-control toothpaste can keep plaque from finding a home. Remember that plaque turns into hard tartar after seventy-two hours—so brush, brush, brush! The combination of the tartar-control ingredient *pyrophosphates* and the antibacterial *triclosan* has been shown to be effective in limiting the amount of new tartar formed on teeth. A great example of tartar-control toothpaste is **Colgate Total.**

Some toothpastes (*Q-Dent*) even add natural antioxidants like *coenzyme Q-10* to their formulas for added protection.

Prescription treatments

Your dentist may prescribe an antibacterial dental rinse called **Peridex** (*chlorhexidine*) to decrease bacteria in the mouth and control plaque accumulation. Be sure to follow the package directions carefully because it can stain your teeth if it is not used correctly.

Oral antibiotics (those taken by mouth in tablet or capsule form), like **Periostat** (*doxycycline hyclate*), are often prescribed to help decrease the mouth bacteria associated with gingivitis.

Lip-Balm Addiction

Q. *Is there such a thing as an addiction to lip balms like ChapStick? My friend swears that she's addicted to it, but there doesn't seem to be anything in the ingredients that is addictive. Am I missing something?*

A. Before receiving this question, I would have laughed if someone told me there was such a thing as a ChapStick lip-balm addiction. Now that I've done quite a bit of research on it, I've changed my tune!

What Is a "Lip-Balm Addiction"?

It seems that there is indeed a real problem out there. Whether it is caused by the ingredients in the lip balm or not has not been determined scientifically. However, if you ask the members of Lip Balm Anonymous (yes, there really is such a thing), you'll be told in no uncertain terms that something in some of the products out there is causing a problem.

The symptoms of "lip-balm addiction" include increasingly chapped lips even though you apply the ointment or stick every few hours. Doctors say that those who become "addicted" to lip balms are simply frequent "lip lickers"; they enjoy the feeling of coolness on their lips from the *menthol* ingredients and the softening effect that the *petrolatum* base has on the lip.

Carmex and **ChapStick** seem to be two of the more common offenders. **Carmex** contains *menthol, camphor, alum, salicylic acid, phenol,* fragrance, *petrolatum, lanolin, cocoa butter, mineral oil,* and a wax base. **ChapStick** is made from *petrolatum, padimate O, lanolin, isopropyl myristate, cetyl alcohol, arachadyl propionate, camphor,* carnuba wax, *D&C Red No. 6 Barium Lake,* flavors, *isopropyl lanolate, methylparaben, mineral oil,* wax paraffin, and white wax.

Nothing terribly scary there. What seems to be happening is that a vicious cycle is created. You apply the lip balm and soon lick it off, then notice that your lips are dry. Apply it again, lick it off again, and the dryness gets worse. Chapping occurs quickly because the enzymes in your saliva are not very friendly to delicate lip tissue.

How Is Lip-Balm Addiction Treated?

Non-drug treatments

There seems to be some truth in the lip-balm addiction story. It's not due to the ingredients in the products, however, but what we do to those ingredients when we put them on our lips. Can you stop using lip balm? You might try going cold turkey—put away all balms in a drawer and see if your lips don't improve on their own. The problem will probably get worse before it gets better, because you're guaranteed to be licking a lot more for the first few days.

OTC treatments

Most lip-balm-addiction experts recommend a more gradual approach to kicking the habit. Use non-menthol or non-camphor balms, rather than trying to stop using them altogether. Lip moisturizers often bridge the gap well.

The Drug Lady Recommends . . .

Often, substituting non-menthol products like *Vaseline Lip Therapy* will give the lips the security of being covered by a balm, but won't have the cooling effect that causes many people to lick their lips more frequently.

Prescription treatments

All it takes to break this addiction is a lot of willpower, and tough lips. The lips will frequently become very red and irritated as the withdrawal begins. If the lips break open and there may be risk of infection, see the doctor. He or she may prescribe an antibiotic cream or ointment to speed healing, but be careful and don't get too attached to the prescription medicines!

Toothache

Q. *I have an awful toothache and I don't have time to see the dentist until later in the week. What can I do for relief until then?*

A. There are few pains that drive us crazier than that of a throbbing and aching tooth. My first recommendation is that you call right now for a dental appointment. If you've already done this, wonderful! Now we'll go into detail about what products will bring the fastest relief for that terrible pain.

What Causes a Toothache?

Toothaches can be caused by trauma to the tooth, an infection around the tooth, or tooth decay. Pain from a tooth also can be caused by new teeth coming in (wisdom teeth), impacted teeth, sinus infections, or grinding the teeth. More often than not, a toothache is a sign that something deeper is going on that should be taken care of by a dentist as soon as possible.

How Is a Toothache Treated?

Non-drug treatments

Natural remedies for tooth pain are generally aimed at decreasing the inflammation (by warm towels on the face) or numbing the tooth (by using SMALL amounts of *clove oil*). With clove oil, it is very important to use just a few drops on a clean cloth, applied directly to the sore area, and only for a maximum of three days. This can cause allergic reactions or small ulcerations in the gum if overused.

Tincture of *echinacea* (one to two teaspoonfuls in water) taken several times a day has been shown to decrease pain as well as protect against further infection.

Rinsing the mouth gently with warm salt water (a half-teaspoonful salt to 8 ounces water) several times daily will soothe the ache.

OTC treatments

Over-the-counter treatments for a toothache include those applied directly to the sore tooth and those taken by mouth to ease the ache. Typically, those medicines that are applied directly to the tooth give only short-term pain relief. However, short-term is better than nothing, especially when you find that you must eat or drink. Topical toothache medicines all contain an active ingredient that completely (and very temporarily) numbs the area; names to look for are **Anbesol Maximum Strength Liquid** (*benzocaine*) and **Red Cross Toothache Medication** (*eugenol*). It is not advisable to eat or drink for one hour after using these products, as your ability to swallow effectively may be impaired.

Medicines that are taken internally, like *aspirin, ibuprofen, ketoprofen,* or *naproxen sodium,* work well to bring down the inflammation and pain of a toothache.

The Drug Lady Recommends . . .

Never, never, never, put an *aspirin* directly on a sore tooth to relieve the pain! Take the aspirin and swallow it, but don't put it against the delicate mucus membranes in your mouth. Very nasty mouth burns have occurred from individuals placing an aspirin (*acetylsalicylic acid*) between their cheek and gum to help a toothache.

Prescription treatments

If the tooth damage is serious, your dentist may have to perform oral surgery to correct the problem. Less-serious conditions may be treated with antibiotics to clear up any infection or abscess, and/or painkillers (like **Vicodin**) to ease the pain until the infection clears.

Pill Humor

Real Names of Dentists and Orthodontists (from Pharmacists' Files)

- Dr. Lips
- Dr. Root
- Dr. Chew
- Dr. Pulley
- Dr. Payne
- Dr. Smiley
- Dr. Yankum

Tooth Whiteners

Q. *What is the best over-the-counter tooth-whitening kit?*

A. Tooth whiteners are quite controversial due to the fact that some years ago the FDA declared them drugs, not cosmetics. Gum and mouth burns that occurred when tooth whiteners were used raised concerns that these products should be used only under a dentist's supervision.

What Are Tooth Whiteners?

Combination products with the ingredients *hydrogen peroxide, carbamide peroxide,* and *perhydrol urea* are used to bleach the enamel on the tooth's surface by oxidizing stains and bubbling them out of the enamel. Unfortunately, they are so strong that they can remove the entire enamel coating of the tooth if you leave them on too long.

How Can Teeth Be Whitened Safely?

Non-drug treatments

To keep tooth stains to a minimum, limit the amount of coffee, tea, or cola that you drink. I live in Seattle, where that statement would be considered sacrilegious, but it doesn't change the truth! Or, if you must drink these delicious but evil beverages, brush with a mildly abrasive thick paste of *baking soda* afterwards. Stopping smoking is another great way to keep your smile brighter.

OTC treatments

The American Dental Association (ADA) advises patients to consult with their dentists to determine if bleaching is appropriate *before* purchasing an over-the-counter tooth-whitening kit. Then treatment in the dentist's office or dentist-supervised home treatment is recommended. The unsupervised use of tooth whiteners (other than those found in FDA-approved toothpastes) may cause damage to the enamel of the tooth. Other safety concerns include soft tissue (gum) and tooth pulp damage, as well as delayed mouth wound healing.

The Drug Lady Recommends . . .

I'll have to stand close to the ADA and not recommend anything (other than ADA-approved toothpastes) for over-the-counter use to whiten your teeth. *Colgate Total Plus Whitening Toothpaste* and *Crest Multicare Whitening Toothpaste* are two excellent choices for at-home everyday tooth-brightening. For extra whitening, ask your dentist about the *Platinum Professional Toothwhitening System* or *Rembrandt Lighten Gel.* These may be purchased from your pharmacy and taken to the dentist's office for proper supervised treatment.

Prescription treatments

If dull teeth are a problem, see your dentist for a consultation. He or she may recommend a gradual bleaching and whitening plan that extends over several weeks. By having the treatments done in the office you can protect your teeth and delicate gum tissue.

Legs, Feet, and Toes: Stand Up for Those Tootsies!

Athlete's Foot ▦ Blisters ▦ Bunions ▦ Corns and Calluses ▦
Diabetic Foot Care ▦ Gout ▦ Ingrown Toenails ▦ Intermittent Claudication ▦
Leg Cramps ▦ Plantar Fasciitis ▦ Plantar Warts ▦
Restless-Leg Syndrome ▦ Toenail Fungus ▦ Varicose Veins

WE DEPEND ON our lower extremities—legs, feet, and toes—for so much. We stand on them for long hours every day, we pound them into hard concrete for the sake of exercise, and when do we ever say thanks? As much as we use our feet and legs, many, many conditions can affect them. Let's take a look at some of the common problems and how to best deal with them before they slow you down.

Athlete's Foot

Q. *I have an awful case of athlete's foot and I'm not the least bit athletic! What can I use to get rid of this quickly?*

A. Unfortunately, you don't have to be athletic to pick up an itchy case of athlete's foot. It can happen to anyone who happens to have his or her feet in the wrong place at the wrong time. It doesn't seem quite fair, does it?

What Is Athlete's Foot?

Athlete's foot is actually a type of ringworm fungus infection. You may also see athlete's foot referred to as *tinea pedis.* The fungus itself goes by the formal names of *Trichophyton* or *Epidermophyton.* It loves the warm, moist areas between your toes, especially when those toes have been around shower or pool areas, where the fungus thrives and can easily be acquired.

The first sign you'll usually notice is itching or a burning feeling between the toes. As it progresses, small blisters may form. When these crack open, it can be quite painful and can leave the feet susceptible to an infection in addition to the athlete's foot—and to top it off, foot odor also can accompany athlete's foot. All in all, this isn't a very pleasant experience. It is also very contagious, so if family members share the shower, there is a good chance they'll be sharing all this unpleasantness as well.

How Is Athlete's Foot Treated?

Non-drug treatments

Keeping the feet dry is the first step to preventing athlete's foot from starting or spreading. Changing your socks daily and wearing different shoes also will be helpful. If you can, wear sandals or at least use cotton socks to let those tootsies breathe.

Tea tree oil in a 100-percent concentration is an excellent anti-fungal for treating athlete's foot. Apply twice a day, morning and night, for best results. Be careful, though, because at this high concentration this oil can really sting irritated skin. It generally takes several days of treatment for the rash to disappear and an additional seven to ten days to ensure that the fungus is completely and totally eliminated.

OTC treatments

Most cases of athlete's foot can be easily treated with OTC products, but you will have to be patient! It can take up to four weeks for a deeply set infection to go away completely. OTC antifungal products are available in a variety of forms, including creams, lotions, powders, and sprays.

Tinactin (*tolnaftate*) is the only OTC product advertised to prevent, as well as treat, athlete's foot. Others that are also effective include *Lotrimin* (*clotrimazole*), *Lamisil* (*terbinafine*), and *Micatin* (*miconazole*). In fact, they cure the infection completely in about 80 percent of sufferers. Put the medicine on in the morning before you don your socks, then again in the evening when you take them off. You may also use both a cream, for direct application between the toes, and a powder to help keep the toes as dry as possible.

Prescription treatments

If your infection doesn't respond to OTC products, or if the condition is severe, you may want to see the doctor for a prescription antifungal. These are taken internally in tablet or capsule form and some of the names you may see are *Nizoral* (*ketoconazole*), *Lamisil* (*terbinafine*), *Sporanox*

The Drug Lady Recommends . . .

For the fastest cure that is available over-the-counter as of this writing, try the new *Lamisil AT* (*terbinafine*) cream. Lamisil was recently available only as a prescription, but now can be bought over-the-counter. Apply the cream between the toes twice a day (morning and night) for one week or as directed by a doctor. For infections on the bottom or sides of the foot, apply twice a day (morning and night) for two weeks, or as directed by a doctor. That is a considerably shorter time of treatment than for other antifungals. You don't need to suffer any longer than necessary!

(*itraconazole*), or **Grifulvin V** (*griseofulvin*). There may be a higher potential for side effects with these medicines because they work from the inside (systemically) rather than from the outside (topically).

Blisters

Q. *I got an awful blister on my heel when I went hiking last week. Every time I walk it hurts. What can I do to heal it faster, besides going barefoot all the time?*

A. While going barefoot might be a great idea when it's warm and sunny, in the winter it could get a little chilly! What we have to do is heal that blister quickly so you can get back to hiking.

What Causes Blisters?

Plain and simple, blisters are caused by the friction of something rubbing against your skin. That "something" can be the back of your shoe, socks that slip and slide, even the handle of a rake in your hand (especially when your hands haven't done anything more strenuous for several months than type). The skin forms a liquid-filled bubble for protection. Unfortunately, this bubble or blister can really hurt, especially if it happens to pop.

How Are Blisters Treated?

Non-drug treatments

The best healer for a blister is time and no more friction until the skin underneath has a chance to form and toughen. Going barefoot around the house and soft, non-rubbing shoes at work are a must. Using gloves for most chores will save your hands.

Two pairs of socks with *talcum powder* between them can be effective as blister prevention for those who walk or run a great deal.

A method of toughening skin to prevent a blister is using a *tincture of benzoin.* Apply the liquid tincture before bedtime, and then slip on a sock overnight.

The Drug Lady Recommends . . .

Don't pop a blister! Opening this top layer of skin can allow bacteria to reach the delicate skin under the blister, and an infection could develop. It's tempting, I know, but the fluid inside will be reabsorbed through your skin or will break open on its own. Don't do it yourself! Let the blister heal on its own.

OTC treatments

It's a fact that blisters are caused by friction—the rubbing together of delicate skin against something hard and unyielding. Covering the potential blister area with something soft like moleskin will protect and keep direct friction to a minimum. Don't worry, this doesn't really come from a mole, it's just soft like one! Moleskin is a spongy, flannel material that, when applied directly over and around the blistered area, will pad and protect the skin.

Dabbing a small amount of *Vaseline* directly on the blister can keep it soft. You may try putting a *Band-Aid* over the blister, but if your shoe is rubbing against the bandage, these rarely stay on for long.

If the blister bursts, you should apply a topical skin antibiotic like *Neosporin* or *Polysporin* to the area. This kills existing bacteria and helps keep a bacterial infection from developing,

Prescription treatments

If a blister contains white or yellowish liquid, it could be infected. Call the doctor to have a look. If your blister refuses to go away and looks un-

The Drug Lady Recommends . . .

Blister Relief from *Band-Aid.* It covers the blister completely and protects it from any more irritation. The adhesive seals it completely and when it is removed after forty-eight hours or when the patch becomes loose, *presto!*—the blister is much better!

usually red and angry, you may have an infection that should be treated with oral antibiotics. Over-the-counter topical antibiotics like **Neosporin** (*bacitracin, neomycin,* and *polymyxin B*) should be used only on fresh wounds, not those that are already infected. Call the doctor just to be sure.

Bunions

Q. *My mother has a very painful bunion. Is there anything that I can get for her to try? Is there any cure?*

A. **Bunions can be very painful because they are involved in every step that you take. The joint of the big toe can be aggravated to the point of making walking almost impossible. You should remember this, too: bunions are very often an inherited condition.**

What Is a Bunion?

A bunion is the inflammation of the fluid-filled sac (called a bursa) that is found along the outer joint of the big toe. This inflammation can be caused by many factors, including the way a person sits or walks, tight or ill-fitting shoes, inherited foot structure, and even corns and calluses. (See "Corns and Calluses," page 195.)

Generally, once started, bunions are around for the duration. It is possible to have a bunion that isn't painful, but most hurt. Because the area often constantly rubs the inside of a shoe, a bunion can be swollen and very tender.

How Are Bunions Treated?

Non-drug treatments
Changing shoe styles may be enough to bring relief from bunion pain. Even slipping on more comfortable shoes or slippers while you sit at your desk can bring a nice "Ahhhh!" to irritated feet.

Heating pads or warm footbaths can be a wonderful treat for painful bunions. However, diabetics should avoid this type of treatment because

The Drug Lady Recommends...
Cushy pads like *Dr. Scholl's Cushlin Gel Bunion Guards* have soft gel inside to protect the tender bunion. Its cushioning inner surface molds to the shape of any foot and sticks to your skin without leaving a tacky feeling behind. Its outer surface is tough but smooth, to prevent snags and runs in socks and hosiery.

with decreased sensation in the foot, burns may result. (See "Diabetic Foot Care," page 198.)

OTC treatments

If the pain is simply from the friction against your footwear, using soft moleskin (a soft, spongy, flannel pad) directly on the bunion may be enough. Don't worry. Moleskin isn't really from a mole. It's just a soft, spongy, flannel to pad and protect the skin.

Anti-inflammatory medicine, like *ibuprofen* or *naproxen,* may be effective for short-term pain relief.

Prescription treatments

If the bunion has been around untreated for a long time, the only options may be surgery or long-term treatment with special orthopedic shoes, which should be a good incentive to seek early treatment when bunions first become a nuisance.

Corns and Calluses

Q. *What is the difference between a corn and a callus? Are they treated the same way?*

A. Corns and calluses are often referred to in the same sentence—as in, "I saw him in the 'corns and calluses' department of the drugstore." There are some similarities, but these are two different conditions affecting the feet. Both corns and calluses are areas of toughened skin that form as a result of some type of friction. Unlike a blister (see

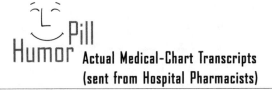

Pill Humor Actual Medical-Chart Transcripts
(sent from Hospital Pharmacists)

- ▥ "On the second day the knee was better and on the third day it had completely disappeared."

- ▥ "The patient has been depressed ever since she began seeing me in 1993."

- ▥ "She was divorced last April. No other serious illness."

- ▥ "I will be happy to go into her GI system; she seems ready and anxious."

- ▥ "Patient was released to the outpatient department without dressing."

- ▥ "Dr. Blank is watching his prostate. The patient was advised not to go around exposing himself to other people."

- ▥ "Patient developed a puffy right eye, which was felt to be caused by an insect bite by an ophthalmologist."

- ▥ "The patient refused autopsy."

"Blisters," page 192), which forms from short-term friction, corns and calluses result from long-term friction.

What Are Corns and Calluses?

Corns can be either soft or hard. A hard corn has a shinier look with a compact core. It has a rough, toughened outer surface. Hard corns appear on the areas of the foot that are in constant contact with shoes, like the tops of toes, the outside of the little toe, and the sole of the foot. Soft corns are fleshier and are usually found between the toes. These are whitish in color and have a thin, smooth center.

A callus may be broad or it may have well-defined edges. It is made up of rough dead skin that has been protecting that area against friction. Calluses typically cover a bony spot, such as a knuckle of a finger or a toe. Plantar calluses occur on the soles of the feet and have a distinctive white center.

How Are Corns and Calluses Treated?

Non-drug treatments

The most effective treatment of both corns and calluses is to stop the friction and pressure that caused the problem in the first place. Well-fitting shoes are a must!

Using an herbal salve with *calendula* can soften and soothe irritated tissue. Warm footbaths in *Epsom salts* can also be helpful for softening the skin and soothing irritated feet.

The FDA recommends a fifteen-minute soak in lukewarm water and mild soap as the treatment of choice for both corns and calluses. The toughened tissue should then be rubbed off with a towel or *pumice stone*. (See the warning for diabetics below.)

OTC treatments

Corn-removal products are available as plasters, pads, or discs, or in liquid form. They use the active ingredient *salicylic acid* to gradually eat through your skin until the core of the corn is exposed and dissolved. ***Dr. Scholl's Corn Removers*** can be cut to fit the precise area of the corn. These may take several weeks of daily use to remove the corn.

A pumice stone or callus file can be used to gently take a callus down to new skin. Remember that this is new skin, so if the original source of the friction that caused the problem isn't removed, the area could become quite painful.

Warning:

Diabetics (and others with poor circulation) should use special care

The Drug Lady Recommends . . .

Just a word of caution about corn removers containing salicylic acid: BE CAREFUL! This is an acid that you are putting on your skin, and it can be very damaging to tender skin that doesn't have a thick layer. Dabbing *Vaseline* around the corn can protect the tender skin that shouldn't be actively treated.

not to injure the feet as healing can take a long time and may lead to infection.

Prescription treatments

Corns and calluses generally don't require medical treatment unless they are very painful or if you have other chronic conditions, like diabetes, that make daily foot care essential (see below).

Diabetic Foot Care

Q. *My dad has diabetes and doesn't see very well. His doctor said that he should pay special attention to his feet. What can I do to help?*

A. **For diabetics like your dad, the goal is to keep an eye on the feet to make sure that any blood-circulation problems aren't doing damage. This is a very real problem for diabetics, since nearly 25 percent will develop a serious foot or leg problem in their lifetime.**

Why Is Diabetic Foot Care Important?

Diseases like diabetes can greatly reduce the amount of blood circulating through the legs. The blood vessel damage from diabetes involves blockage of the major arteries that carry blood and oxygen. Reduced blood flow to the legs means reduced nerve sensation, so the diabetic may not realize it if there is an injury to the foot. This condition, also called diabetic neuropathy, may begin with a burning or tingling feeling in the hands and feet.

The Drug Lady Recommends . . .

DON'T let Dad use a heating pad on his feet. With the lack of good sensory perception in the feet, burns could occur without his being aware of it. Also, ask that he only use footbaths under supervision, because the water temperature may be much higher than he realizes. It is very easy for the feet to sustain a burn from the hot water.

How Should a Diabetic's Feet Be Treated?

Non-drug treatments

A daily foot inspection is very important, to see whether any cuts or sores are present. Foot ulcers (small sores on the soles or toes) are a special danger to diabetics because of the lack of circulation to the feet. Infections can occur quickly and the ulcers may take a very long time to heal; these must not be neglected—even for one day. It is easy for a diabetic to get an ulcer on the foot if shoes don't fit properly or if there is friction on a particular area of the foot.

Washing the feet daily with soap and water is important, but it is even more important to be sure the feet are thoroughly dry afterwards. This keeps bacteria and fungus from finding a hospitable home between the toes.

Massaging or rubbing the feet daily can help stimulate blood flow—and it usually feels pretty good, too!

OTC treatments

Keep dry, callused skin as pliable as possible. Apply **Vaseline** to calluses and keep the feet covered and warm whenever possible.

The Drug Lady Recommends . . .

RX Comfort Socks for diabetics are wonderfully soft socks made with a special Teflon fiber that decreases the friction that can occur while walking. The fibers also act to reduce foot moisture and counter any bacterial growth that may cause problems. These socks are designed to give support, but not to cut off the blood circulation that's so important to diabetics' feet.

Prescription treatments

Any type of sore or cut that doesn't seem to be healing properly should be shown to your doctor promptly. The FDA has reported some startling statistics: Approximately 25 percent of persons with diabetes will develop severe foot or leg problems, and nearly 50 percent of all leg amputations are performed on persons with diabetes. Don't wait! Your feet are too important to take any chances.

Gout

Q. *I get a pretty bad case of gout about twice every year. Is there anything I can do to avoid this? What about the fastest treatment when I get it?*

A. That's one thing about gout. When it occurs, there is little else as necessary as stopping the pain FAST! In past centuries, it was thought that gout was caused by dietary excess only affordable by the rich and thus was associated with nobility and royalty. Today, unfortunately, with our excessive diets we "commoners" know that it is a condition that can affect us all.

What Is Gout?

Gout is a type of arthritis in which a crystallized form of uric acid accumulates in the joints if the kidneys become overloaded and cannot filter it from the blood. Gout can be triggered by certain foods (like alcohol or meals high in fat or protein), sickness, or stress. It occurs most often in the joint of the big toe, but it can affect any major joint in the body. The pain generally increases quickly and soon the affected joint is swollen and very tender. Because the pain is so severe, you may also feel as though you have flulike symptoms (fever, chills, body aches).

How Is Gout Treated?

Non-drug treatments

Paying attention to what triggers your gout is one way to avoid gout attacks. If you know that large amounts of alcohol cause pain, ease up at that wedding reception. Ditto for the steak dinner. In fact, a healthy, low-fat diet may be one of the best ways to find welcome relief from gout pain.

Drinking lots of water also will help flush the excess uric acid from your system.

OTC treatments

Over-the-counter anti-inflammatories like **Motrin** (*ibuprofen*) and **Aleve** (*naproxen*) are very helpful in bringing down inflammation and easing joint pain.

Prescription treatments

The prescription medicine *colchicine* is effective for bringing down joint inflammation within twelve to twenty-four hours. *Allopurinol* is the drug of choice for prophylaxis (preventing gout attacks from occurring). It works by stopping uric acid from forming in the body.

If left untreated, gout can lead to long-term joint damage.

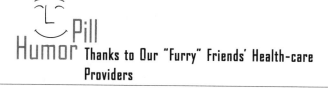

Humor Pill Thanks to Our "Furry" Friends' Health-care Providers

A woman told the veterinarian that something was wrong with her dog. He examined the animal and told her that her dog was dead.

"I don't believe you," she said, "I'd like a second opinion."

The vet said that would be fine. He went into the other room and got a cat. He put the cat up on the table with the dog. The cat sniffed the dog and jumped down. The vet then got a black Labrador retriever, put him on the table, and the lab sniffed and jumped down.

The vet tells the lady again, "I'm sorry, but your dog is definitely dead. That will be six hundred dollars for the exam."

"Six hundred dollars!! That's ridiculous! What for?" she exclaimed.

"Well, that breaks down to fifty dollars for my fee and five hundred and fifty dollars for the cat scan and Lab work."

Ingrown Toenails

Q. *I have an ingrown toenail. What can I do to make it stop hurting?*

A. An ingrown toenail can cause agony. Trying to stuff your swollen, throbbing toe into a tight shoe for a day of standing and walking isn't a pleasant experience. Fortunately, painful ingrown toenails can be corrected quickly. And, by taking some simple preventative steps, there are very effective ways of ensuring that they don't come back.

What Is an Ingrown Toenail?

An ingrown toenail occurs when a hard section of the edge of the toenail pushes into the soft, tender skin of the toe. Often the nail can break the skin, causing ulcerlike sores in addition to the pain and swelling. An ingrown nail can be caused by wearing tight shoes that push the toes together or by cutting the nail into a curved shape rather than straight across.

How Are Ingrown Toenails Treated?

Non-drug treatments

Warm soaks with *Epsom salts* can soften the nail and relieve the pressure. For most people, cutting the nail straight across with clippers that have a straight edge will help avoid ingrown toenails.

The Drug Lady Recommends . . .

The FDA has determined that there are no effective over-the-counter treatments for removing ingrown toenails. They did, however, approve of OTC remedies for ingrown toenails that generally focus on relieving the pain rather than removing the nail. An example is the *OutGro Pain Relief Formula*, which contains 20 percent *benzocaine* as a numbing agent. Applied directly to the nail, it eases discomfort quickly, but the effect may last only a few hours.

OTC treatments

Anti-inflammatory medications like *ibuprofen, aspirin,* and *naproxen* are often very effective for fast pain relief.

Prescription treatments

If the surrounding nail area becomes warm and has pus, it's time to see the doctor. If the nail can't be trimmed in the office, the doctor may numb your toe to remove the part of the nail that is causing the problems.

Intermittent Claudication

Q. *My father was diagnosed with what the doctor wrote down as "intermittent claudication." What is this?*

A. This does sound like something scary, doesn't it? Take heart—this is a fairly common condition that, while painful at times, isn't as frightening as the name suggests.

What Is Intermittent Claudication?

This strange-sounding condition occurs when blood flow to muscles in the legs is interrupted. A narrowing of the major arteries that bring blood into the legs (a form of atherosclerosis) can cause this interruption of blood flow. This narrowing of the vessel is generally caused by the build-up of fatty plaques under the artery wall lining. Intermittent claudication can actually be one of the first symptoms that this narrowing is occurring. The calf muscles may ache or cramp with any type of exercise or walking uphill. The veins in the lower leg may be painful and bulging. This type of leg pain is commonly referred to as "claudication." Because it occurs only periodically, this condition is referred to as "intermittent claudication" or IC. Rest makes the pain go away.

IC can get progressively worse, even to the point that the leg aches all the time. Propping the leg up makes it even more difficult for the blood to flow into the constricted vessels, and the pain may increase. In advanced stages, the foot can go completely cold and numb.

How Is Intermittent Claudication Treated?

Non-drug treatments

The doctor may tell your father to try to walk at least thirty minutes a day, even if it hurts. This is a common treatment. When pain is felt during the walk, he should stop until it eases before starting again. The muscle contractions while walking force the other blood vessels in the leg to expand to compensate for the narrower one.

Stopping smoking, improving diet, and mild daily exercise may also be helpful.

Herbal medicines like *hawthorn* (160 mg per day) and *gotu kola* (30–60 mg per day, triterpenic acids) are said to promote circulation by dilating blood vessels and are used in many natural preparations for strengthening and toning blood vessels.

The Drug Lady Recommends . . .

The herb *ginkgo biloba* has also had some success with circulatory disorders, especially those in the extremities (arms and legs) and the brain. The generally recommended dose is 40–60 mg three times daily. However, ginkgo should not be used with blood thinners like *Coumadin* (*warfarin*) or *aspirin* because of the potential for serious bleeding disorders to occur.

Prescription treatments

The prescription medicine **Trental** (*pentoxifylline*) acts as a blood-flow enhancer and is used to improve blood circulation in the legs. This gets more oxygen to the muscles of the lower leg and relieves the pain significantly.

Leg Cramps

Q. *I get leg cramps often at night. Is there any medicine that I can take for this?*

A. Leg cramps are one way to get your heart racing in the middle of the night! Getting a leg cramp can get even a normally non-athletic person up and out of the bed in a very speedy manner.

What Causes Leg Cramps?

Leg cramps are an involuntary, violent, and painful spasm of the muscle, usually in the calf area. This quick tightening and shortening of the muscle causes a knot or a "charley horse" to form.

These nighttime visits can occur after long periods of inactivity or even after a very strenuous workout. According to medical research, it looks as though cramps are usually caused by a combination of an overstimulation of nerves leading to the muscles and an electrolyte imbalance within the body.

Certain medicines like *diuretics* (water pills) can deplete your body of important minerals (*sodium, calcium, potassium,* and *magnesium*) the muscles need to work more efficiently. Hormonal and weight changes with pregnancy can also trigger leg cramps. Smokers often carry less oxygen in their blood, and so are more prone to excruciating cramps when the leg muscles are stressed.

How Are Leg Cramps Treated?

Non-drug treatments

It's easier said than done, especially when you're hopping up and down and yelling in the middle of the night, but the fastest way to relieve a cramp is to RELAX. Gently massage the area, then slowly—slowly—stretch it out. Ahhhh . . . much better! Heat can be soothing to cramps, too.

For preventing leg cramps, first try a daily multivitamin. If your body is missing a certain essential mineral or vitamin, this should provide what your body needs. Give this a try for at least two weeks. If this isn't enough, adding an extra *vitamin E* supplement has been shown to help some individuals.

Electrolyte-replacement drinks, like **Gatorade,** work in the body at a cellular level to replace the *potassium* and *sodium* salts that may be missing. Before you try Gatorade, however, try just drinking lots more water. It's better for you and has fewer calories and less sodium.

Since the FDA took *quinine sulfate* off the market for leg cramps, there has been a tremendous void for those individuals who really felt that it worked for them. The FDA could not find any medical studies that proved its effectiveness. If my customers are any indication, the FDA did not speak to them directly. Commercial soda water with quinine is one option. The homeopathic remedy called **Hyland's Leg Cramps with Quinine** is a product that has a VERY tiny amount of quinine. The dose is so small, in fact, that the FDA doesn't consider it an active ingredient.

The Drug Lady Recommends . . .

Adding a glass of orange juice or a banana to your day adds *potassium* to your diet to help prevent the leg cramps. Many people find that avoiding milk or milk products before bedtime will also help decrease their cramps.

OTC treatments

There are products on the market advertised specially for leg cramps, like **Legatrin,** that contain only the antihistamine *diphenhydramine* as a sleep aid. These medicines are effective for helping you sleep, but really don't have any effect on the leg cramp itself. The **Legatrin PM** product contains the pain reliever *acetaminophen* (found in **Tylenol**) in addition to the *diphenhydramine.*

Prescription treatments

Unfortunately, there aren't any prescription medicines to prevent leg cramps. If you are taking a *diuretic* (water pill) like *furosemide,* and are having severe cramps, tell your doctor. There may be a different type of medicine that won't change your body's salt balance as drastically.

Pill Humor — Medical Terminology 101

Sometimes it seems as though individuals in the medical profession have a language all their own. Here is an attempt by some of our patients to get back at us!

▓ ANTIBODY—against everyone

▓ ARTERY—the study of fine paintings

▓ BACTERIA—the back door to a cafeteria

▓ BANDAGES—the rolling stones

▓ BARIUM—what you do when the patient dies

▓ BENIGN—what you be after you be eight

▓ BOTULISM—tendency to make mistakes

▓ BOWELS—letters like *a, e, i, o,* or *u*

▓ CAESAREAN SECTION—a district in rome

▓ CARDIOLOGY—advanced study of poker playing

▓ CAT SCAN—to search for one's lost kitty

Plantar Fasciitis

Q. *I have a very painful condition called plantar fasciitis. What can I do for the most effective relief?*

A. I can't pronounce its name very well, but I certainly can sympathize with anyone who has this condition. Imagine waking up each morning and putting your feet on the floor and being greeted by pain. No, it's not an ice-cold floor—it's plantar fasciitis.

What Is Plantar Fasciitis?

Plantar fasciitis is a painful inflammation and irritation of the tissue covering the bottom of your foot from the middle of your foot (the ball) to the back (the heel). This tough tissue, called the plantar fascia, contracts during periods of inactivity, and causes pain when it is stretched. Heel pain is the most common symptom. It is worse with the first step out of bed in the morning due to the inflamed fascia being stretched out. You'll be more susceptible to this if you are a serious runner, wear high heels, or have experienced rapid weight gain. (I don't mean that all plantar fasciitis sufferers are overweight runners who wear high heels—any ONE of these can make you more susceptible.)

How Is Plantar Fasciitis Treated?

Non-drug treatments

Staying off the heel as much as possible when you have a flare-up is the best (though arguably not the most convenient) way to ease the pain. Weight loss often will decrease the pressure and resulting pain.

Night splints (devices fitted to the calf and foot to keep the foot stretched out) can be used to keep the fascia from contracting during the night. Ice also may help decrease the inflammation.

OTC treatments

Anti-inflammatory medicines like **Motrin** (*ibuprofen*) or **Aleve** (*naproxen*) can be very effective in reducing the swelling and pain when the heel is very irritated.

The Drug Lady Recommends . . .

Change your shoes! Ease up on the high heels! Change worn heels or heel pads in running shoes. Give those feet a break whenever possible. This is one foot condition that is almost entirely preventable.

Prescription treatments

If this continues to be a problem even after changing shoes and losing weight, your doctor may prescribe special orthopedic inserts for your shoes. He may even diagnose a bone misalignment that can be cured with surgery.

Plantar Warts

Q. *What can I use to get rid of plantar warts?*

A. Plantar warts can be very annoying! Of course, anything on the bottom of your foot that causes pain when you walk is not very pleasant. These tender but stubborn growths can be overcome, but it does take patience and perseverance.

What Are Plantar Warts?

Plantar warts (*verrucae plantaris*) are small growths on the soles of the feet that are caused by a virus, like regular warts, but which have tiny blood vessels inside that look like small black dots. The warts may be flat against the bottom of the foot, or slightly bumpy and painful when you step on them. Since it's difficult not to take a step if you ever want to get anywhere, the key is to get rid of them. Even if you don't do anything, they will go away—but this could take anywhere from months to years. You don't have to wait that long to get relief.

How Are Plantar Warts Treated?

Non-drug treatments

Tea tree oil has been shown to decrease the size of some plantar warts. It seems to have very mild antiviral properties, which help eliminate the cause of the wart.

Home remedies that some of my customers have used with success are raw garlic or a raw potato applied directly to the wart, or soaks in warm water with vinegar. While I didn't find any scientific evidence on how these remedies work or how long the treatment should last, they do seem to benefit some people. It certainly won't hurt to try.

OTC treatments

While no OTC treatment is available for curing plantar warts completely, *salicylic acid* applied to the skin has been FDA-approved to help in removal, and in turn to decrease the pain these warts cause.

Salicylic acid may be used in patches, liquids, or pads that gradually dissolve the wart. Remember that salicylic acid is a potent acid and may burn other areas of the skin, so it is a good idea to protect the surrounding skin area with a dab of **Vaseline.**

The Drug Lady Recommends . . .

Trans Ver Sal PlantarPatch Wart Remover Kits provide a simple and convenient overnight application of *salicylic acid.* They are sized for the bottom of the foot and can be worn easily. Each patch provides a controlled, continuous delivery of medication; when used as directed, this form is gentler on surrounding skin than using salicylic acid alone.

Use of salicylic acid or any product that could be damaging to the skin is not recommended for individuals who have diabetes or circulatory problems or have diminished immune systems. The reasoning behind this is that it is difficult enough for these individuals to get proper circulation to the feet without adding an injury that could take a very long time to heal. (See "Diabetic Foot Care," page 198.)

Prescription treatments

The most effective way of removing plantar warts is in your doctor's office. Here the doctor can freeze, cauterize (burn), or cut them off surgically. This is the fastest way of getting rid of the warts, but there is still a possibility that they may return.

Pill Humor Thanks to the Psychiatrists Who Keep Us Sane

A guy goes to a psychiatrist. "Doc," he says, "I keep having these alternating recurring dreams. First, I'm a teepee, then I'm a wigwam, then I'm a teepee, then I'm a wigwam . . . it's driving me crazy! What's wrong with me?"

"It's very simple," the doctor replies, "you're two tents."

Restless-Leg Syndrome

Q. *My mother has restless-leg syndrome. I heard that vitamin supplements could help this. Is it true? What else will work?*

A. Because medical science knows so little about what causes restless-leg syndrome, taking supplements would definitely be worth a try, especially if she's tried everything else. Restless-leg syndrome (RLS) should first be diagnosed by a doctor to rule out other conditions.

What Is Restless-Leg Syndrome?

Restless-leg syndrome, or RLS, is the uncomfortable and overwhelming sensation of having to move the legs, especially at night. Those who have RLS report a tingling, twitching, numbness, or "crawling" feeling in the leg muscles. Moving the legs by flexing and unflexing will relieve this feeling temporarily, but it sometimes takes getting up and walking around to make it stop. Sleep can be very difficult, especially when this continues night after night.

It is thought that RLS is caused by a slight chemical imbalance in the brain or in the muscle tissue itself. Low blood-iron levels appear to be related to this condition in many individuals. Alcohol, caffeine, smoking, and stress can aggravate the condition. Even with as much information as medical science has about RLS, the cure remains elusive.

How Is Restless-Leg Syndrome Treated?

Non-drug treatments

The herb *valerian* has been shown to be an effective sleep aid that may also allow you to sleep deeply enough not to be disturbed by RLS. Common dosages are from 150 to 300 mg in capsule form of dried powder extract, taken twenty-five minutes before normal bedtime.

Since many who suffer from RLS also have been shown to have lower-than-normal iron levels, adding a multivitamin with iron may be helpful.

Some individuals have also found relief by adding 400 IUs of *vitamin E* daily to their diet. Most multivitamins contain at least this much, but check your labels to be sure.

OTC treatments

While there are no OTC products specifically for RLS, certain sleep aids are helpful in getting you through some of the tougher nights. **Legatrin PM** (500 mg *acetaminophen* and 50 mg *diphenhydramine*) and **Nytol** (25 mg of *diphenhydramine*) are two names to look for when short-term sleep aid is needed.

The Drug Lady Recommends...

A good choice for a short-term sleep aid is *Tylenol PM*. It has both the antihistamine *diphenhydramine* (for sleep) and *acetaminophen* (for pain relief). You may notice a slightly groggy feeling the next morning (I know I do!). However, it does let you sleep well and this may be enough to avoid being troubled by RLS as you sleep.

Prescription treatments

In severe cases your doctor may want to try an anti-anxiety drug like **Xanax** (*alprazolam*) to help you overcome RLS and get some sleep. **Klonopin** (*clonazepam*) may help stabilize the conduction of nerve impulses along the muscle fibers. The drug commonly used for Parkinson's disease, called **Sinemet** (*carbidopa* and *levodopa*), also shows good results in some patients. Talk with your doctor to see which might be most appropriate for you.

Toenail Fungus

Q. *What can I use to get rid of toenail fungus? I'm going on vacation and want to wear sandals!*

A. First, I hope that your vacation isn't coming up in the next few days! Because the nail grows so slowly, it can take up to eighteen months for a toenail fungus to go away completely, and the fingernail can take up six months for a complete turnover. Let's see what we can find to get this process under way.

What Is Nail Fungus?

The *tinea ungulum* fungus causes the fungal condition. When the fungus finds a home, the nail can become very thick, discolored, and rough (also referred to as **onychomycosis**). This isn't a good thing for the over 70 percent of sandal-wearing adult American men and women who suffer from this condition. But all is not lost.

How Is Nail Fungus Treated?

Non-drug treatments
While there aren't any good scientific studies to prove this, many of my customers have found that applying the powerful antifungal *tea tree oil* twice daily for several months has helped lessen their cases of nail fungus. Some have even seen the fungus clear up completely. It is certainly worth a try if you are looking for a more natural alternative.

OTC treatments
While there are several products available OTC for the treatment of nail fungus, none of these has been approved by the FDA for that purpose.

The Drug Lady Recommends . . .

Dr. Scholl's Fungal Nail Revitalizer is a cream to be scrubbed into the surface of the infected nail, applied daily for three weeks. It is advertised to reduce nail discoloration and to smooth out thick, rough nails, helping them look more natural again while your prescription medication takes effect. This works cosmetically to aid the appearance of the nail, but doesn't treat the underlying fungus.

That doesn't mean that you won't get some benefit from them, it just means they haven't been proven to be very effective. Because they do not penetrate the nail, they work best in infections of the skin or the nail surface. Once the fungus has found a home deep in the nailbed, it is usually too late for OTC products.

Some products to look for are **Fungi-Nail** and **FungiCure.** You'll see them available as liquids, solutions, or creams. They contain *undecylenic acid* as their active ingredient. Undecylenic acid has mild fungistatic, or fungus-killing, properties.

Prescription treatments

Prescription medicines are by far the most effective (maybe the only truly effective) way to completely eliminate a nail fungus. Because the nail takes so long to grow out, prescription medicines often have to be taken orally (by mouth) to work from the inside out. Some medicines your doctor may prescribe include **Sporanox** (*itraconazole*) or **Lamisil** (*terbinafine*). These can cure 80 to 100 percent of fungal infections with one course of treatment, but this treatment can be VERY expensive. It costs up to $400 for a full course of medicine, and it still usually takes three months of taking this medicine for any effect to be seen. Ouch!

For those who aren't into taking pills, the newest prescription treatment for nail fungus is a nail polish—yes, really. **Penlac Nail Lacquer** contains the antifungal *cicloprox.* Because it is used topically on the nail, rather than taken by mouth, there is a smaller chance of side effects. Unfortunately, the studies done by the manufacturer show only a 12 percent cure rate after using it daily for one year. See? I told you nail fungus would be difficult to get rid of!

Varicose Veins

Q. *Is there anything I can use for treating my varicose veins? I'm so embarrassed to wear shorts or skirts.*

A. I remember the first time I noticed varicose veins when I was a child. I thought, "Wow! Those must really hurt!" Now that I have them myself, I know better—no pain, but they are something that I'd rather not have.

What Are Varicose Veins?

Varicose veins are veins close to the skin which have lost elasticity, so that now they bulge and appear swollen. Some varicose veins resemble very intricate road maps, criss-crossing and twisting. (I've seen what looks like several major highways on my legs when I stand.)

The reason we have varicose veins instead of varicose arteries is because our veins must use the muscles in our legs to return blood against the flow of gravity. Arteries have it easy; the heart pumps blood through them and gravity does the rest. Veins have tiny one-way valves to prevent the blood from backing up or pooling in our legs, but as we age, these valves get leaky. Extra weight from pregnancy or from standing up for many hours at a time can contribute to their development. Lifestyle, hormones, and possibly genetic predisposition determine whether or not you will have this condition. One day you just wake up and *presto!*—you've got varicose veins!

How Are Varicose Veins Treated?

Non-drug treatments

Herbal remedies like *ginkgo biloba* (40 to 60 mg three times daily) and *bilberry* (20 to 40 mg three times daily) have been used historically for strengthening circulation. Remember: Ginkgo may interfere with blood-

The Drug Lady Recommends . . .

Venastat Leg Health is advertised as a natural way to support leg-vein health and protect against lower-leg swelling by promoting circulation in the leg veins. The active ingredient is 300 mg of *horse chestnut*. There are some good scientific studies that show this herb is very effective for toning veins while decreasing swelling. This is an herbal product, but you may see it on the OTC drugstore shelves, too.

thinning medicines like **Coumadin** (*warfarin*) or *aspirin*. The potential for serious bleeding complications is an important factor to consider for those already taking medications to thin the blood. Individuals taking these medicines should avoid this herb unless specifically advised by their doctor.

OTC treatments

Support hosiery or support stockings are a must for everyone who stands on his or her feet all day. (Are you listening out there, pharmacists?) These help push the blood back up toward the heart and prevent pooling and bulging in the veins. Companies like **Futuro** carry a large selection of stockings and hosiery in knee-highs and full leg support.

Prescription treatments

The more complete (and drastic) methods for eliminating varicose veins are done in your doctor's office. **Sclerotherapy** involves injecting a sclerosing agent into the veins. This irritating liquid causes the vein to collapse and forces blood through the healthier veins. Varicose veins may also be stripped or removed from the legs. None of these remedies, however, can guarantee that the varicose veins won't eventually come back. Varicose veins seem to be just one of nature's unpleasantries that we may have to live with.

NINE

Men's Good Health:
Direct from the Planet Mars

Benign Prostatic Hyperplasia (BPH) ▦ Contraception and Condoms ▦

Erectile Dysfunction (ED) and Viagra ▦ Hair Loss ▦ Jock Itch ▦

Penis Enlargement ▦ Premature Ejaculation ▦ Prostate Cancer ▦

Sexually Transmitted Diseases

WHEN YOU LOOK at magazine covers promoting today's men's-health topics, it may seem that they focus around one thing—sexual function. In my work as a pharmacist, I've found that men's questions tend to center around many other health issues as well. Moreover, men have just as great a need as women for accurate, up-to-date information. Why speculate or accept half-truths when you can get the real scoop here?

Benign Prostatic Hyperplasia (BPH)

Q. *What exactly is BPH (benign prostatic hyperplasia)? Is it a form of prostate cancer? What symptoms should I be on the lookout for?*

A. Despite its somewhat daunting name BPH, or benign prostatic hyperplasia (also called hypertrophy), is a common condition. In fact, over 50 percent of men will have to deal with it by the time they are age sixty. Medical science hasn't quite pinpointed the exact cause, but it could be related to the hormonal changes that come with getting older.

What Is Benign Prostatic Hyperplasia (Hypertrophy)?

Here is one less thing to worry about: BPH is NOT cancerous. BPH (benign prostatic hyperplasia) is a swelling of the prostate gland ("benign" means non-cancerous; "prostatic," meaning it involves your prostate gland; "hyperplasia," meaning a growth or swelling).

The prostate is the walnut-sized gland that helps produce semen; it encircles the urethra (the tube that carries urine from your bladder and out through your penis). So when the prostate swells, it makes it very difficult to urinate or it can cut off the flow of urine. The first symptoms include difficulty in starting to urinate, then feeling like you're not quite "finished," even after the stream has stopped. Nighttime trips to the bathroom become more common. Urinary incontinence (dribbling) may develop along with bladder infections or kidney stones. If you notice any of these symptoms, it is important to contact your doctor right away. Letting this condition go untreated could cause bladder and kidney damage.

How Is Benign Prostatic Hyperplasia Treated?

Non-drug treatments

Avoid alcohol, over-the-counter **decongestants, antihistamines,** and caffeine, all of which tend to cause urine retention. While it may be tempting, DON'T limit the amount of fluids you drink. Fluids are very important, to flush out the bladder and prevent infections from developing. Drink lots of water to decrease the likelihood of kidney stones and bladder infections.

Studies show that *saw palmetto* taken in a dosage of 160 mg twice daily provided improvement in urinary flow for 90 percent of the men taking it for mild-to-moderate benign prostatic hypertrophy. This herb decreases the ability of receptors in the prostate to take in more testosterone; in effect, this slows the growth of prostate cells. Results were seen after just four to six weeks on the standardized extract (85–95 percent fatty acids and sterols). It appears that only the capsule or tablet forms are effective; teas were found to be ineffective.

The Drug Lady Recommends...

 Before trying to self-treat the symptoms of BPH, please see a doctor first. The very same symptoms of this benign condition may be the body's way of telling you that something more serious, like prostate cancer, is going on (see "Prostate Cancer," page 234). Talk to the doctor FIRST, then try the herbal alternatives if that's advised.

OTC treatments

You can find the herbals listed above on the OTC medicine shelves. This is a good thing, as more awareness is shifting to the natural alternatives that are available for some conditions. There are no non-herbal OTC medications specifically for the treatment of BPH.

Prescription treatments

If BPH has gone unchecked for some time and urine is backed up in the bladder, it may be necessary to insert a catheter to release the pressure. Prescription medications also may be needed. Your doctor may prescribe **Hytrin** (*terazosin*), **Flomax** (*tamsulosin*), or **Cardura** (*doxazosin*) for short-term relief. These medicines act to relax the bladder sphincter and let the urine flow more freely. **Proscar** (*finasteride*) shrinks or halts the enlarging prostate by blocking an enzyme (*5-alpha reductase*) that causes the prostate cells to divide more rapidly. It relieves symptoms for up to 50 percent of the men who take it, but it must be taken for at least six months before it takes effect.

Contraception and Condoms

Q. *What's the best type of condoms to buy? Are they all the same?*

A. No, condoms aren't all the same. In fact, picking the right one can be quite a challenge, especially with that line of people just getting home from church standing just behind you while you're trying to figure out the difference between latex, lubricated, and ribbed!

What Are Condoms?

Basically, as you probably already know, a condom is a thin rubber sheath. For the male, the condom slips on and snugly covers the erect penis; for the female, the condom is inserted into the vagina. The condom catches sperm during ejaculation and prevents them from entering the vagina. Because condoms also prevent some skin-to-skin contact, they provide significant protection against pregnancy, sexually transmitted diseases, and HIV/AIDS.

How Do You Choose a Condom?

The success rate for avoiding pregnancy with condoms is about 90 percent, but for protection against sexually transmitted diseases (STDs) the

The Drug Lady Recommends . . .

Don't buy the "Super-Size" condoms unless you truly are super-sized! So many young men (and some older ones, too) come into the pharmacy and purchase these large condoms to impress themselves or their partners. It is very easy for these condoms to slip off if they don't fit properly. Believe me, your partner will be much more impressed if the condom stays on than if it comes off during lovemaking.

The Drug Lady Recommends . . .

Buy new condoms and do not rely on the one you've kept in your wallet for the past few weeks. Condoms should be kept away from heat (out of back pockets and glove compartments). Those with spermicide have expiration dates. So, if it's been around for a while, toss it and buy some with new expiration dates. Also, do NOT use oil-based lubricants (*Vaseline,* baby oil, or lotion) with condoms. These products weaken the latex and may cause the condom to break. Use a water-soluble lubricant, like *K-Y Jelly,* specifically designed for use with all condoms.

rate goes up to nearly 100 percent. However, latex condoms are the ONLY types considered "protective" against both bacteria AND viruses. Some individuals who suffer from latex allergies (see "Latex Allergies" chapter 2, page 47) find that they get protection and allergy relief by using a lambskin condom under the latex one. But please, PLEASE don't use a lambskin condom alone! There are tiny microscopic holes in the condom's material that allow viruses to pass through easily.

How Are Condoms Used?

An important part of the effectiveness of a condom is that it is used correctly. Here are a few of the basics.

1. Carefully tear the package along one side.

2. Be careful not to tear the condom with fingernails or other sharp objects.

3. Put the condom on before having any intimate contact with your partner (oral, vaginal, or anal). There are fluids that can spread disease (or that contain live sperm) present before ejaculation.

4. Place the rolled-up condom on the tip of the erect penis, making sure that the rolled-up condom ring is on the OUTSIDE.

5. Squeeze the tip of the condom between your fingers to remove any air and unroll it slowly until the condom ring is resting firmly against the base of the penis. Leave enough space at the tip of the condom to hold the semen.

6. Immediately after ejaculation, withdraw the penis while holding on to the base of the condom so that the semen does not spill out and to make sure the condom stays on.

7. Throw out the condom in the garbage when finished. Do not flush it down the toilet.

8. Use a new condom each time you have sex.

You can increase your chances of avoiding pregnancy by using condoms with the spermicide *nonoxynol-9*. Some condoms even advertise the spermicide as a lubricant. You may also use lubricants made especially for condoms, like **K-Y Jelly,** but other lubricants should be avoided because they may weaken the latex.

The only side effect to be aware of is a possible latex or nonoxynol-9 (spermicide) allergy. If you're allergic, you may experience a burning sensation or irritation of the vagina or penis, caused by an allergic reaction to the latex or the lubricant used in the condom.

Erectile Dysfunction (ED) and Viagra

Q. *I saw a commercial for Viagra and they mentioned a condition called "ED." What is ED? How does Viagra help? Is Viagra safe?*

A. With the large amount of direct-to-consumer advertising being shown on television about prescription drugs, it's no wonder that you have questions. It's difficult to put several pages of important information into a thirty-second TV spot. "ED" is short for "erectile dysfunction." We'll go into a lot more detail about Viagra (sildenafil) under "Prescription treatments" for this condition in a minute.

What Is Erectile Dysfunction (ED)?

Erectile dysfunction is also referred to as impotence. This condition is characterized by the inability to get or keep an erection long enough for satisfying intercourse. Erectile dysfunction affects more than forty million American men, so if you have this problem, you're certainly not alone. In

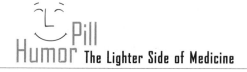

Pill Humor The Lighter Side of Medicine

Are you ready for the *Viagra* jokes?

- A man at the pharmacy to pick up his Viagra prescription exclaimed over the $10-per-pill price. His wife, who was with him, had a different opinion: "Oh, $40 a year isn't too bad."

- A bank sign in Texas during a heat wave complained: "Who put Viagra in the thermometer?"

- Bread with Viagra as an added ingredient is being marketed through a Boston bakery under the name "Pepperidge Firm."

- Q: How many doses of Viagra does it take to change a lightbulb? A: One little tablet and it's a whole new bulb.

- The Viagra computer virus turns your floppy disk into a hard drive.

---

fact, studies have shown that nearly ALL men have experienced ED at one time or another in their lives.

ED can be caused by several different factors. Nervousness, fatigue, stress, too much alcohol, or even being angry with your partner are common external factors leading to erectile dysfunction. ED caused by these external factors is typically not treated directly with medication. However, as you get older, internal or physical factors become much more likely to be the cause of the problem. Chronic conditions like diabetes, hypertension, or narrowing of the arteries are responsible for the majority of cases in men over the age of fifty; these causes respond best to prescription therapy for ED.

How Is Erectile Dysfunction Treated?

Non-drug treatments

Many herbalists recommend the use of the amino acid *l-arginine* and the oat extract *avena satvia* for impotence. While these have been used for centuries to promote increased sexual responsiveness and prowess, there are no modern scientific studies that back up these claims. Several of my customers who have tried these remedies claim to have found improvement, though.

Asian ginseng is sold and advertised as an aphrodisiac, based on its properties as a vasodilator, meaning it opens up blood flow. Historically many, many people have used ginseng with great success. Standardized root extracts are taken in dosages of 100 to 200 mg daily.

While *ginkgo biloba* is showing success in increasing circulation to the brain and the arms and legs, I have not found any good studies that show it is useful in treating ED. However, since ED is often caused by a circulatory disorder, the use of ginkgo may provide an alternative. Remember that ginkgo should be avoided by those taking blood thinners like *aspirin* or *Coumadin* (*warfarin*) because uncontrolled bleeding can result when the two drugs are combined.

For ED caused by the external factors listed above, often simply relaxing and not putting so much pressure on yourself will take care of the problem. If it continues, you and your partner may want to see a third party (like a therapist) to discuss any underlying causes.

OTC treatments

For severe cases of ED, a pump device is a safe way to achieve an erection. The pump draws blood into the penis and a ring is placed around the base to help maintain the erection. The ring should be removed after thirty minutes so normal circulation can be restored.

Prescription treatments

Viagra, Viagra, Viagra! Who hasn't heard about this "wonder drug" that has revolutionized the sexual climate of America? *Viagra* (*sildenafil*) news stories, anecdotes, and jokes abound. In some countries in which this medication is not yet legalized, or is difficult to obtain, a very lucrative black market has developed. For example, a Viagra tablet that costs $10 in the United States was sold in some Far East countries for as much as $500!

Viagra acts as a vasodilator, allowing a greater flow of blood into the penis and therefore a stronger erection. Viagra works by blocking the enzyme *PDE5,* and at the same time promotes blood flow to the penis. This allows a normal erection to occur as long as there is stimulation. But all this fun can't be had without some risk. Because of its action in increasing blood flow away from the heart, Viagra has a tendency to cause a mild lowering of blood pressure. When used with certain heart medications, it can lead to a dangerous and severe drop in blood pressure.

Another concern is that older users with severe heart disease may die from the strain of sexual exertion, from the chemical effects of the drug, or from a combination of the two. The drug is capable of interacting with some nitrate cardiac medications like **Nitro-Dur** or **Imdur.** The result can be a rapid and dangerous drop in blood pressure. The FDA published a statement saying that doctors should be cautious about prescribing it to whole groups of men, including those who recently have had heart attacks or have very high blood pressure. Since impotence often is a symptom of underlying heart disease or high blood pressure, or even a side effect from drugs used to treat those conditions, the manufacturer, Pfizer, stresses that men seeking Viagra first need a full and complete medical exam.

Patients with liver or kidney disease should take lower dosages of 25 mg, because they tend to eliminate the Viagra more slowly (it stays in the body longer). Some medications, such as certain antibiotics (*erythromycin*) or anti-fungal medications (*ketoconazole*), also interfere with the breakdown of Viagra, and patients taking them should also take the lower dosage. On the other hand, other drugs like **Rifampin** (an anti-tuberculosis drug) increase the breakdown of Viagra, and therefore the men taking them may require higher dosages to get a full effect. Your doctor is the expert to consult in all these situations.

So what can the "average" man expect in regard to side effects? The most common adverse reactions associated with the use of Viagra (in 4 to 16 percent of patients) are headaches, facial flushing, indigestion, and nasal congestion. Other, less-frequent side effects include diarrhea, rash, dizziness, and abnormal vision, including increased sensitivity to light and a disturbance in the perception of blue and green colors. Most of the adverse reactions are mild and quite well tolerated by healthy patients.

The Drug Lady Recommends...

Here is a thumbnail sketch of what NOT to do if taking *Viagra*.

Do not take this medicine if you are allergic to *sildenafil* (the active ingredient) or if you are taking nitrate medicines such as *nitro-glycerin* (**Nitro-bid, Nitro-Dur, Transderm Nitro, Nitrol** ointment, **Nitrolingual** spray) or *isosorbide* (**Imdur, Monoket, Ismo, Isordil**).

Viagra (*sildenafil*) in combination with any nitrate medicines can cause very low blood pressure, and increase the risk of fainting and possible heart attacks. Every drug has side effects, some very serious, and Viagra is no exception. If given for the proper condition as determined by a medical exam, and if the proper precautions are taken with regard to medication interaction and underlying health problems, Viagra can greatly improve the quality of life for many couples.

Hair Loss

Q. *I have heard that certain drugs can stop baldness. What works best?*

A. The prevention of baldness is one of the most commonly asked questions I receive from men. There are many, many treatments advertised to "cure" this condition. Some are useful, while others are not. Let's separate what works, from what will simply part you from your hard-earned funds.

What Causes Hair Loss?

Male-pattern baldness is the most common type of hair loss seen in men. It begins on the sides, near the front, and proceeds over the top of the head toward the back. It can be caused by your genetic makeup, or by the fact that you produce a higher than normal amount of testosterone. (Tell that to anyone who dares say anything about your head!)

We are all born with 100,000 to 150,000 hair follicles and we have them all our lives. As youngsters we have the soft, fine, almost colorless strands called vellus hair. At puberty, many of these vellus follicles become terminus (or finish growing) and leave you with thicker, coarse, and darker hair.

The increased levels of testosterone (androgens) that cause these changes are also responsible, in part, for pattern baldness in men and the general thinning of hair in women. The scientific term is **alopecia.** People with androgenic alopecia are more sensitive to androgens. As a result, hair follicles shrink and new hairs are finer and grow for a shorter time. The factors of heredity, aging, hormones, and even stress levels can decide whether or not we're predetermined to lead a hairless life.

The classic pattern baldness seen in men can begin as early as the twenties and continues with age. The first hairs begin to disappear from the top of the head, with a gradual spread to the temple areas, leaving the typical fringe or crown of hair. Unfortunately, the earlier the hair loss begins, the more hair will be lost. Some individuals experience several short, intense periods of hair loss, followed by longer, stable periods. Some studies have shown that the hair follicles themselves are not dead, but merely choked off by these high androgen levels (testosterone). The thicker, full-grown terminus hair falls out and is not replaced as in a normal state. It comes in finer and only grows for a short amount of time.

There are other types of baldness and other causes for hair loss. Vitamin deficiencies (especially the *B vitamins*) or use of some prescription drugs can cause hair loss. Chemotherapy for treating cancer, thyroid disease, poor circulation, and even stress also may temporarily decrease the active production of hair. A sudden, unexpected hair loss can also be the warning sign of a medical problem. And environmental factors like application of large quantities of follicle-clogging hair products (like gels, dyes, or sprays) may contribute to the destruction of the terminus hair.

How Is Hair Loss Treated?

Non-drug treatments

Baldness is a normal part of aging but if it is something that you still can't accept, there are other options. Many men have found cosmetic satisfaction with hairpieces or hair-transplant operations.

Beware of products on the market "guaranteeing" to restore your hair just as it was before. Creams and shampoos may be very effective at unclogging follicles, and ridding them of residues that plug the pores. Shampoos like *Progaine,* from the makers of *Rogaine,* make hair look fuller by cleaning out follicles and exposing the suffocated hair shaft, but they can't help the follicles that have stopped producing.

Some people have claimed to see increased hair growth from the use of scalp massage or other stimulation techniques. I can see where this idea comes from: The hair follicle is nourished by many tiny blood vessels; if these are stimulated, it makes sense that the hair in the follicle may grow as a result.

OTC treatments

So, are the over-the-counter hair-restoration products for you? Only if your hair loss is of the hereditary variety; if your family has a history of pattern baldness, then perhaps you should give them a try. The drug *Rogaine* (*minoxidil*) has been shown to slow down and even reverse baldness in some men. You must use it religiously—twice a day, every day, for three to four months—before you'll see results. You should see an increased growth primarily of the vellus hair (the fine, thin, colorless variety we all have as children).

The Drug Lady Recommends . . .

As for using *Rogaine* to PREVENT balding, it won't work. The *minoxidil* works by stimulating those follicles that have almost given up. They have already stopped producing the terminus hair, but if caught before the follicle completely dies, it can still produce the vellus hair. If you haven't lost the hair yet, there is no reason to use minoxidil.

Prescription treatments

Propecia (*finasteride*) is a tablet that works by blocking the body's conversion of testosterone to dihydrotestosterone, the "active" form of testosterone. It is responsible for masculine characteristics like a deep voice and a hairy face. Because the drug brings down the levels of dihydrotestosterone, the male-pattern baldness slows down too. Fortunately, your voice shouldn't get higher or your beard diminish from taking this medicine. The side effects that have been reported, however, include erectile dysfunction (ED) (see "Erectile Dysfunction," page 222), decreased sex drive, and decreased volume of ejaculate.

It has been shown that with a dosage of 1 mg daily, some hair will grow back. The amount varies quite a bit from person to person. Like the over-the-counter product **Rogaine** (*minoxidil*), it has to be used indefinitely in order to keep working.

Jock Itch

Q. *What can I use to get rid of jock itch? I'd like something that works fast.*

A. I understand your urgency. Having jock itch is no picnic! When the skin is moist and one surface rubs against another, conditions are right. Damp gym shorts, working outside in warm weather, and restrictive clothing all contribute to the problem. Getting rid of it fast is a top priority.

What Is Jock Itch?

Jock itch is a fungal infection of the ringworm variety. Both women and men can get it. Women typically get this from the spread of a vaginal yeast infection (*candida*), and men from the irritation of the moist groin area and the growth of the *Trichophyton rubrum* fungus. Jock straps and tight pantyhose both contribute to the problem (separately, of course!).

The rash may look like small, red, ringlike bumps that cover the groin area and the external genitalia (sex organs). These bumps may be very itchy and can produce blisters. Thankfully, jock itch usually can be taken care of at home.

How Is Jock Itch Treated?

Non-drug treatments

I have talked to herbalists who recommend the use of the antifungal *tea tree oil* or the use of a solution of dilute fresh *lemon juice* to be applied directly to the rash. I can't say that I would recommend this myself because these would sting very badly! Especially on the already irritated and sensitive skin of your groin area. You're welcome to try it and it may be helpful, but there are far less painful ways of taking care of jock itch.

OTC treatments

Antifungal medicines can be purchased as powders, sprays, creams, or lotions. Active antifungal ingredients include *miconazole* in **Micatin,** *clotrimazole* in **Lotrimin AF,** *tolnaftate* in **Aftate,** and now *terbinafine* in **Lamisil AT.** The way you apply it is a personal choice. Powders are good for places where sweating is a problem, like in folds of skin or where your underwear is in constant contact. Sprays are easiest to apply, but may be cold and may waste medicine unless you have great aim. Creams or lotions can be applied directly to the rash and are generally thought to be most effective; unfortunately, they are also messy.

The Drug Lady Recommends . . .

Lamisil AT (*terbinafine*) was recently approved for over-the-counter use as an antifungal. In the past it has been available only as a prescription. It seems to work significantly faster than most of the other products on the OTC market. You apply this product to the affected area once or twice daily. The advertising claims to clear up the infection in a week (half the time of other products). With jock itch, that one week saved can feel like a very long time.

Most OTC antifungals require that you use them twice a day for at least two weeks (except Lamisil AT, which advertises a one-week cure). Also, during this time it is important that you keep the groin area as dry as possible. If you are wearing a jockstrap and briefs, you might consider switching to boxers until the infection clears up. This will give your groin area more opportunity to stay dry.

If the itching becomes severe, applying a light coating of *hydrocortisone* cream or ointment to the rash could help.

Prescription treatments

For jock itch that just won't die, there are always prescription antifungals like *griseofulvin, fluconazole,* or *ketoconazole.* If there is the possibility of a secondary bacterial infection, the doctor may also prescribe an antibiotic until the infection clears.

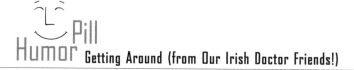

Pill Humor Getting Around (from Our Irish Doctor Friends!)

An Irishman had been drinking at a pub all night. The bartender finally said the bar was closing. The Irishman stood up to leave and fell flat on his face. He tried to stand one more time—same result. He figured he'd crawl outside and get some fresh air to sober up. Once outside, he stood up and fell again flat on his face. So he decided to crawl the four blocks to his home.

When he arrived at the door, he stood up and—again—fell flat on his face. He crawled through the door and into his bedroom. When he reached his bed, he tried one more time to stand up. This time he managed to pull himself upright, but he quickly fell right into bed and was sound asleep as soon as his head hit the pillow.

He was awakened the next morning to his wife standing over him, shouting, "So, you've been out drinking again!!"

"What makes you say that?" he asked, putting on an innocent look.

"The pub called—you left your wheelchair there again."

Penis Enlargement

Q. *I've read that there are some products that will make your penis larger. Is this true? Which ones do you recommend?*

A. You wouldn't believe how many guys ask this same question. It's no wonder that people selling "natural" or OTC products that "guarantee" to increase penis size are doing so well!

What Determines Penis Size?

Here is the real scoop: The size of your penis is determined by your genetic makeup. Once you've gone through puberty and all that testosterone has done its job, you will have the size penis nature intended you to have.

Are Treatments Available to Increase Penis Size?

Non-drug treatments

So, are there any herbal products out there that can increase penis size? No. In fact, some of the anabolic-type muscle builders, like *androstenendione,* may actually shrink normal sex organs by converting to the female hormone *estradiol.*

Wild oats (*avena satvia*), *garlic,* and *ginseng* are sold in many combinations claiming to be an "herbal **Viagra.**" There have been no studies showing these supplements have ANY effect on increasing penis size.

OTC treatments

Are there any products, like "The Pump," that will increase your penis size? Not permanently. "The Pump" works by using a vacuumlike device to forcefully pull blood into the penis. While this may temporarily increase penis size, once the circulation has returned to normal, size does too.

You may see advertisements for weights to wear to gradually stretch the penis. Worn on the penis, these are painful and uncomfortable at best, and no long-term size increases have been shown.

The Drug Lady Recommends . . .

You should not worry too much about your penis size. But if you are really into knowing whether you're on track with everyone else, read on; if not, then just skip the next few sentences. In 1996 a study was published in the *Journal of Urology* by researchers at the University of California San Francisco. They studied eighty normal men and found that the average soft penis was 3.46 inches long. With an erection the average length was 5.08 inches.

Prescription treatments

If your penis size is of great concern, there are surgical techniques that may add some permanent length. One type of surgery releases ligaments from the groin area at the base of the penis and gives a "natural" extension. There is also the "liposuction" method that takes fat from another area of the body and injects it into the penis. Side effects can include swelling, pain, and scarring. Typically, sexual relations can be resumed two to three weeks after the operation.

Premature Ejaculation

Q. *I have a problem with "coming too soon," or premature ejaculation. What can I do to stop this embarrassing problem?*

A. First you should realize that you're not alone; this is a very common problem among men. If you think about it, there is often a tremendous amount of anticipation in this event and the stress of worrying about this condition just seems to make it happen more frequently.

What Is Premature Ejaculation?

Premature ejaculation is the condition in which a man ejaculates (or comes) just before or soon after entering his partner. While the cause of this problem is usually psychological, there have been cases linked to swelling of the prostate gland.

How Is Premature Ejaculation Treated?

Non-drug treatments

Let's start with some techniques and products that have worked very well for others. Chances are, they'll work for you too.

One easy technique is the "squeeze" method. You or your partner can squeeze the base of the penis tightly for several seconds or until the feeling of impending ejaculation passes. This can be repeated as often as desired to stretch out the lovemaking.

A second technique is to wear a condom, or even two condoms, in order to decrease stimulation. This may reduce stimulation long enough for sex to be more satisfying for both of you.

A third technique is the "stop and start" method. Your partner stimulates you just to the point of ejaculation, then stops and waits twenty to thirty seconds before resuming. With practice, this can help in 95 percent of cases.

It's essential to discuss this problem with your partner, and then experiment with ways to increase sexual pleasure for the both of you. This will take off the pressure to perform.

OTC treatments

One product you might try is called **Detane.** It is a cream with a numbing agent (*benzocaine*) to decrease the sensation on the penis. However, some people (either the man or his partner) may have an allergic reaction to the chemicals. Also, as the cream rubs off on the woman's clitoris and vagina, her sensation may be diminished as well. Wearing a condom after you've put on the Detane may be helpful to avoid this problem.

Prescription treatments

If premature ejaculation continues to be a problem, there are also prescription alternatives. Antidepressants like **Prozac** (*fluoxetine*) or **Zoloft** (*sertraline*) have been shown to work well in many men to increase the time it takes to ejaculate. Your doctor may recommend taking these either on a daily basis or an hour before lovemaking is planned.

Prostate Cancer

Q. *What should I be looking out for with prostate cancer? Are there any particular symptoms?*

A. Prostate cancer is a big deal, and it's a good idea that you're being proactive. In men over the age of fifty, there are 200,000 new cases diagnosed each year. As you get older, the chances of developing prostate cancer increase dramatically; it is the second-leading cause of cancer deaths among men. If you have a family history of prostate cancer, you are three times more likely to get it.

What Is Prostate Cancer?

The prostate is the walnut-sized gland that helps produce semen and is regulated by the male hormone testosterone. It surrounds the urethra (the tube that carries urine from your bladder through your penis to the outside world).

Early prostate cancer typically doesn't cause any symptoms because the cancer is slow to grow. While most older men experience enlargement of the prostate (see "Benign Prostatic Hyperplasia," page 218), this does not seem to correlate with prostate cancer; only in the later stages of the cancer does the prostate swell. At this time the symptoms will be often the same as those of BPH.

How Is Prostate Cancer Treated (and Avoided)?

Non-drug treatments

The best thing you can do if you are over fifty is to have a yearly rectal exam. Some prostate tumors can be found this way, but it is also recommended that the PSA (prostate-specific antigen) test be done at the same time. This test measures the level of the protein PSA, which increases when

---

Signs and Symptoms of Prostate Problems

If you notice any of the following symptoms, it is a good idea to give your doctor a call. Symptoms of BPH or possible prostate cancer include

- ▨ difficulty starting or stopping urinating
- ▨ weak or interrupted urinary stream
- ▨ pain or burning with urination
- ▨ frequent nighttime urination

The Drug Lady Recommends . . .

From the most recent medical studies, it appears that there is a connection between a high-fat diet and prostate cancer. Fats produce higher levels of testosterone, and this level of testosterone may trigger the prostate cancer cells. So if you haven't heard it enough—EAT WELL! That means occasionally substituting chicken or veggies for that steak or burger. Taking care of yourself now is much easier than fighting prostate cancer (or other maladies) later.

prostate cancer is present. Early detection is the very best treatment of prostate cancer.

OTC treatments

As with any type of cancer, this treatment is best left to the medical experts. Treating with over-the-counter products is NOT recommended for prostate or other cancers.

Prescription treatments

Surgery is one option for prostate cancer treatment. Unfortunately, there are some risks to this type of surgery. Impotence or urinary incontinence may result. If the cancer is small and slow-growing, you and your doctor may opt for "watchful waiting" to avoid the potential side effects.

For more advanced prostate cancer, the testosterone blocker *Lupron* (*leuprolide*) is often used to decrease testosterone, which seems to feed the tumor.

Sexually Transmitted Diseases

Q. *What are the more common sexually transmitted diseases to be worried about?*

A. If you are sexually active, you should be worried about ALL of the sexually transmitted diseases (STDs), not just the more common ones. Here are a few on the A-list, as in keep "*a*-way" from these—they are serious health risks.

Young people are most at risk for STDs. Of the millions of Americans with STDs, nearly two-thirds of the cases are among young adults under the age of twenty-five!

Humor Pill

A young man goes into a drugstore to buy condoms. The pharmacist says the condoms come in packs of three, nine, or twelve and asks which the young man wants.

"Well," the man says, "I've been seeing this girl for a while and she's really something special. We're having dinner with her parents, and then we're going out. I think tonight's 'the' night. I want to be prepared, so you'd better give me the twelve-pack." The young man makes his purchase and leaves.

Later that evening he sits down to dinner with his girlfriend and her parents. He asks if he might give the blessing and they agree. He begins the prayer, but continues praying for several minutes.

The girl leans over and says, "You never told me you were such a religious person."

He leans over to her and says, "You never told me that your father is a pharmacist!!"

What Are Sexually Transmitted Diseases?

The name is pretty self-explanatory. You get these diseases from having sex with someone who is infected. Risk factors increase with the number of partners you have and when you don't wear a condom. The only sure way not to ever be exposed to an STD is to totally abstain from sex, or to be in a monogamous relationship with someone who is disease-free; the next-best way is to always use a latex condom.

There are more than twenty STDs, all transmitted by bacteria or by virus. Bacterial STDs include gonorrhea, syphilis, and chlamydia. Some viral STDs are genital herpes, genital warts, hepatitis B, and AIDS.

Bacterial STDs

Here are some general symptoms to be on the lookout for with bacterial STDs.

- vaginal, anal, or penile discharge with an odor or unusual consistency
- flulike aches
- burning or pain when urinating
- any unusual rash, blisters, or growths in the genital area
- pain or swollen glands in the genital or groin area

Gonorrhea

This STD wins the award for being one of the most common in the world. Caused by the *Neisseria gonorrhoeae* bacteria, this infection is transmitted through fluids in the mouth, penis, and vagina. Men may notice a discomfort when urinating, then a thick, yellowish discharge from the penis. This typically occurs from two to fourteen days after the infection. For women, the symptoms take longer to appear (seven to twenty-one days) and may or may not include vaginal discharge or discomfort when urinating. Over half of women with gonorrhea show no symptoms until the disease has progressed to an acute inflammation, called pelvic inflammatory disease (PID).

Syphilis

Syphilis is caused when the bacterium *Treponema pallidum* finds a home in the moist mucus membranes of the mouth, vagina, urethra, or anus. The symptoms usually appear in three to four weeks after exposure and are divided into four stages: (1) "Primary"—when a red but painless sore appears at the site of infection. (2) "Secondary" appears about two months after the sore has healed; symptoms include a skin rash, nausea, loss of appetite, and mouth sores. (3) The disease now enters a latent stage that may last for years. (4) The final, or tertiary, stage of syphilis may produce tumors or even damage to the heart, brain, and nervous system.

Chlamydia

The parasite *Chlamydia trachomatis* is the culprit behind the STD we know as chlamydia. While gonorrhea wins world honors as being the most common internationally, chlamydia takes the prize as the most common STD in the United States.

For women, the symptoms may include a vaginal discharge that is frothy and of a slightly greenish hue. The entire vaginal area may be painful and you may feel as though you have the burning of a urinary-tract infection. (See "Urinary-Tract Infections," chapter 13, page 329.) For men, a discharge that is puslike or frothy may appear from the penis. It may burn when you urinate or you may feel the need to urinate more frequently. This STD is easily diagnosed in a doctor's office where they will look at the secretions under a microscope. Antibiotics for BOTH partners (see below) generally clear it up quickly.

The Drug Lady Recommends . . .

Chlamydia is the leading cause of infertility in women—take it very, very seriously. Get prompt medical attention and be sure that you and your partner take the FULL course of the antibiotics prescribed. Your future children's lives could be at stake!

Viral STDs

Genital herpes

The *herpes simplex* virus, either Type 1 or Type 2, causes genital herpes. This virus finds a way into your body through a cut or tear in the skin. The first symptoms appear as a rash of small, watery, very itchy blisters anywhere in the genital area. These blisters break open, leaving an ulcerated area that, as you can imagine, is very painful. This is considered the "active outbreak" stage and this is when you are most contagious.

Other symptoms include a tingling or numbness in the genital area, especially just before the rash appears. You may notice a burning feeling as you try to urinate, or pain with urination. When the "active" phase is over, the blisters begin to heal and the virus travels to nerve bundles in your spinal cord. The virus lies dormant there until the next outbreak. Stress, heat, or even certain foods can trigger an outbreak.

Genital warts

Genital warts are very common. In fact, ten to twenty million Americans have these small growths on their bodies. The human papilloma virus (HPV) is also responsible for the same warts (the non-genital variety) that you always thought were from unfriendly frogs. Genital wants are painless and have a fleshy or almost cauliflower-like appearance and are very contagious. For women, genital warts have been linked to a higher incidence of cervical cancer; in fact, 90 percent of women who have cervical cancer have had genital warts!

Hepatitis B

While technically an inflammation of the liver, hepatitis B may also produce arthritis-like inflammation of the joints, and skin rashes. This type of hepatitis is one of the more serious forms of the virus and can be transmitted through sexual contact, blood transfusions, and the use of contaminated intravenous needles.

AIDS (HIV)

The human immunodeficiency virus (HIV) is a retrovirus (an RNA-containing virus) that attacks the immune system and causes acquired immunodeficiency syndrome (AIDS). HIV enters the body through contact with blood, semen, or vaginal fluids. Once the HIV virus has entered the body, it takes over the genetic material of healthy white blood cells (T-lymphocytes) that we count on to fight infections, and makes itself over again and again. This cellular takeover progresses until the body is unable to defend itself against other invaders. AIDS is a condition defined as having a T-cell count of less than 200 (as opposed to the healthy count of 1,000–1,500) cells per microliter of blood, or when an opportunistic infection (one that would not normally harm a healthy person) takes over. Opportunistic infections may include *candida* yeast, certain pneumonias, and chronic bacterial and viral attacks.

How Are Sexually Transmitted Diseases Treated?

Non-drug treatments

Prevention is obviously the best course of action to avoid STDs. Taking a good multivitamin and eating a healthy diet will give your body the best chances of fighting these infections. There have been reports that *glycyrrhizic acid,* found in licorice, may actually deactivate the herpes virus. Ask your doctor about specific recommendations.

For hepatitis B, the herb *milk thistle* has shown excellent results as a liver protectant. It helps to increase bile secretion in the liver, allowing for better processing of fats.

OTC treatments

Sexually transmitted diseases are very serious conditions that require close medical attention. Talk to your doctor FIRST. For genital herpes, OTC creams that help the itch (**Benadryl**) and dry up the blisters (*calamine* lotion) may be used. Also, antibiotic creams (**Neosporin**) may be used to prevent a bacterial infection from the open blisters. Pain relievers like **Tylenol** (*acetaminophen*) are a good choice for pain relief.

Prescription treatments

Bacterial STDs often can be treated successfully with a course of antibiotics.

Gonorrhea is typically treated with an injection of **Rocephin** (*ceftriaxone*) and a week of the antibiotic *doxycycline* for BOTH partners.

The Drug Lady Recommends . . .

If you even suspect that you might have genital herpes (or any other STD), please, please, PLEASE don't have sex until you've been to the doctor for a diagnosis. There is no cure for herpes, so if you are having an outbreak (even if you use a condom), you could be passing it along.

Syphilis is still treated by the old standby *penicillin*. For those allergic to *penicillin*, the choices are *tetracycline* or *doxycycline*.

Chlamydia treatment may include a single dose of the antibiotic **Flagyl** (*metronidazole*) or **Zithromax** (*azithromycin*). It is VERY important that your partner is treated at the same time or the infection will continue to be passed back and forth.

Viral STDs can't be cured, but the new protease inhibitors and antivirals can manage the symptoms much better than before. Hepatitis B has a vaccine, but it isn't effective once you already have the disease.

With genital herpes, antiviral medicines like **Zovirax** (*acyclovir*) can decrease the recurrence of outbreaks up to 90 percent.

For genital warts, your doctor may prescribe medicines like **Aldara** (*imiquimod*), a cream that you apply directly to the warts three times a week. It may take up to sixteen weeks of treatment for the warts to disappear. Aldara eliminates genital warts in about 50 percent of people treated. **Condylox** (*podofilox*) is another prescription gel or liquid that you apply directly or "paint" on the genital warts twice a day, three times a week, for up to four weeks. Condylox clears up genital warts in about 65 percent of people treated. Pregnant women should not use the podophyllin "paint." Injections of **Intron-A** (*interferon alpha*) have eliminated the warts in about 50 percent of people treated. Doctors may also remove genital warts with chemicals, freezing (cryosurgery), or surgery. The best way to prevent the contraction of genital warts is to use a condom.

TEN

Senior Health:
Getting Older—Getting Better!

Alzheimer's Disease ■ Diabetic Eye Disease ■ Insomnia ■ Macular Degeneration

■ Osteoarthritis ■ Rheumatoid Arthritis ■ Strokes and TIAs

A S WE GET older, it's common to experience aches, pains, and things that just don't quite work right. If we think of our bodies as being like cars, we can see how lots of mileage can wear us out. Our belts and hoses become worn, our headlights dim, and our engines sometime stutter or stop. But getting older doesn't have to be something to dread. As long as we take care of all of our parts and pieces, there is no reason the "golden years" shouldn't be the very best years of all.

Alzheimer's Disease

Q. *My father was recently diagnosed with Alzheimer's disease. How can we help Dad? What are the best treatments?*

A. **What your dad (and your family) is experiencing is shared by nearly seven million Americans and the number is growing each year. Named for Dr. Alois Alzheimer, a German physician, Alzheimer's disease (AD) is the most common cause of geriatric dementia, a decrease in normal mental facilities.**

What Is Alzheimer's Disease?

Alzheimer's disease is a puzzling condition of the brain with no known cause. With AD, progressive damage to the brain cells in certain areas causes a gradual and complete change in the personality of those we love. Nerve impulses become jumbled and protein deposits (plaques) build up in the brain. As a result, areas of the brain responsible for memory and emotional response begin to deteriorate. It is thought that Alzheimer's disease may be related to our genetic makeup, or even due to damage from free radicals (highly destructive oxygen molecules) found in pollution, pesticides, and even in the air that we breathe.

Early symptoms may be subtle, like forgetting details (especially of recent events), or asking again and again for someone to explain something that was just clarified. As the disease progresses, the sufferer may become suspicious or lash out angrily for no apparent reason. Eventually, even simple tasks like remembering one's children or a spouse become impossible. This is especially difficult for the family to deal with. Before these changes start to occur, it's best to arm yourself with as much information as possible to plan for the future with your loved one.

How Is Alzheimer's Disease Treated?

Non-drug treatments

Antioxidants serve the purpose of decreasing the damage potential of free radicals. *Coenzyme Q-10,* at a dose of 50 mg twice daily, is one herbal antioxidant that is showing promise in its ability to increase oxygen supplies to the brain.

Ginkgo biloba has shown outstanding results in several studies. Given in a divided daily dose of 240 mg, this herb may slow the progression of the disease in its early stages. Ginkgo biloba also shows promise for improving memory and increasing circulation in the brain.

There are excellent community resources for both the individual who has AD and his or her family. The Alzheimer's Disease and Related Disorders Association, out of Chicago, is a good place to start. You can find information about local AD adult day-care centers and support/education groups for the whole family. You can find this organization on the Internet at www.alz.org.

OTC treatments

Anti-inflammatory drugs, like **Motrin** or **Advil** (*ibuprofen*), *aspirin*, **Aleve** (*naproxen sodium*), and **Orudis KT** (*ketoprofen*), may provide both a slowing of the disease and protection against further damage. The downside of these drugs is always possible stomach upset and even GI bleeding, so always make sure they are taken with food.

The Drug Lady Recommends . . .

Avoid sleep aids and cold remedies containing **antihistamines** like *diphenhydramine, chlorpheniramine,* or *brompheniramine.* These can depress the nervous system and actually make the symptoms of AD worse.

Prescription treatments

There are two drugs currently approved for treatment of Alzheimer's: **Cognex** (*tacrine*) and **Aricept** (*donepezil*). They do not cure Alzheimer's disease, but help in chemical nerve-impulse conduction, which allows more of the memory to remain intact.

Medical studies are also finding that women who take estrogen after menopause have a much lower incidence of AD. If you're female, talk to your doctor about hormone-replacement options.

Diabetic Eye Disease

Q. *I see that my pharmacy is holding a vision and glaucoma screening next week. As a diabetic, would that be something I should take advantage of?*

A. Absolutely! And if your local pharmacy doesn't have regular eye screenings, run to your local eye doctor or clinic ASAP. Before becoming a pharmacist, I had no idea how devastating diabetic eye disease could be, and this is a PREVENTABLE condition! Over 25,000 diabetic Americans lose their sight needlessly each year, because they were too busy or thought they felt too well to go to an eye doctor. Diabetic eye disease can be deceiving since often the damage is occurring with few or no symptoms until it is too late to save your precious vision. If this book just gets one person to make that appointment, it will be worth every scolding!

What Is Diabetic Eye Disease?

Diabetic eye disease is a combination of problems, all leading to the eventual dimming of sight, and often blindness. Three of the more common conditions are diabetic retinopathy, glaucoma, and cataracts, with the retinopathy occurring exclusively in diabetics. Even the glaucoma and cataracts are seen twice as often in those with diabetes as in those who don't have the disease. It seems pretty clear: If you have diabetes, take care of those eyes!

With **diabetic retinopathy** there are often no symptoms, no pain, no changes in vision. But what happens is that the blood vessels that supply the retina begin to swell, or grow out of control and cover the retina. The swollen blood vessels can leak, causing vision to blur—a condition called macular edema.

If you have **glaucoma,** the internal pressure of the fluid in the eye (aqueous humor) builds up and irreversibly damages the interior nerve fibers. With the more common "open-angle glaucoma," the liquid that fills the eye goes in at the regular rate, but can't drain out of the eye fast

Warning Signs of Diabetes

According to the American Diabetes Association (ADA) symptoms of diabetes include

- frequent urination

- increased hunger

- increased thirst

- weight loss despite increased appetite

- feeling edgy, tired, sick to the stomach

- blurred vision

- dry, itchy skin

- tingling or loss of feeling in hands and/or feet

If you notice any of these symptoms, call your doctor right away.

There are two different types of diabetes, Type I and Type II. Type I diabetes is usually detected in childhood, but can be diagnosed later in life; the symptoms are usually more severe and have a sudden onset. Type II diabetes, on the other hand, develops slowly. Symptoms can be mild and go unrecognized for a long time.

If your doctor checks your blood glucose (sugar) level and finds that it is higher than 140 mg/dl two hours after eating, this is considered a high reading. Before eating, the levels usually range from 70–110 mg/dl. It is very normal for the blood sugar level to fluctuate during the day.

enough. The pressure builds up gradually over time, slowly killing the optic nerve. Vision becomes narrower and more tunnel-like, often without you even being aware of the changes until it is too late. It doesn't take long for the damage to occur, sometimes within just a few years! Glaucoma can't be cured, but it can be treated very effectively.

In the glaucoma screenings that your local pharmacy or clinic hosts, the pressure inside the eye is measured with a quick burst of air blown at the eyeball. This is just a screening test, however, and even if the results are good, it is still a good idea to follow up with a more complete examination. This is especially true if you are a member of the "high-risk glaucoma

The Drug Lady Recommends . . .

It's a good idea to have your doctor check every year for diabetes or if you notice any unusual symptoms like those above. Diabetes can be serious—don't take any chances!

group": are over forty; are African-American; or have high blood pressure or diabetes, or a family history of glaucoma. Since over two million Americans have glaucoma—and it, like diabetic retinopathy, often occurs without any warning signs—it is definitely in your best interest to be checked.

A more dangerous condition is "narrow-angle glaucoma." Some individuals have a tiny angle between the iris and cornea where the fluid drains from the eyeball. This angle is so small that it can close off easily, causing a rapid increase in pressure in the fluid in the eye. If this path is closed off completely, then pain, nausea, redness of the eye, and blurred vision can be the precursors to blindness within days. Screenings and regular eye exams can detect this condition and prevent damage.

Cataracts are a condition in which the lens or the capsule of the eye becomes cloudy and impairs vision. Diabetics are twice as likely as the rest of the population to develop cataracts—and at an earlier age. The key, as with retinopathy and glaucoma, lies with early detection. The cloudy lens of the eye, through which we view the world, can be surgically removed and replaced with an artificial one. Clearer vision is restored quickly.

Vision loss from diabetic eye disease is very preventable. It is up to you to make that appointment with your eye doctor, attend that vision screening, learn what you can about your diabetes, and keep on looking at all the beautiful things out there to enjoy.

How Is Diabetic Eye Disease Treated?

Non-drug treatments

The very best treatment for diabetic eye disease is close control of blood glucose levels. High glucose levels may cause temporary blurriness, and studies have shown that those with closely controlled glucose levels have FOUR TIMES LESS of a chance of ever developing retinopathy. It may mean the difference between clearly seeing your grandchild's smile or not.

Since high blood pressure can cause those already-swollen vessels in the eye to expand and leak even more, it is very important to monitor your blood pressure and to take your medication regularly, as directed by your physician.

Also, the American Diabetes Association has cited studies finding that those individuals who smoke are more likely to get **diabetic retinopathy.** Part of this may be due to the damaging effects of the free radicals found in cigarette smoke. There are many different types of **antioxidants** that help squelch the free radicals found in pollution, UV rays, and cigarette smoke. Look for both supplements and food high in *beta-carotene, lycopene, zeaxanthin,* and *lutein. Carotenoids* are found in bright-colored foods like egg yolks, corn, spinach, red grapes, oranges, and bell peppers. The minerals *zinc* and *selenium* are also powerful antioxidants that may protect the eye tissue from damage.

OTC treatments

While proper nutritional support is an important way to get your antioxidants, sometimes it's just not feasible to get those five servings of fruits and veggies each day. This is when supplements become very important.

The Drug Lady Recommends . . .

A vitamin and mineral combination called *Ocuvite* by eye-product experts—Bausch and Lomb. This particular brand is especially useful to diabetics because in addition to *zinc* and other key antioxidants to protect the eyes at a cellular level, it is both sugar-free and lactose-free. Other key minerals are *selenium* and *copper* with *vitamins A C,* and *E.*

Prescription treatments

If you experience any sudden changes in your eyesight, like blurriness, double vision, painful pressure, or decreased vision on either side, go see your eye doctor. Floating spots or flashes can also be a good reason to pick up the phone. Your ophthalmologist will take a closer look at what's going on inside the eye by putting in drops that dilate or enlarge the pupils, and looking at the retina to see how the blood vessels are doing. If there is a problem, you can discuss treatment options to prevent any further damage. Laser surgery to seal off leaky blood vessels can reduce the risk of blindness by 90 percent!

The Drug Lady Recommends . . .

 Sometimes it is difficult to focus for a while after having your pupils dilated, so have someone drive you home from your doctor's appointment. Remember that it may take hours for your eyesight to return to normal—so be careful!

With **glaucoma,** the key is to bring down the pressure within the eye as quickly as possible. Eyedrops like **Timoptic** (*timolol maleate*) and **Betoptic** (*betaxolol hydrochloride*) lower the pressure by slowing down the rate that fluid gets into the eye. The oral medication **Diamox** (*acetazolamide*) controls fluid secretion in the body and is widely used for open-angle glaucoma. Diamox is most often prescribed in addition to other glaucoma drugs. It is in the sulfa family, so if you have a history of allergic reactions to sulfa drugs, be sure to tell your doctor.

Insomnia

Q. *I'm having a lot of problems getting to sleep. I think I have insomnia. What can I do?*

A. Getting enough sleep at night is very important to good health and high energy. Without a good night's sleep, your body and mind work at less-than-optimal productivity. Many factors can cause this disorder, and it affects nearly everyone at one time or another. Let's see what we can do to get you snoozing again!

What Is Insomnia?

Insomnia is the inability to get enough quality sleep to feel rested. This includes being unable to fall asleep or to stay asleep, waking up very early, and/or not feeling refreshed after sleeping. Certain medicines, excessive stress, medical conditions, or poor sleeping or bedtime habits affect sleep quality. While the majority of cases can be directly traced to stressful or anxiety-producing life events, there are also insomniacs with depression, vitamin and mineral imbalances, and breathing difficulties.

Non-drug treatments

Developing good sleep habits is often one of the best treatments for this condition. Going to bed at a regular time and avoiding stimulation (like exercise or caffeine) before bedtime may be enough to break the pattern of sleeplessness. Relaxation techniques, changes in your diet to foods high in the amino acid *tryptophan* (such as bananas, turkey, cottage cheese, and milk), and a healthy lifestyle that includes exercise can often help you sleep more soundly.

The leading herb used for sleeplessness is *valerian*. Valerian root makes getting to sleep easier and increases deep sleep and dreaming. It does not cause a morning "hangover"—a side effect common to some prescription sleep drugs. Many people use 300 to 400 mg of a concentrated valerian-root preparation thirty minutes before bedtime.

Melatonin has also shown some success in getting sleep patterns back on track after jet lag, but not for general insomnia.

OTC treatments

Sleep aids like **Sleepinal** and **Nytol** contain the antihistamine *diphenhydramine* and may be effective in the short term. Although over-the-counter sleep aids may be helpful for occasional treatment of insomnia, it is not a good idea to use these products on a regular basis. These do not help with the cause of insomnia and may become less effective after a few days of use.

The Drug Lady Recommends . . .

Tylenol PM works well for insomnia accompanied by any sort of aches and pains. The active ingredients are *diphenhydramine* as a sleep aid, and *acetaminophen* as a pain reliever. The downside is that it might make you feel a little groggy the next morning, but that's a problem with all diphenhydramine products.

Prescription treatments

For cases of insomnia that last longer than one month, prescription medications may be called for. Common medicines for insomnia are **Restoril** (*temazepam*) or **Halcion** (*triazolam*), but these have a tendency to make you sleepy during the day. There is a new medicine called **Sonata** (*zaleplon*) that shows promise for those who have difficulty falling asleep, but not for those who wake up and can't go back to sleep. For the best effect, it should be taken just before going to bed, as it starts to work very quickly.

Macular Degeneration

Q. *My grandmother is losing her eyesight due to a condition called "macular degeneration." What can she do to help this condition? How can I prevent the same thing from happening to my eyes?*

A. The type of vision loss that your grandmother is experiencing is shared by many people over the age of sixty. In fact, age-related macular degeneration (AMD) is one of the most common reasons that seniors lose their sight.

What Is Macular Degeneration?

Macular degeneration is a progressive condition that affects a tiny area of the back of the retina, called the **macula.** The macula is where our sight sensibilities of light and sharpness are found in the highest concentrations.

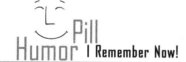

Humor Pill I Remember Now!

A retired pharmacist was having trouble with his memory. One evening he read in the paper about a doctor who could help restore memory by using ordinary things you see every day. After seeing the doctor for about six weeks, the pharmacist and his wife went down to the senior-citizen center and ran into one of their old friends.

The friend said, "I understand you're going to the memory doctor."

"Yes, that's right—we're both going," the pharmacist said.

His friend asked, "Is he any good?"

"Is he any good?" said the pharmacist. "He's the best doctor we've ever been to; he's really good!"

His friend said, "You know, I'm having trouble with my memory, too. I think I ought to see that doctor. What's the doctor's name?"

The pharmacist hesitated. "What's the doctor's name? . . . What's the doctor's name?" He said, "Look, there's a flower with a real long stem, the stem has little green leaves and there are thorns sticking out of the stem. At the top of the stem is a big bulb flower that comes in all different colors. What do you call that?"

"Why, that's a rose," his friend said.

The pharmacist said, "Yeah, that's right—rose." He turned to his wife and said, "Hey, Rose, what's the name of that doctor we've been going to?"

Irreversible macular degeneration occurs when this area of the retina is damaged. This damage is classified as either "wet" or "dry." "Wet" is the most damaging type of AMD and is characterized by fluid or blood leaking into the retina. Scar tissue often forms around the leaked fluid and destroys the macular tissue. "Dry" AMD is the most common type, and is characterized by age-related breakdown or thinning of the tissues in the macula or a dark pigment deposit in the retina.

The first symptom of macular degeneration is often a noticed waviness in lines that used to appear straight. A dark spot in the middle of the normal field of vision is also a telltale sign of progressing macular damage.

As the nerves and tissue become more damaged, the field of vision is reduced greatly. It becomes very difficult to distinguish faces, to drive, or to perform normal daily tasks that require seeing objects clearly. While this condition often leaves peripheral (or side vision) intact, it makes it very difficult to perform daily routines and maintain a good quality of life.

How Is Macular Degeneration Treated?

Non-drug treatments

Because there is a clear relationship between macular degeneration and cellular damage caused by free radicals, one of the most important ways to prevent this condition is to arm the body with an arsenal of antioxidants. "Eye-friendly" antioxidants include the carotenoid family: *beta-carotene, lycopene, zeaxanthin,* and *lutein.* These may be purchased in supplement form at your local pharmacy or you can naturally increase the amount of brightly colored fruits and vegetables—corn, spinach, red grapes, oranges, and bell peppers—that you eat.

Lutein alone or in combination with other vitamins and minerals is showing great promise as both a protector of vision and a nutrient that may actually reverse eye damage. A common dose is 5 mg up to three times daily. *Zinc* (15–35 mg) and *selenium* (200 mcg) are powerful daily doses of antioxidants that protect eye tissue from age-related free-radical damage. An herbal supplement with at least 160 mg of *bilberry* uses the active chemical ingredients called anthocyanidins to deactivate free radicals.

Vitamin C serves double duty as an anti-inflammatory nutrient that helps prevent capillary hemorrhaging and one that is necessary for the proper formation of connective tissue throughout the body. Stock up on your citrus fruits for fighting those free radicals trying to harm your eyes!

Ginkgo biloba is another natural product showing promise for AMD. This herb has properties that increase circulation to the extremities and the brain. Dosage for ginkgo is 40 to 80 mg of the standardized extract (flavone glycosides 24%/terpenes 6%) taken three times daily.

OTC treatments

While proper nutritional support is an important way to get your antioxidants, supplements are a perfectly good substitute.

The Drug Lady Recommends . . .

A product that I like very much is called *Icaps-Plus Antioxidant for Healthy Eyes.* It has a great blend of important vitamins and minerals to support and protect delicate eye tissue. The ingredients are *vitamin A* (as *beta-carotene*), *vitamin C, vitamin E, riboflavin* (*vitamin B-2*), *zinc, copper, manganese,* and *selenium.*

Prescription treatments

Laser therapy is the treatment of choice for "wet" AMD. This laser surgery seals the leaky blood vessels in the retina and prevents more damage from occurring. However, even surgery doesn't remove damage that is already done, so vision may still be diminished if surgery isn't done early enough.

Osteoarthritis

Q. *My knees ache from some type of arthritis. I played lots of sports in my youth and wonder if I'm paying for that now. What can I do about my painful joints?*

A. Aging adults often don't like to think about their bodies wearing out, but with some forms of arthritis this fact of life becomes painfully clear. There are actually different forms of arthritis that can manifest as the painful inflammation of the joints, which stiffen and limit movement. (See "Rheumatoid Arthritis," page 259.)

The type of arthritis described above is called osteoarthritis, or the condition affecting the weight-bearing joints, like the knees and hips. This is the most common form of arthritis, seen to some degree in nearly 80 percent of adults over the age of fifty. Because we are born with a finite amount of cartilage to protect our bones from rubbing together, it gradually wears away through years of playing sports, or may just be the result of getting older. This degenerative condition, osteoarthritis, can be helped a great deal with both modern and natural medicines.

What Is Osteoarthritis?

In the body, a joint is where two bones come together. We have joints in our knees, elbows, wrists, and fingers. In a healthy joint there is a nice cushioning of liquid (synovial fluid) and a layer of thick cartilage that covers the ends of bones as they come together. In healthy joints, the bones move over each other with very little friction and no pain at all. When osteoarthritis strikes, the cartilage begins to wear off the bones at a much faster rate than normal. Without the protective covering, the ends of the bones grind together and inflammation occurs. Over time, this grinding action breaks off small pieces of bone that float in the synovial fluid. The bone ends become ragged and joint movement feels rusty and painful.

As this disease progresses, it becomes harder to move, and when you do move, pain results. Osteoarthritis can come on gradually and before you know it, your body hurts when you stand up or try to walk across the street. Or it can come on suddenly, with a great deal of pain and inflammation. In either case, because the body can't reproduce cartilage naturally, the treatment options consist of making the pain more bearable, or helping the body produce more protective cartilage.

How Is Osteoarthritis Treated?

Non-drug treatments

Within the past few years there has been a tremendous upsurge in the use of natural products for the treatment of osteoarthritis pain. Here are some natural options that are showing great promise, even when compared directly to prescription-strength products.

▓ *Glucosamine sulfate.* This amino acid–and–carbohydrate supplement works by providing a building block for the body to make more cartilage. If this supplement is taken at a dosage of 500 mg three times daily, studies have shown dramatic results in as little as four weeks. In fact, medical studies compare it directly to the pain-relieving power of anti-inflammatories like *ibuprofen.* This supplement worked as well or better for many with osteoarthritis pain and had few stomach-related side effects.

■ *MSM—methylsulfonylmethane.* This sulfur compound forms a building block of new connective tissue and cartilage around arthritis-damaged joints. Take 500 mg of this supplement 3–4 times daily with meals to prevent stomach upset.

■ *Vitamin E.* This amazing antioxidant seems to exert a protective effect on the joints, even as they begin to degenerate. Doses of 400 to 600 IU of *vitamin E* daily for three weeks have been found to result in a decrease of osteoarthritis pain. However, if you are taking a blood thinner (like **Coumadin** or *aspirin*), talk to your doctor before adding vitamin E.

■ *D-phenylalanine.* While I feel that more studies need to be done on this one before I recommend using it exclusively for pain, there have been some interesting results with the use of this amino acid. In one study, doses of 250 mg were given to individuals three to four times per day. They reported significant pain relief within four to five weeks.

OTC treatments

Anti-inflammatories like *ibuprofen, aspirin,* or *naproxen sodium* help a great deal in bringing down painful joint, muscle, or tendon inflamma-

The Drug Lady Recommends . . .

SAM-e. This is one of my favorites because I have talked to so many people for whom it has worked well. No one seems to know exactly how it does it, but SAM-e (*S-adenosyl methionine*) seems to increase the formation of cartilage in the joints and reduces pain, stiffness, and swelling. It also has an anti-inflammatory property that benefits arthritis sufferers. Studies show it equal in pain-relieving capability to drugs such as *ibuprofen* and *naproxen* for some individuals. The dosage for most studies using SAM-e has been 400 mg taken three times per day.

tion. Remember that they can be upsetting to your stomach, so always be sure to take these medicines with a meal or a snack.

If you have ever experienced an allergic reaction to aspirin, especially one that caused difficulty in breathing, it is advised to avoid all anti-inflammatory medicines, too. Any of these may trigger the same (or a more severe) reaction in allergic individuals.

With long-term use of these medicines, there is the potential for stomach bleeding, ulcers, or even perforations. Alcohol can increase this bleeding risk, so limit or discontinue alcohol while on this type of medicine. Your doctor can keep an eye on this bleeding possibility for you with regular checkups, but if you ever begin to vomit blood or material that looks like coffee grounds or notice blood in the stool, call the doctor immediately.

Prescription treatments

The most commonly prescribed medicines for this disease are anti-inflammatories (yes, they're in the same family as those in the "OTC" section, but are stronger). You'll also see these referred to as **non-steroidal anti-inflammatory drugs** (**NSAIDs**). Prescription NSAID brand names to look for are **Daypro** (*oxaprozin*), **Orudis** (*ketoprofen*), **Naprosyn** (*naproxen*), or **Voltaren** (*diclofenac*).

A troublesome side effect of NSAIDs is stomach upset, so much so that many people can't take them at all. However, there are some newer medicines called COX-2 inhibitors that provide alternatives. The manufacturers claim fewer cases of stomach upset than with other NSAIDs. Names to look for are **Celebrex** (*celecoxib*) and **Vioxx** (*rofecoxib*).

The Drug Lady Recommends . . .

While the advertisers of the COX-2 inhibitors promote them as having fewer stomach-related side effects than their older counterparts, please use caution when first giving them a try. Nausea, burning throat, heartburn, and ulcers may still occur even with the new COX-2 inhibitors. If you are sensitive to the older **NSAIDs**, use care when starting the new medicines like **Celebrex** (*celecoxib*) and **Vioxx** (*rofecoxib*).

Rheumatoid Arthritis

Q. *Is there anything at all that will help the pain of rheumatoid arthritis? My mother seems to be in almost constant pain, and I would do anything to help her feel good again. She won't go to a doctor because she says it's just old age. Please help!*

A. I can understand your concern. We never like to see our loved ones in pain. While there is no cure as yet for rheumatoid arthritis (RA), there are treatments that can give your mother more freedom from pain, as well as a greater range of movement. It is important that she get to her doctor for an evaluation as soon as possible. Early treatment may give her many pain-free years.

What Is Rheumatoid Arthritis?

Rheumatoid arthritis is a bewildering condition in which the body begins to attack its own joint systems. Called an autoimmune disease, RA causes the joints of the hands and feet to become swollen and extremely painful and stiff. The body begins to perceive its own joints as "foreign" and attempts to break down the fluid sac that cushions the bone-to-bone joint. This sac becomes swollen, the bone ends enlarge, and ligaments and tendons start to disintegrate. RA typically affects the same joints on both sides of the body, like fingers or hips, and the pain is usually much worse first thing in the morning.

How Is Rheumatoid Arthritis Treated?

Non-drug treatments

Gentle exercises like swimming or stretching may keep joints more pliable and prevent long-term tissue damage. Exercise releases chemicals from the brain, called endorphins, that increase the body's threshold of pain. The pain may still be there; you just don't feel it as severely.

Vitamin E levels in those with RA are typically lower than normal. Adding 400–600 IU of vitamin E daily may be beneficial as a protective antioxidant. Vitamin E can interfere with blood clotting, so only use vitamin E with **Coumadin** or *aspirin* with a doctor's supervision.

Low levels of certain fatty acids in the diet have been linked with RA in several studies. Adding a daily dose of 3 grams of the Omega-3 fish oils *EPA* and *DHA* has shown promise in decreasing the pain and inflammation of RA in as little as three weeks (but it may take twelve weeks for the full effect to be seen). *Evening primrose oil* (EPO) in combination with fish oils has also been shown to have an anti-inflammatory effect, providing some relief for RA. In fact, morning stiffness was greatly decreased by a dose of 6 grams of EPO given daily.

OTC treatments

The over-the-counter drugs of choice to treat RA are **non-steroidal anti-inflammatory drugs** (**NSAIDs**) like *aspirin, ibuprofen, ketoprofen,* and *naproxen,* which are effective in relieving pain and inflammation. The topical pain-relieving cream **Zostrix** (*capsaicin 0.025 percent*) and **Zostrix-HP** (*capsaicin 0.075 percent*) are powerful products for arthritis pain-relief. Please be aware that these may cause a burning sensation or sting the skin quite a bit when first applied, especially the high potency (HP) product. It is derived from the cayenne pepper plant, so use gloves or wash your hands thoroughly with vinegar or soap and water before the hands find their way into the eyes or other sensitive areas. Capsaicin works by decreasing Substance P, the transmitter that tells the brain when to feel pain from the joints. Less Substance P equals less pain. Use 3–4 times daily for the best spectrum of relief. Unfortunately, the OTC products often do not provide enough pain relief for the sufferers of RA.

The Drug Lady Recommends . . .

Talk to your doctor first. Because rheumatoid arthritis can be relieved or sent into remission with prompt and proper medicines, it should be treated with stronger prescription products as a first resort. If you are looking for a less expensive short-term alternative on the OTC shelves, you might look for one of the non-steroidal analgesics or their generic equivalents, like *Aleve* (*naproxen sodium*) or *Orudis KT* (*ketoprofen*).

Prescription treatments

For short-term pain relief, your doctor may want to try a prescription corticosteroid to reduce inflammation. There are also other groups of medications that appear to alter the course of the disease. Included are *gold compounds, methotrexate,* or *hydroxychloroquine.* For appropriate patients who aren't responding to other medicines, some doctors are using the new recombinant DNA drug **Enbrel** (*etanercept*) with quite a bit of success. There are many side effects to all of these drugs, so they should only be used short-term and under very close medical supervision.

New, stronger prescription **non-steroidal anti-inflammatories** called COX-2 inhibitors are also showing some promise for RA pain relief. Look for names like **Celebrex** (*celecoxib*) or **Vioxx** (*rofecoxib*). These appear to have fewer stomach-related side effects than their other NSAID counterparts; however, it is a good idea to use caution when first giving them a try—especially if you've had problems with other NSAIDs. Nausea, burning throat, heartburn, and ulcers may still occur.

Strokes and TIAs

Q. *My husband had a small stroke that the doctor called a "transient ischemic attack." What is this, and how does it differ from a "real" stroke? Can strokes be prevented?*

A. This question really hit home with me, because I received a phone call a few years back from the hospital where my mother had suffered a similar attack. She was unable to stand up or communicate, and the entire side of her face was paralyzed. Fortunately, by the time I arrived at the hospital, she was just fine. All motor control had returned and she was sitting up chatting with the nurses! She had suffered a TIA or transient ischemic attack. The doctor in charge referred to it as a "small stroke" with no apparent lasting damage.

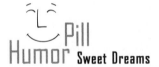

Pill Humor — Sweet Dreams

An elderly woman went into the doctor's office. When the doctor asked why she was there, she replied, "I'd like to have some birth-control pills."

Taken aback, the doctor thought for a minute and then said, "Excuse me, Mrs. Smith, but you're seventy-five years old. What possible use could you have for birth-control pills?"

"They help me sleep better," the woman responded.

The doctor thought some more and continued: "But birth-control pills contain no medicine for sleep. How would they help?"

The woman said, "I put them in my granddaughter's orange juice and I sleep much better at night."

What Causes a Stroke or a TIA?

A stroke results from a temporary lack of blood supply to the brain, usually caused by a small blood clot blocking an artery. It is a terrifying experience for all concerned. The patient has most cognitive, or "thought," faculties, but no motor control. She knows she wants to tell you something, but the words will not form. She loses her balance for no apparent reason and is unable to get back up. Often these symptoms are accompanied by a sudden and very severe headache, with the head pain occurring near the clot that blocks blood flow.

Strokes are a leading cause of death in older individuals, but are an even greater cause of permanent disability. If you notice any unusual weakness, lose feeling on one side of the body, have difficulty forming words, feel dizzy, or experience an excruciating headache that comes on without warning, call 911—fast.

A transient ischemic attack (or TIA) is characterized by the same symptoms as a stroke, but it only lasts a few minutes to a few hours, then just as quickly disappears. Being the incredible machine that it is, the human body uses a TIA as a frantic warning sign that a major stroke may occur. Some people have several TIAs over an extended period of time before a major stroke and, thankfully, others never have a stroke at all—a lot of it depends on the individual. What you may not know is that many strokes are preventable! A TIA is a wakeup call that things in the body are not working quite right.

Since strokes occur due to a sudden disruption of blood flow in the brain, the conditions that could cause a blockage or burst artery need to be carefully evaluated. High-risk factors include high blood pressure, **athero-sclerosis** (clogged arteries), heart disease, diabetes, smoking, and being overweight. It's easy enough to greatly reduce your chance of a stroke.

- ▦ Take your blood pressure medication regularly, even if you feel fine.

- ▦ Stop smoking.

- ▦ Manage your diabetic condition carefully, since the body's blood vessels may already be weakened.

- ▦ Eat a healthy, low-fat diet and watch your cholesterol level.

- ▦ This one is especially important: Exercise. Regular exercise has been proven to strengthen the heart and improve circulation. The arteries of people who exercise regularly, regardless of age, have been shown to be less stiff and hard than their counterparts. Stiff arteries can mean trouble, either as arteriosclerosis (hardening of the arteries) or a thickening of the heart muscle, which can increase the risk of heart attack.

How Are Strokes and TIAs Treated?

Non-drug treatments

If you could prevent a stroke, wouldn't you do it? Of course you would. So, resolve to make some changes for the better. If you're overweight, the heart has to work much harder to pump blood up into the brain, increasing the chance of a major stroke. Just dropping a few pounds at a time will greatly decrease the workload put on the heart muscle.

Types of Strokes

The largest percentages of strokes are of the **thrombolytic** variety. These occur when fatty deposits or plaques build up in the brain arteries and eventually form a clot or lump (a thrombus) that blocks all blood flow. An **embolic stroke** results when a clot breaks away from another part of the body and travels to the brain. A **hemorrhagic stroke** occurs when a blood vessel bursts in the brain, damaging the tissue.

Ditto for high cholesterol. Just bringing down high levels a little at a time can prevent the fatty plaques from breaking loose and blocking vessels in the brain.

For those who have suffered a stroke, there are many options available for rehabilitation. Physical therapy begins in the hospital and continues until the progress meets the needs of the patient. Often extensive therapy is needed for rehabilitation of speech, language, and occupational skills, but in many cases the results are amazing.

The Stroke Connection of the American Heart Association (1-888-4STROKE) provides a valuable resource for patients and families who have suffered a stroke. Their national publications allow extensive sharing of new information for medications and therapy. (See "Resources," page 355.)

OTC treatments

Today's physicians and pharmacists are also recommending an *aspirin* a day for preventative care. The 81 mg strength of *Half-prin* has been shown to give adequate anticoagulant control while reducing the stomach upset often found with aspirin.

The Drug Lady Recommends . . .

Use *aspirin* therapy only if your doctor approves and if you ARE NOT taking prescription anticoagulants like *Coumadin* (*warfarin*). Combining the two could cause decreased clotting problems for surgery, dental care, or everyday mishaps.

Prescription treatments

Strokes definitely must be taken seriously, whether you've suffered a TIA or just want to prevent one from occurring. When a large area of the brain is damaged, the brain cells are either injured or die. If injured, the cells can regenerate and the motor functions of speaking and walking will be regained. But if the cells are left without oxygen for a long period of time, they will die and the damage becomes irreversible.

The doctor who specializes in disorders of the brain is a **neurologist,** and he can run the tests needed to determine whether a stroke has occurred or is still in progress. The **electrocardiogram** (**EKG**) measures the electrical activity of the heart, since a stroke can be the direct result of a heart attack when the heart muscle can't pump enough blood to the brain. An **electroencephalogram** (**EEG**) measures nerve-cell activity in the brain, and a tomography scan can see what damage has occurred. An MRI (magnetic resonance image) shows the doctor pictures of the brain and whether or not the stroke is still going on. Prompt treatment can also decrease the long-term disability associated with strokes.

There are very powerful medicines to break down the clots that cause both **thrombolytic** and **embolic strokes;** these are thrombus or clot-dissolving agents, like *streptokinase.* They have to be injected quickly and must go directly into the vein that supplies the clot, where they dissolve

The Drug Lady Recommends . . .

Since high blood pressure is a major risk factor in **hemorrhagic strokes,** taking the proper medication to bring it down is very important. The hemorrhagic type is one of the most severe forms of stroke, when a blood vessel bursts in the brain. The tissue is damaged from both the pressure of built-up blood (hematoma) and the inadequate blood flow to other areas of the brain. High blood pressure accounts for the largest percentage of this type of stroke. Take your medication as prescribed! Very often you'll feel fine, but there may be a time bomb ticking inside you. Check your pressure regularly and if it's high, sit down with your doctor, pharmacist, or nurse to develop a good plan to manage it.

it and open up blood flow before too much irreversible damage has occurred.

For those who have suffered a TIA or who may be at high risk for stroke, the doctor can prescribe an anticoagulant like **Coumadin** (*warfarin sodium*) to stop the clots from getting larger or forming in the first place.

ELEVEN

Skin Conditions: "It's Red, It Itches, and It Burns!"

Acne Rosacea ▨ Acne Vulgaris ▨ Burns ▨ Contact Dermatitis ▨ Eczema ▨

Poison Ivy, Oak, and Sumac ▨ Psoriasis ▨ Scabies (see Chapter 5) ▨ Scars ▨

Stretch Marks (see Chapter 13) ▨ Sunburn ▨ Wrinkles (see Chapter 13)

THE SKIN IS our largest organ. Conditions that affect it—from itches to burns to little bugs that like to call it home—make life tough sometimes. Skin conditions can vary from mild annoyances to life-threatening emergencies (wrinkle removal is NOT a reason to call 911!). Some of these skin conditions can be treated at home, while others require a visit to the doctor or hospital. Keeping medicines on hand for quick treatment, and knowing when to call the doctor, are equally important.

Acne Rosacea

Q. *My wife is almost forty years old and has been diagnosed with acne rosacea. Shouldn't her acne be finished by now?*

A. Just when you think it's safe to put away the Stridex Medicated Pads! What your wife is experiencing is commonly called "adult acne." We usually associate acne with raging hormones and pimples before the prom, but it is actually much more complex. "Rosacea" refers to "redness" and this is what makes this type of acne so distinctive. It has no cure, but can often be treated to the point that it's hardly noticeable.

Tell your wife she's in good company. Over four million adults will develop acne long after their prom dress or tuxedo no longer fit.

What Is Acne Rosacea?

Acne rosacea is a condition characterized by redness of the nose, facial flushing, and tiny spider veins in the face. Rosacea is not related to the pimply type of acne (see "Acne Vulgaris," page 269), but it may occur in people who have acne.

At first you'll experience frequent blushing. You'll often notice either bumps or pustules on the cheeks and nose, but no blackheads. Over time the reddened nose may begin to take on a bulblike appearance. The skin can also start to have an orange-peel–like texture.

Because acne rosacea responds so well to antibiotics, the theory is that it is caused by a bacterium, but we don't actually know what causes it. It is important to have any condition that you suspect is rosacea looked at by a physician. A doctor will commonly make the diagnosis based on the appearance of the redness and spider veins.

How Is Acne Rosacea Treated?

Non-drug treatments
Because the redness and facial flushing can trigger an attack of breakouts, minimizing the chances for flushing can decrease outbreaks. Hot

The Drug Lady Recommends . . .

Always wear a sunscreen or a hat to shade your face if you have to be out in the sun. Sunlight (and sunburn) may worsen the appearance of acne rosacea.

drinks, alcohol, spicy food, and hot or cold temperatures can stimulate the skin to turn red.

OTC treatments

Because so little is known about the cause and progression of this skin condition, it is not recommended that you try to treat it with over-the-counter medicines. Sunscreens are a good idea once the condition has been diagnosed.

Prescription treatments

The most common treatment for acne rosacea is an oral antibiotic regimen of *erythromycin* or *minocycline.*

The topical (to put on the skin) antibiotic *metronidazole* is also very effective for controlling this type of acne. Metronidazole (found as the brand names **MetroLotion, MetroGel,** and **MetroCream**) is now available as a lotion, gel, or cream. The lotion is designed for patients with normal-to-dry skin; the gel is great for those with normal-to-oily skin; and a cream works best for those with dry skin.

For more severe cases of rosacea, **Accutane** (*tretinoin*) may be prescribed to speed up the sloughing-off of skin cells.

Acne Vulgaris

Q. *Help! We have two preteenagers and one is already starting to have acne breakouts. What can we do to minimize the trauma that acne brings? Are there certain foods they should avoid? Are certain products better than others for treatment?*

A. Oh, no! A houseful of teenagers with acne? Your life will never be the same. As if puberty weren't enough—now you've got to deal with acne. Before you roll your eyes when your teenagers complain that their life is over due to the appearance of a pimple, remember how traumatic acne was for you when you were a teen.

There are things you can do to help keep harmony. Teach your children the facts, not fallacies, about acne. Let them know that nearly 85 percent of people will develop acne in some form by the time they are twenty-five years old. It's not caused by what they eat and drink and it can often be treated effectively. Acne is a fact of life—not a pleasant one, but something that nearly all of us go through.

What Is Acne Vulgaris?

"Acne vulgaris" is the scientific term for the condition we affectionately know as "zits." Very simply, it is an inflammation of the skin. In puberty the body goes overtime producing oil and stimulating hair follicles. If this excess oil plugs up the pores, you get whiteheads (total blockage) and blackheads (partial blockage). To make matters even worse, a strain of bacteria called *Propionibacterium acnes* thrives on this oil. If this blockage of oils and bacteria irritate the surrounding tissue, that's when you will see redness and inflammation. In severe forms, cysts or nodules can develop in the oil-plugged pores.

Unfortunately, the ducts that become plugged are located mainly on the face and on the upper chest and back—right where everyone can see! And acne usually occurs just at the time when everything is a sensitive issue to an adolescent.

Girls may begin to see signs of breakouts around the age of eleven, while for boys the average age that acne starts is thirteen. Acne is seen more often in teenage boys, possibly due to the higher levels of hormones (androgens like testosterone) present at that time. The 40 to 50 percent of adult women who experience low-grade persistent acne have higher-than-normal levels of this same androgen.

How Is Acne Vulgaris Treated?

Non-drug treatments

While the following tips won't always prevent acne, good treatment can begin anytime. Washing your face daily with ordinary bath soap (like **Ivory**) and water is effective for control of mild production of oil. Also, keeping your hair off your face can be one way of keeping the skin free of extra oils from your hair or hair-styling products.

Moderate doses of natural sunshine have cleared up many breakouts. Eating fruits and vegetables to nourish the body—and not indulging in the fats and oils found in chips and fries—can also help clear the skin.

OTC treatments

There are literally hundreds of acne products on the market today, but just a few active ingredients for you to keep track of. The most common OTC acne ingredient is *benzoyl peroxide.* You'll find this in strengths as high as 10 percent. Benzoyl peroxide works by irritating the skin to such a point that the pores are not able to close. This irritation causes a higher turnover of cells and sloughs out extra oil. The downside to this ingredient is that it can cause temporary stinging, burning, drying, and redness. Because its effectiveness depends on a complete turnover of skin, it may take four to six weeks before the full effects are seen.

Salicylic acid is another effective ingredient for acne treatment. Yes, it really is a mild acid, and it works by penetrating skin oils and opening up blocked pores. It has a keratolytic action, which means that it takes off the

The Drug Lady Recommends . . .

A product that I like very much is the *Neutrogena Oil-Absorbing Acne Mask.* It has a clay base in addition to *benzoyl peroxide* as the active ingredient. Applied once a day, the clay soaks up the oils and dirt that may find a home in your pores, while the benzoyl peroxide works to turn over new skin cells.

entire top layer of skin. You can also expect redness, stinging, and burning with salicylic acid.

If you are using both of these products for your acne treatment, it is important that you wait twelve hours between applying one on top of the other. Using an anti-bacterial wash in addition to benzoyl peroxide and salicylic acid may keep the bacteria normally found on the skin from getting trapped in plugged pores and causing an infection.

Prescription treatments

The treatment of your acne depends on how severe it is. For mild cases, the doctor may use an extraction tool to physically open up the plugged pores. As the acne gets worse, there are more choices. Antibiotics, like **Cleocin-T** (*clindamycin*) or **T-Stat** (*erythromycin*), are available in gel, solution, or pad forms; these are used on the skin rather than taken internally. **Benzamycin Gel** (*benzoyl peroxide 5%/erythromycin 3%*), used as a topical (applied directly on the skin) antibiotic, is also available by prescription.

The oral (taken by mouth) antibiotics *tetracycline, minocycline,* and *doxycycline* are good choices to kill the *Propionibacterium acnes* bug responsible for the redness and inflammation of your skin. Side effects of these antibiotics are stomach upset and a drastically increased sensitivity to the effects of sunlight (**photosensitivity**). Tetracycline should be taken on an empty stomach, and not within two hours of ingesting any dairy, iron, or antacid products (these substances have a tendency to bind with the drug, lowering or eliminating its effectiveness).

Minocycline and doxycycline may be taken with food to reduce stomach upset. *Erythromycin,* also to be taken with food, is another effective antibiotic given by mouth. There are no sun-exposure cautions with erythromycin, but the bacteria are more resistant to it than to the others listed. If the acne still shows resistance to all of these, the combination products **Bactrim** or **Septra DS** (*trimethoprim* and *sulfamethoxazole*) may be used. Again, beware of stomach upset or sensitivity to sunlight. Keep in mind that these medications may take four to six weeks before they start to be effective.

A few more that your doctor may choose from to treat more severe forms of acne are in the retinoid family, including **Retin-A** (*tretinoin*),

Retin-A Micro (with a microsponge delivery system), **Differin** (*adapalene*), and the new **Zorac** (*tazarotene*). The retinoids loosen up and push out the stuff inside your pores and help to prevent more pimples from coming back. But here come the disclaimers: Topical retinoids can cause some serious problems if not used correctly. At first the skin may look worse instead of better, possibly for up to eight weeks! It will, however, eventually look normal again. The medicine should be applied at bedtime and you should avoid any type of sunlight while you're using it; the skin will become ultrasensitive and direct sunlight (real or artificial) can cause serious burns. Use protective clothing as well as high-numbered sunscreens (over SPF 30). You may also notice greater susceptibility to windburn and cold. Begin treatment with the lowest-strength cream or gel, using cream for dry skin types and gel if your skin type is oily.

Accutane (*isotretinoin*) is a retinoid that you can take in capsule form. Accutane has one of the longest lists of side effects and cautions that you will find. This drug is very tightly regulated by the FDA, and with good reason: The incidence of miscarriages and birth defects in children born to women taking Accutane is notable. Doctors should only prescribe it to women who have passed a negative pregnancy test, do not intend to become pregnant while taking it, and sign a consent form that they have been fully informed of the side effects involved. This is serious stuff! Also, 90 percent of men and women taking Accutane will experience inflammation of the lips and, less frequently, the eyes. A drying of the skin around the nose and mouth is observed in 80 percent of cases. This medication is also the most expensive of all acne medications—sometimes costing well over several dollars for each capsule!

If your skin doesn't react well to the retinoids, **Azelex** (*azelaic acid*) may be an option. It generally takes longer to work than retinoids, but may cause less skin sensitivity. It can be used under makeup and with moisturizers. Azelex is both bacteriostatic (slows bacterial growth) and bactericidal (kills the bacteria) and is indicated for mild-to-moderate acne. Applied twice daily, this cream has proven as effective as Retin-A and benzoyl peroxide.

Burns

Q. *My mother used to keep an aloe plant by the kitchen sink for family burns. She would just pinch a piece off and apply it directly to the burn. It seemed to work well, but is this safe? Is it the best treatment for burns?*

A. I remember the aloe plant in the kitchen, too—that wonderfully cool, green, gooey, sticky stuff from inside of it seemed to make the pain of a burn go away instantly. It almost made getting burned not so bad! *Almost.*

I understand your concern for your family. Burns can happen quickly and bring with them a great deal of pain and discomfort. Fast relief is imperative. There are many different ways to cool a burn, but before you treat it yourself, be certain that it is only a minor burn. Cooling is important, but if there is tissue damage, a doctor's care is needed to prevent infection and other complications.

What Causes Burns?

Burns can be caused by moist heat (like steam or hot water), chemicals, electricity, or dry heat (like sunburn or directly from a flame). When a burn damages tissues, the extent of the damage determines the degree of the burn. First-degree burns (like mild sunburn) involve only the top layer of skin (epidermis); redness and pain, but no blisters, characterize this type of burn. Second-degree burns go deeper into the tissue and are accompanied by blisters; the pain may be severe. Third-degree burns go through all layers of the skin and destroy nerves, too—there is no pain because the burn consumes the nerves. The skin may look charred or it may appear bright cherry red.

Fortunately, 85 percent of most burns are of the minor, or first-degree, variety. This doesn't mean they don't hurt—only that there is less risk for infection and scarring. The doctor should treat any burns that involve the face, the palms of the hands, or the soles of the feet. Also, medical supervision is required for anyone suffering from a burn who is under the age of two and over the age of seventy.

How Are Burns Treated?

Non-drug treatments

The *aloe* plant (and the even handier jar of aloe gel) seems to be making a comeback in kitchens and homes all over the United States. Aloe isn't something new—in fact, it's been used historically, since the fourth century B.C., when Greek doctors used it for both fighting disease and fighting evil.

The *aloe vera* species is what you commonly see today, a squatty little shrub with about twenty-five fleshy, fluid-filled leaves. The gel can be applied directly to the skin. Aloe has been used internally as an aid for digestion and as a laxative. That's a pretty versatile plant!

Aloe gel, the jellylike material found within the leaves of the plant, is thought to work in two ways: First, the compounds in the gel limit the effects of *bradykinin,* a pain-producing agent in our bodies. Second, it stimulates skin-cell growth, immune response, and regeneration of some types of nerve cells. This is pretty amazing, especially considering that we don't yet know exactly how the compounds in aloe work their wonders.

If you are looking for a commercial aloe product, look for "pure gel" rather than "aloe extracts," which may be very diluted and not as helpful when they are needed. Pure products do tend to break down fairly quickly, however; it may be necessary to replace these periodically to ensure that you have the highest potency possible.

If you want fresh aloe, keep a little plant or two around the house. They are inexpensive and you're always assured of the very freshest and most natural aloe gel. As for safety, unless you have a rare aloe vera allergy, you

What NOT to Do

Even though Grandma might have done it, putting butter, grease, or oil on a burn is NOT a good idea. This is a good way to seal in bacteria and cause an infection. In addition, these oils on the skin will hold in heat and make the burn feel warmer.

and your family will be just fine. Aloe applied to the skin has no other side effects. It's good stuff to have around!

Taking extra vitamins and minerals after a burn is also very important. *Vitamin A, beta-carotene,* and *zinc* aid in healing skin. *Vitamin C* also helps give the body extra immune support while healing.

A quick "icing" brings fast relief for minor burns. Grab an ice cube and put it in a plastic sandwich bag, so that when it melts it won't get all over everything (it also makes it easier to hold on to the slippery cube). Hold it directly on the minor burn for several minutes or until the heat subsides.

OTC treatments

Anti-inflammatory pain relievers like *ibuprofen, aspirin,* or *naproxen sodium* can help ease the pain while the burn heals.

Cooling sprays, like **Americaine,** contain the numbing agent *benzo-caine.* These are wonderful for those burns when there is no way you can bear to actually touch them.

The Drug Lady Recommends . . .

A product that I like very much for minor burns (especially sunburns) is *aloe vera* with *lidocaine.* The aloe vera does its job well, and there is the added bonus of lidocaine to act as numbing agent. You get cooling and numbing relief at the same time! Be sure to wash your hands thoroughly after you apply this; I had an incident with a bag of potato chips that resulted in numb lips for several hours. (Don't ask!)

Prescription treatments

More serious burns can be treated with the cream **Silvadene 1%** (*silver sulfadiazine*). Just a small layer (one-sixteenth of an inch) of this cream protects the skin against bacteria and some forms of yeast. However, this cream shouldn't be used if you have had a previous sulfa allergy. Your doctor or pharmacist can advise how often and what type of dressing to use over the burned area. Some prescription dressings are available that are already treated with silver sulfadiazine.

Pill Humor

Three pharmacists died and went to Heaven, where Saint Peter met them at the Pearly Gates. To the first, he asked, "So, what did you do back on Earth? Why do you think you should be allowed to come into Heaven?"

"I was a pharmacist at a children's hospital," she replied. "I worked to bring medicine and smiles to many sufferers, especially poor, helpless children."

"Very noble," said Saint Peter. "You may enter." And in through the Gates she went.

To the next, he asked the same question: "So, what did you do?"

"I was a pharmacist at a missionary hospital in the Amazon basin," he replied. "For many years before, I worked in research to develop a cure for many of the world's illnesses."

"How touching," said Saint Peter. "You, too, may enter." And in he went.

Peter then came to the last pharmacist, whom he asked, "And, what did you do back on Earth?"

After some hesitation, she explained, "I was a pharmacist with a well-known HMO. You know, a health-maintenance organization."

Saint Peter pondered this for a moment, and then said, "Okay, you may enter, too."

"Whew!" said the pharmacist. "For a moment there, I thought you weren't going to let me in."

"Oh, you can come in," said Saint Peter, "but you can only stay for three days, and your wings and harp aren't covered by your plan!"

Contact Dermatitis

Q. *I tried a new laundry soap and now three members of my family (and myself!) have a horrible rash. I looked up our symptoms on the Internet and it looks like we might have a contact rash. How can I be sure? Should we see the doctor or will this go away on its own?*

A. Well, one thing is for sure. You'll certainly be able to tell if it's a contact rash (dermatitis) if you remove what you think is causing the problem and see if the rash goes away. The key to this type of rash is contact. When the irritating substance touches the body, the skin revolts by breaking out into a red, itchy mess. Typically these rashes will go away on their own, but you may be surprised at just how many ways laundry that has come into contact with the detergent will keep showing up!

What Is Contact Dermatitis?

A contact **dermatitis** is a rash that occurs when your skin comes into contact with something it sees as very unfriendly—this can be a laundry detergent, aftershave lotion, moisturizing cream, jewelry, and even the dyes used to color clothes.

Contact dermatitis is usually very easy to identify because once the substance touches the skin, redness, swelling, small blisters, and itching begin. Once the substance that causes the rash is removed, the rash generally goes away in a few days. Still, that's a long time to be in itchy misery.

The hardest thing about contact dermatitis is that sometimes it can be very difficult to determine exactly what is causing the rash, especially if you've been exposed to the substance before without a reaction. The location of the rash may give good clues as to where it is originating—for example, if you try a new laundry detergent and the next day all areas that touch clothes are red and itchy; or if you try that nifty new cold cream before bed and the next morning you're beet-red. If it isn't possible to determine the cause of the rash quickly, your doctor may do a patch test. This is where small patches containing irritants that commonly cause a rash (like detergent or lotion) are placed directly on the skin to see what happens. If a rash develops under the patch, you've identified the irritant.

How Is Contact Dermatitis Treated?

Non-drug treatments

If you notice the beginning of what could be a contact dermatitis, it is a good idea to wash the area thoroughly with a mild soap and water. However, this can be dangerous if you're not sure whether the soap is to blame for the rash. Use only a soap that you're very familiar with, or avoid soap entirely and just use plain water.

Cool, moist cloths are great for easing the itch. A half-cup of cornstarch in tepid bathwater can bring a smile and great big "Ahhhh" to a contact-dermatitis sufferer.

OTC treatments

Once the offending irritant is removed, the task is to stop the itch and to prevent skin infections. Over-the-counter *hydrocortisone* creams and ointments should be first in line when the itching starts.

Antihistamines like **Benadryl** (*diphenhydramine*) may be taken by mouth when sleep becomes a necessity. This medicine is also available in a cream form for putting directly on the itchy rash. If the itching results in broken skin, a topical antibiotic like **Neosporin** can help ensure that bacteria do not find a happy home. The drying action of *calamine* lotion is a good choice if the blisters start to ooze a bit.

The Drug Lady Recommends . . .

Not only do you not have to touch the itchy, blistered skin, but the product *Rhuli Calamine Aerosol Spray* also acts as a numbing, an anti-itch, and a drying agent for weepy rashes. It contains *calamine, camphor,* and *benzocaine.* I love these combination products!

Prescription treatments

If the rash becomes unbearable or if you feel there may be something more going on than just a contact dermatitis, pack yourself and the family up for a trip to the doctor. Prescription steroid medicines like *prednisone* or *methylprednisolone* (**Medrol**) may be given for a very short course to stop the inflammation.

Eczema

Q. *My daughter and I both have eczema and the itching is driving us crazy. What can we do to make it go away?*

A. Not the dreaded *e*-word!! If you're looking for a cure here, please go look somewhere else. Since we don't actually know what causes eczema, we don't have a clue as to what will cure it; all we can do is to make the symptoms easier to live with. Fortunately, there are excellent medications that do offer some relief.

What Is Eczema?

Eczema is also called **atopic dermatitis.** The skin around the face, knees, elbows, and wrists is most commonly affected, with itchy, dry, thick, and scaly patches. Eczema is very often a gift you give your children—in fact, over 70 percent of cases run in families. You'll also see more cases of eczema in people who already have allergies or asthma. It's as if the body sees the entire outside world as one giant **allergen.**

Babies are especially sensitive to eczema, but normally grow out of it by the age of three. For adults, it's a sadder story. Stressful conditions (everyday life?), temperature extremes, and allergies are often to blame for the intense itching, which can be maddening. Eczema also can be very unsightly, with the scaly areas turning a different color from the normal skin tone; as if it wasn't annoying enough, now it has to be visible, too.

Other concerns to be aware of are the infections that can occur from scratching. Because your body is already busy fighting other invisible foes, these infections can become quite severe.

How Is Eczema Treated?

Non-drug treatments

We must first be aware that treating a condition when we don't know the cause is very difficult. Sometimes it is impossible. The key to treating eczema is to make the symptoms more bearable. The first step in controlling the itch from eczema is to eliminate what is causing the body to fight so desperately.

Relaxation techniques, breathing exercises, and stress-reduction techniques are a good first choice. When the body doesn't see itself as being threatened, it begins to relax. This relaxation can often bring about a much faster remission of the condition.

To reduce the number of things the body is fighting may also include avoiding certain allergy-provoking foods like milk, eggs, and wheat. Many people find that if they cut back on red meat, their eczema retreats; it is thought the fatty acids in meat are seen by the body as an allergen that must be attacked.

The herbal product *evening primrose oil* has shown quite a bit of promise as an effective eczema reliever. Adult dosages of 500 mg taken two or three times daily have shown improvement after three to four months of use.

OTC treatments

There are mild corticosteroid creams available over-the-counter (like *hydrocortisone*) that are great for mild eczema attacks. This will control the itching for a short time.

Using plain **Vaseline** petroleum jelly can serve to keep the skin moist and decrease scaling. Also, it's wise to keep baths to a minimum too; certain soaps and even warm water can dry the skin out, making eczema even worse.

Coal tar products like **Balnetar** or **Neutrogena T-Derm** actually form a seal over the skin. Coal tar also has the properties of being an antiseptic (kills germs) and anti-pruritic (stops the itch). Unfortunately, coal tar can be messy and may cause the skin to be supersensitive to the sun.

The Drug Lady Recommends . . .

Patients like the *coal-tar*-based product *Exorex* because it does not exhibit many of the traditional disadvantages of other coal tar products—like being smelly, sticky, and staining. It is absorbed into the skin quickly, and becomes colorless and virtually odorless. It is designed not to stain clothing when properly applied. Most important, Exorex is completely non-steroidal and does not have the potential side effects of other treatments used for these illnesses. It comes in a scalp-and-body formula for psoriasis and a regular or gentle formula for eczema.

Prescription treatments

Prescription products for eczema are almost exclusively steroid creams or those with steroidlike actions. These should be used very cautiously even though they work very well. It's tempting to ignore the doctor's warnings to use this for only a very short period of time (usually no more than two weeks), especially when this is the only thing you've found that will ease the itch.

New studies are showing the immuno-suppressant *tacrolimus* (in a cream form) to be effective for treating eczema. The way it seems to work is by decreasing the body's natural allergic tendencies. At this writing, it hasn't yet been approved by the FDA, but the studies look very good.

Keep It Short

Please *do* listen to your doctor and your pharmacist when they tell you that steroid medicines can do long-term damage to your body if used for longer than the prescribed time. Also, don't cover the area when using steroid creams, as your skin can become thinner and white spots may appear. Because steroids interfere with the body's immune response, long-term use can lead to acne, glaucoma, and obesity.

Poison Ivy, Oak, and Sumac

Q. *I was clearing the backyard and somehow came in contact with some very itchy bushes. Now I have a rash all over my arms and legs. How would I tell exactly what I have and is there any difference in treatments?*

A. Not the dreaded itchies! This is something every would-be gardener dreads. It's easy to remember the old adage "leaflets, three . . . let it be" AFTER you start itching. Here are a few tips on both recognizing the culprits and treating what's causing the itching.

How Do You Get Poison Ivy, Oak, and Sumac?

Blame **urushiol.** No, that's not someone's name. Urushiol is the potent oil found inside the leaves of plants from the poison ivy, oak, and sumac families. Coming into contact with this oil (it may be yellowish, but it's usually clear) is the fastest way known to start itching. If you are allergic to this substance, and over 85 percent of people are, just a very minute amount will be enough to trigger an allergic reaction.

A really sneaky thing about this oil is that it has a tendency to hang around—on your gardening gloves, shoes, clothes, and even in the air if you are burning the pesky plants!

Often you won't start itching right away, even if you've been exposed to

Recognizing the Plants

Sure, sure, leaflets three and all that, but what about the other plants?

■ Poison oak can appear as a low shrub or a vine and can have leaves of different shapes, sizes, and even colors depending on where it is growing.

■ Poison ivy typically has glossier leaves with a distinctive three-leaflet pattern.

■ Poison sumac grows in moist areas and resembles a small tree. Its branches can have seven to eight leaflets on each stem.

the oil directly. It can take from a few hours to up to one week for a full reaction to be seen. Typically the first exposure takes the longest time to develop. Second or third exposures can start itching within hours. This reaction can begin as a redness and swelling of the skin. Soon the intensely itchy rash sets in, followed closely by small, oozing blisters. Not very pleasant at all!

It usually takes fourteen to twenty days for the rash to run its course. That's a very long time to be itching, oozing, and miserable.

How Are Poison Oak, Ivy, and Sumac Treated?

Non-drug treatments

Before the itch: If you even suspect that you might have been exposed to poison ivy, oak, sumac or any other itchy plant, wash the area with water as soon as possible. Soap and water are better, but use plain water if there is no soap available. Wash long! Take as long as necessary, keeping in mind that you are washing off a very tenacious oil. *Isopropyl rubbing alcohol* is very effective for neutralizing the urushiol oil.

Wash everything (including shoes, gardening tools, gloves, and clothes) separately from everything else. It's a good idea to protect your hands while doing this. Gloves or even socks over your hands will do. Don't forget to toss the socks in to wash, too!

After the itch: A cool compress of baking soda and water can be soothing to the prickly, itchy rash. Taking a bath in a tub of lukewarm water can bring a big "*Ahhhh*" for poison plant rashes. And not too hot! Hot water may actually release more histamine. Also be careful not to do this before you've thoroughly washed off the oil or you may spread the oil even more widely. Toss a cup of oatmeal into the bath—this helps the skin feel less fiery and comforts the sufferer. Be careful getting out of the tub, as it can be *very* slippery.

OTC treatments

Calamine lotion is the old standby for drying up poison ivy blisters. A combination product called *Caladryl* combines calamine and the topical antihistamine *Benadryl* (*diphenhydramine*).

Other over-the-counter remedies for itch relief include mild steroid

The Drug Lady Recommends . . .

Don't they think of everything? There is a product called *Ivy Block* (*bentoquatam*) that will actually protect you from exposure to poison ivy. It is applied to the skin and forms a barrier. When the urushiol touches the Ivy Block, it can't penetrate the skin and cause a reaction. If you are severely allergic, you may still get some itching, but nothing like what would happen without the Ivy Block.

creams and ointments like *hydrocortisone*. The highest over-the-counter strength is 1 percent hydrocortisone, which you may see as the brands **Cortisone-10, Lanacort 10,** and **Cortaid Maximum Strength.**

For an allover body relief, you can try an **Aveeno** bath. The oatmeal bath soothes the skin and eases the itchies. When the itching becomes too intense for words, an antihistamine that you take internally (like diphenhydramine) can help.

For severe cases, you may also be saddled with flu-like symptoms of fever, aches, and pains in addition to the itches. The general body aches, fever, and pains from this battle your body is fighting can be treated with a pain reliever, like **Tylenol** (*acetaminophen*).

Prescription treatments

When the itching gets unbearable or it spreads to your eyes, face, mouth, or genital areas, it's time to call the doctor. Higher-strength prescription steroid creams (like *triamcinolone*) may be required to control the swelling, itching, and the spread of the rash. In severe cases, steroid pills or shots, like *prednisone* and **Medrol** (*methylprednisolone*), can bring quick relief from the inflammation and itch.

Psoriasis

Q. *My mother has very unsightly psoriasis on her arms. She's embarrassed for the grandchildren to see it and is worried that it is contagious. What can I do to help her?*

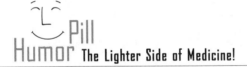

Pill Humor — The Lighter Side of Medicine!

The pediatrician walks into the nurse's lounge with a rectal thermometer tucked behind his ear. One of the RN's asks why he has a thermometer behind his ear. In a frantic motion, he grabs it and looking at it, exclaims, "Uh-oh! I bet I know where I put my pen!"

A. Poor Mom! Please ease her mind that psoriasis is *not* contagious, although she might have passed it on to her relatives through their genes. It does seem to be hereditary, just not contagious. It may look unattractive, but her best course is not to worry about it. I know—easier said than done, but worry (or emotional stress) is often a trigger for the condition. Psoriasis is another one of those baffling, but intense, skin conditions. Thankfully, there is little itching, just patches of skin she wants to hide. We don't know the cause and we don't have a cure. All medical science can do is try to make her less embarrassed with her own skin.

What Is Psoriasis?

Psoriasis appears as pink, raised patches of skin that usually starts as a small area that becomes progressively more flaky and itchy. It is most often seen on the head, elbows, knees, and back. The strange thing about psoriasis is that skin samples show the affected area has skin cells that are multiplying at ten times the normal rate! These cells push up through the skin layers and appear as whitish-pink areas of brand-new skin. A strep infection can be a psoriasis trigger. As can certain medicines, like *ibuprofen*. And an overwhelming 80 percent of people report a not-so-coincidental occurrence of a very emotionally stressful event before an outbreak.

How Is Psoriasis Treated?

Non-drug treatments

Again, the key is eliminating the cause of the problem to bring about a change. Keeping the skin moist is very important. Plain **Vaseline** can help seal in the much-needed moisture.

Diets high in protein and alcohol, but with low fiber, have been shown to have a direct correlation with psoriasis outbreaks. So ease up on the meat and alcohol, and eat more fiber!

Fish oil, in doses of 1.8 grams of *EPA* (*eicosapentaenoic acid*) daily, has been shown to improve psoriasis. It may take up to eight weeks to see results, but for some people the results have been amazing. Read your product labels carefully, as it may be difficult to find EPA in that high a dosage. Look for high-potency gelcaps, as many fish oil products have low concentrations of EPA, and this is the important component to look for.

Doses of pure sunshine have also been shown to have dramatic results, both for psoriasis and for smiles.

OTC treatments

Psoriasis is a condition that should be first diagnosed by your doctor. Most OTC remedies are only useful for mild cases and should be used only under a doctor's supervision.

Mild corticosteroid creams (like *hydrocortisone*) will often help keep the plaques at bay.

Shampoos containing *selsun, coal tar,* and even *salicylic acid* are effective treatments for scalp psoriasis, but the most important thing to re-

The Drug Lady Recommends...

The over-the-counter, coal-tar-based *Exorex* seems to be working very well for many psoriasis sufferers. Coal tar can be tricky, though. It binds to the skin and can cause your skin to burn much more easily than normal. This effect can last after the coal tar has been removed—even up to twenty-four hours later!

member is to keep it on for the recommended time. Contact time can determine whether or not the psoriasis responds.

Prescription treatments

Once your condition has been diagnosed, there are several options your doctor may choose from for treatments. Here are just a few of the many, many choices.

Light therapy, using ultraviolet-A light (UVA) in combination with the medications **Oxsoralen** (*methoxalen*) or **Trisoralen** (*trioxsalen*), can be a fast way to clear the plaques of psoriasis. These medicines are called psoralens and they make the skin supersensitive to the ultraviolet light. **Calcitriol** (a vitamin D derivative) is also effective in many cases.

Florone-E (*diflorasone*) and **Tridesilon** (*desonide*) are strong steroid creams that help control the inflammation of psoriasis. As with all steroids, read the package instructions very carefully!

Dovonex (*calcipotriene*) is a synthetic vitamin D3 cream that has been shown to be effective for psoriasis treatment. Try the sunshine first, it's a good source of vitamin D!

Scabies

(See Chapter 5, page 146.)

Scars

Q. *I have a scar on my leg that I've had for many years. It's very unsightly and I would do anything to get rid of it. What can I do?*

A. The skin is really an amazing thing! When it's injured it quickly repairs itself and a scar is often what's left after the healing. Some consider their scars a "badge" to be proudly displayed, but most of us would rather they weren't so visible. While scar treatments are a big business, there are definitely facts to be aware of before starting this often expensive and time-consuming process.

What Are Scars?

Normal skin is composed of many, many layers of cells. When the skin is injured from a burn, a cut, or surgery, these cell layers are disrupted and as a result the tougher, more fibrous tissue comes in to repair the damage. Scars can start out a vivid red color as the skin heals and then fade to a lighter tone over a period of time. Different skin pigments determine how obvious the scar appears. **Keloids** are scar formation in the skin following an injury or surgical incision. These are difficult to treat because the scar tissue formed is out of proportion to the amount needed to do the job. These raised, thickened scars are more common in African-Americans.

How Are Scars Treated?

Non-drug treatments

If your scar is in the early stages (within the first several days to a week), *vitamin E* or *cocoa butter* can help keep the skin soft and pliable and aid in a more uniform healing pattern. During these early stages, keeping the skin as moist as possible is most effective in preventing hard, fibrous tissue from forming. This is also something to keep in mind if you are worried about stretch marks. (See "Stretch Marks," Chapter 13, page 327.)

OTC treatments

I'd like to pass on just a word of warning regarding over-the-counter scar-removal products. When the skin has worked this hard to heal itself and protect the underlying tissue, it isn't going to be easy to get the skin back to its original smooth consistency. It can be done to some degree, but don't expect miracles.

OTC scar faders and levelers can be effective for lessening the appearance of scars. You can find these as creams, gels, and even sheets to be applied directly on the scar tissue. These are especially effective for new scars and those caused by stretch marks. Please remember that these products will not make scars disappear. However, some individuals have noticed dramatic results in scar softening, leveling off, and filling in, as well as the recovery of a more natural color tone.

The Drug Lady Recommends . . .

An OTC product called *Mederma* may help soften scars and make them less noticeable. This is a unique combination of onion extract and *allantoin* in a gel base that is applied directly to the skin. The onion extract acts as a natural fiber replacement and allantoin is an **astringent** (removes moisture) and keratolytic (it gradually takes off the top layer of skin). Mederma can help improve the appearance of both new and existing scars, but new scars generally respond much better than the older, tougher scars. For new scars, begin treatment as soon as the wound heals. Mederma should be used three to four times a day for eight weeks. For older scars, apply the product three to four times daily for up to six months.

The downside? These are often *very* expensive and can require treatment for several months or more before any beneficial effect is seen. Also, I haven't seen any data on long-term effects. We just don't know if the effects are long lasting or if the scar will come back once you stop treatment.

Prescription treatments

While no scar can be removed completely, plastic surgeons may be able to improve the appearance of very unsightly scars. For raised scars, **dermabrasion** may be an option. Dermabrasion is a way to smooth scar tissue by scraping or shaving off the top layers of the skin. This leaves a smoother surface to the skin, but it won't completely erase the scar.

There are new artificial skin replacements in development that might bring a very close resemblance to normal skin, even for severely scarred areas. Ask your dermatologist about these latest medical miracles.

Stretch Marks

(See Chapter 13, page 327.)

Pill Humor The Lighter Side of Medicine!

Good News—Bad News A man gets a telephone call from a doctor. The doctor says: "About this medical test I did for you. I have some good news and some bad news." The man asks for the good news first. "The good news is that you have twenty-four hours to live," says the doctor. Horrified, the man asks: "If that is the good news, then what is the bad news?"

"I couldn't reach you yesterday."

Sunburn

Q. *We've all come back from the beach with sunburns. Help! Obviously, I'm confused about sunscreens and SPFs. What about for children—which products do you recommend for them?*

A. Getting a sunburn is no fun! Especially when it's your first day of a very much-needed vacation. So unless you're planning on spending all of your Florida vacation sitting in the room and watching TV, it's a good idea to do a little planning in terms of the right sunscreen for the whole family.

Picking a good sunscreen is a little like picking apples: the perfect one depends on what you are looking for. What looks good for Mom and Dad may not be the best for the little guys. When picking a sunscreen, you should keep in mind that factors like the amount of time you are in the water, the amount of activity you are engaged in, and the time of day you go out in the sun all contribute to finding the "perfect" sunscreen. You may find that your sunscreen arsenal consists of several different types, but that's OK. It's better to be prepared than to be miserable while in the sun.

Choosing the Right Sunscreen

A sunscreen is a way to maximize the amount of time you can spend in the sun, while still protecting your skin from damage. The choice of which one ultimately depends on where you live (or visit), your skin tone, and how much time you plan to be in the sun. It's important to pick the right SPF (sun protection factor) for everyone in the family. The SPF is a very individual type of ranking. If you have very fair skin (or skin that hasn't seen the sun in a while) and normally start to burn in about fifteen minutes, an SPF of 2 would allow you to stay in the sun for twice as long or thirty minutes. If you have darker skin tone and don't start cooking until forty-five minutes, then the same SPF of 2 would give you an hour and a half in the sun.

The American Academy of Dermatology and the National Institutes of Health recommend that everyone start out with an SPF of 15, and possibly higher. The higher the SPF, the more protection from sun damage you can expect—or is there a limit? I have seen sunscreens on the market with SPFs as high as 50, but is that much protection really necessary? If you need to keep your skin from the sun completely, a total block like zinc oxide or a good hat and T-shirt are in order. The FDA has not yet found that SPFs over 30 are any more effective than those with an SPF of 30. The reasoning behind this is that even if you burned in fifteen minutes, there would not be enough sun time to warrant the seven plus hours of protection the 30 SPF gives. We all know that one application (even of a 30 SPF) doesn't stay on all day, so it must be reapplied to avoid getting burned.

What Causes a Sunburn?

While most of us know the dangers of sun exposure, it is very difficult to curb the urge to run out and soak up as much of the golden light as possible, especially on vacations. We want everyone to see that "little color." Unfortunately, when we stay out too long or when we choose the wrong strength of sunscreen, a sunburn can result.

The sun naturally produces ultraviolet light in both the A and B spectrums (UVA and UVB), but it's the UVB rays that cause most of the burns. Typically, the redness and pain will appear in one to twenty hours after the exposure. In more serious cases, fever, nausea, prickly sensations, and chills often come with a sunburn. Small blisters and a lizardlike peeling of the skin as the burn begins to heal are also common.

The very best treatment of a sunburn is preventing it from happening in the first place.

How Are Sunburns Treated?

Non-drug treatments

Cool baths and cool compresses are wonderfully soothing for sun-reddened skin. Taking extra vitamins and minerals after a burn is very important. *Vitamin A, beta-carotene,* and *zinc* aid in skin healing. *Vitamin C* also helps to give the body extra immune support while healing.

The *aloe* plant (and the even handier jar of aloe) is as good for sunburn as for other burns (see "Burns" earlier in this chapter). Aloe gel, the jellylike material found within the leaves of the plant, is thought to work in two ways. First, the compounds in the gel limit the effects of bradykinin, a pain-producing agent in our bodies. Second, it stimulates skin cell growth, immune response, and regeneration of some type of nerve cells.

If you are looking for a commercial aloe product, look for "pure gel" rather than "aloe extracts" that may be very diluted and not as helpful when they are needed. Pure products do tend to break down fairly quickly, however. It may be necessary to replace these periodically to ensure that you have the highest potency possible.

If you want fresh aloe, keep a little plant or two around the house. They are inexpensive and you're always assured of the very freshest and most natural aloe gel. As for safety, unless you have a rare "aloe vera allergy," you

Mixing Sunscreens and Water

Waterproof, water-resistant, and sweatproof are terms that are commonly attached to sunscreens. Waterproof simply means that it won't wash off as readily when you or the kids are in the water. Water-resistant formulas don't repel water, but give a small amount of protection before washing off. The directions still recommend reapplying every fifteen minutes while you're actively in the water. Remember—just because it says waterproof doesn't mean you can swim indefinitely without putting more on! Waterproof technically should stay effective for up to eighty minutes in the water. A water-resistant product should maintain its SPF for up to forty minutes in the water.

Sweatproof sunscreens typically are a little more binding to the skin. People who play sports in the sun use these because even after a grueling game of beach volleyball, the sunscreen is (for the most part) still there. Sweatproof sunscreens have a greater tendency to clog the pores and prevent you from sweating. Be aware of this and be sure to keep your body as cool as possible when using a sweatproof sunscreen. Even this type of sunscreen requires that you reapply it at least hourly for maximum protection. To avoid skin irritation, try the sunscreen on a small area of the skin first, especially if you have had skin allergies in the past.

and your family will be just fine. Aloe applied to the skin has no other side effects. It's good stuff to have around!

OTC treatments

Help for sunburn pain is probably already in your medicine chest. Anti-inflammatory pain relievers, like *ibuprofen, aspirin,* or *naproxen sodium,* work well to ease the pain. **Tylenol** (*acetaminophen*), while not an anti-inflammatory, is effective for simple pain relief.

Cooling sprays, like **Americaine,** contain the numbing agent *benzocaine.* These are wonderful for those burns when there is no way you could bear to touch them.

The Drug Lady Recommends . . .

A product that I like very much for minor burns (especially sunburns) is *aloe vera* with *lidocaine*. The aloe vera does its job well, and there is the added bonus of lidocaine to act as numbing agent. You get a coolness and numbness at the same time. Two very important things when your skin feels as though it's on fire. I put the entire bottle in the refrigerator for a few minutes before applying to sunburned skin.

Prescription treatments

A doctor should treat some sunburns. If it lasts over a week and has spreading redness (a possible sign of infection) or large blisters, call the doctor. If the pain becomes too intense, the doctor may prescribe a pain-reliever like **Vicodin** (*hydrocodone/acetaminophen*). Intense swelling can be brought down quickly with steroids, like *prednisone*.

Wrinkles

(See Chapter 13, page 339.)

Teenage Good Health: "Dude, Like, What Do I Do About This?"

Acne ▩ Body Odor ▩ Eating Disorders ▩

Sweating (see Chapter 5) ▩ Underweight

THE TEENAGE YEARS—yes, those wonderful, wacky times when the body does such strange things! As we grow up, some of these bodily changes can be a nuisance, embarrassing, just plain confusing—and exciting. With them comes a new degree of responsibility for our health and well-being. As with so many of the health issues this book discusses, it's important to remember that you're not alone. As hard as it may be to believe, everyone older than you has been through it and survived. You will too—especially now that you have some of the answers to those burning questions about what's really going on with your body.

Acne

Q. *One hundred forty-three dollars for my prescription acne medicine? Are you kidding?! What is the difference between this and those products on the shelf over there?*

A. For any teenager who has ever suffered with acne, $143 seems a mere pittance to pay for social acceptance, but the teen (or the parent) who has to hand over the money has good reason to question the difference in acne products. Since over 80 percent of all teenagers develop acne between the ages of eleven and eighteen, the cost of treatment can be a big shock to an unsuspecting budget.

A great deal of the difference in the costs of treating acne lies in the severity of the acne problem. And the severity is not something you can control; most experts agree that heredity plays the largest part in whether or not a teenager will experience a bad case of acne. In effect, if your parents had acne, you will probably have it too. That's not too encouraging except to remember that they eventually got over it.

Common misconceptions that eating chocolate, nuts, french fries, and colas cause or worsen acne have been laid to rest by most health professionals. But what does cause acne? And, most important, what can you do about it?

What Is Acne?

"Acne vulgaris" is the scientific term for the condition we affectionately know as "zits." Very simply, it is an inflammation of the skin. In puberty the body goes overtime producing oil and stimulating hair follicles. If this excess oil plugs up the pores, you get whiteheads (total blockage) and blackheads (partial blockage). To make matters even worse, a strain of bacteria called *Propionibacterium acnes* thrives on this oil. If this blockage of oils and bacteria irritate the surrounding tissue, that's when you will see redness and inflammation. In severe forms, cysts or nodules can develop in the oil-plugged pores.

Unfortunately, the ducts that become plugged are located mainly on the face and on the upper chest and back—right where everyone can see! And acne usually occurs just at the time when everything is a sensitive issue to an adolescent.

Girls may begin to see signs of breakouts around the age of eleven, while for boys the average age that acne starts is thirteen. Acne is seen more often in teenage boys, possibly due to the higher levels of hormones (androgens like testosterone) present at that time. The 40 to 50 percent of adult women who experience low-grade persistent acne have higher-than-normal levels of this same androgen.

How Is Acne Vulgaris Treated?

Non-drug treatments

While the following tips won't always prevent acne, good treatment can begin anytime. Washing your face daily with ordinary soap (like **Ivory**) and water is effective for control of mild production of oil. Also, keeping your hair off your face can be one way of keeping the skin free of extra oils from your hair or hair-styling products.

Moderate doses of natural sunshine have cleared up many breakouts. Eat fruits and vegetables, which will nourish your body and allow it to spend less time processing fats and oils such as those found in chips and fries.

OTC treatments

There are literally hundreds of acne products on the market today, but just a few active ingredients for you to keep track of. The most common OTC acne ingredient is *benzoyl peroxide.* You'll find this in strengths as high as 10 percent. Benzoyl peroxide works by irritating the skin to such a point that the pores are not able to close. This irritation causes a higher turnover of cells and sloughs out extra oil. The downside to this ingredient is that it can cause temporary stinging, burning, drying, and redness. Because its effectiveness depends on a complete turnover of skin, it may take four to six weeks before the full effects are seen.

Salicylic acid is another effective ingredient for acne treatment. Yes, it really is a mild acid, and it works by penetrating skin oils and opening up

The Drug Lady Recommends . . .

A product that teens (and adults) seem to like very much is the *Neutrogena "On-the-Spot" Acne Patch.* These are hydrogel patches filled with *2% salicylic acid* for overnight use. The handy package has both large- and small-sized discs to cover up and control flare-ups. These are great for those times when an enormous pimple appears on your forehead just before the homecoming dance.

blocked pores. It has a keratolytic action, which means that it takes off the entire top layer of skin. You can also expect redness, stinging, and burning with salicylic acid.

If you are using both of these products for your acne treatment, it is important that you wait twelve hours between applying one on top of the other. Using an anti-bacterial wash in addition to benzoyl peroxide and salicylic acid may keep the bacteria normally found on the skin from getting trapped in plugged pores and causing an infection.

Prescription treatments

The treatment of your acne depends on how severe it is. For mild cases, the doctor may use an extraction tool to physically open up the plugged pores. As the acne gets worse, there are more choices. Antibiotics like **Cleocin-T** (*clindamycin*) or **T-Stat** (*erythromycin*) are available in gel, solution, or pad forms; these are used on the skin rather than taken internally. **Benzamycin Gel** (*benzoyl peroxide 5%/erythromycin 3%*), used as a topical (directly on the skin) antibiotic, is also available by prescription.

The oral (taken by mouth) antibiotics *tetracycline, minocycline,* and *doxycycline* are good choices to kill the *Propionibacterium acnes* bug responsible for the redness and inflammation of your skin. Side effects of these antibiotics are stomach upset and a drastically increased sensitivity to the effects of sunlight (**photosensitivity**). Tetracycline should be taken on an empty stomach, and not within two hours of ingesting any dairy, iron, or antacid products (these substances have a tendency to bind with the drug, lowering or eliminating its effectiveness).

Minocycline and doxycycline may be taken with food to reduce stomach upset. Erythromycin, also to be taken with food, is another effective antibiotic given by mouth. There are no sun-exposure cautions with erythromycin, but the bacteria are more resistant to it than to the others listed. If the acne still shows resistance to all of these, the combination products **Bactrim** or **Septra DS** (*trimethoprim* and *sulfamethoxazole*) may be used. Again, beware of stomach upset or sensitivity to sunlight. Keep in mind that these medications may take four to six weeks before they start to be effective.

A few more that your doctor may choose from to treat more severe forms of acne are in the retinoid family, including **Retin-A** (*tretinoin*), **Retin-A Micro** (with a microsponge delivery system), **Differin** (*adapalene*), and the new **Zorac** (*tazarotene*). The retinoids loosen up and push out the stuff inside your pores and help to prevent more pimples from coming back. But here come the disclaimers: Topical retinoids can cause some serious problems if not used correctly. At first the skin may look worse instead of better, possibly for up to eight weeks! It will, however, eventually look normal again. The medicine should be applied at bedtime and you should avoid any type of direct sunlight while you're using it; the skin becomes ultrasensitive and sunlight (real or artificial) can cause serious burns. Use protective clothing as well as high-numbered sunscreens (over SPF 30). You may also notice greater susceptibility to windburn and cold. Begin treatment with the lowest-strength cream or gel, using cream for dry skin types and gel if your skin type is oily.

Accutane (*isotretinoin*) is a retinoid that you can take in capsule form. Accutane has one of the longest lists of side effects and cautions that you will find. This drug is very tightly regulated by the FDA, and with good reason: The incidence of miscarriages and birth defects in children born to women taking Accutane is notable. Doctors should only prescribe it to women who have passed a negative pregnancy test, do not intend to become pregnant while taking it, and sign a consent form that they have been fully informed of the side effects involved. This is serious stuff! Also, 90 percent of those men and women taking Accutane will experience inflammation of the lips and, less frequently, the eyes. A drying of the skin around the nose and mouth is observed in 80 percent of cases. This medication is also the most expensive of all acne medications—sometimes costing well over several dollars for each capsule!

If your skin doesn't react well to the retinoids, **Azelex** (*azelaic acid*) may be an option. It generally takes longer to work than retinoids, but may cause less skin sensitivity. It can be used under makeup and with moisturizers. Azelex is both bacteriostatic (slows bacterial growth) and bactericidal (kills the bacteria) and is indicated for mild-to-moderate acne. Applied twice daily, this cream has proven as effective as Retin-A and benzoyl peroxide.

Body Odor

Q. *I'm eleven and have started to notice that I smell a little. You know, body odor—B.O. or whatever else it is called. I shower every day. What should I do?*

A. **It looks like your body has decided it's time to grow up! While inside you already feel pretty old, your body is starting some amazing changes. Some of these changes you'll like and others you'll hate, but they are all part of the process.**

What Causes Body Odor?

Several things can cause body odor. Foods that you eat can cause your skin to have a peculiar smell. You can usually tell if someone has eaten lots of garlic, onions, or fish because the smell seems to be attached to them—in a way, it is. When the body perspires (or sweats), it is simply getting rid of waste that it can't deal with. We all have two different types of sweat glands, the **eccrine glands,** which are all over the body, and the **apocrine glands,** which are found only in the hairy areas of the body. Eccrine sweat glands are the body's way of keeping cool when things get toasty. They produce a perspiration that doesn't smell (unless of course, you just ate a double-garlic pizza with anchovies and onions). Normal perspiration (or sweat) doesn't have any odor; it's just there.

Kids don't normally smell bad when they sweat, because their bodies haven't yet formed the apocrine glands. When you start to get older and begin to grow hair under your arms and in the pubic area, you may start to notice a smell. What's happening now is that your body is forming bacteria to break down the proteins in your perspiration from the apocrine glands. By fifth period, when you've been going full speed all day, bacteria are working overtime to break down the perspiration. When the bacteria levels are high, you can bet the smell level will be, too.

How Is Body Odor Treated?

Non-drug treatments

The most effective way to wipe out body odor is to wipe out the bacteria. You don't smell bad right after a shower, right? That's because your body is clean. Wiping your underarms with a damp cloth, or even better, with soap and water, will ensure that no one wrinkles their nose when you walk by.

OTC treatments

An even easier way to control this problem is to ask your parents about a teen antiperspirant/deodorant combination like **Teen Spirit;** they've got scents from "Caribbean Cool" to "Berry Blossom." Adult antiperspirant/ deodorant combinations are fine too. The antiperspirant part of the product has aluminum in it. The aluminum works by actually decreasing the amount that you perspire, so bacteria don't have as much to feast on. Antiperspirants are also good for those times when you have to get up in front of the class and you feel like there are buckets of water running down your sides.

Deodorants are the "good scents" part of the combination. They also help hide the odor by killing bacteria as it grows in the warm, moist areas under your arms. Deodorants alone don't decrease the amount that you sweat, they only cover up what's there.

Using an antibacterial deodorant soap like **Dial** can do the double-duty of getting you out of the shower smelling good and giving your body a jump on killing bacteria that are waiting to take over when you start to perspire.

The Drug Lady Recommends...

For problem areas that aren't under your arms, you might try a body powder, like *Shower to Shower,* that absorbs moisture and has *baking soda* to neutralize odor. *Cornstarch powder* is another way to help keep the perspiration to a minimum.

Prescription treatments

If your body odor is caused by excessive sweating (see "Sweating," chapter 5, page 148), your doctor might try the prescription medicine called **Drysol** (*aluminum chloride hexahydrate*). This may be a good choice for teens who do not get relief from OTC antiperspirants. **Drysol** is reported to work in 80 percent of the people who use it for excessive sweating.

Eating Disorders

Q. *One of my girlfriends has a problem with her weight, but it's not what you think. She's too skinny. I think she might have a problem, but I'm not sure how to ask if she's okay. Could you tell me what to look for?*

A. Sometimes it's much easier to go on with your own life and not take the time to notice that someone close by might need your help. Or you may feel that you don't want to interfere—but you are doing a good thing by paying attention and wanting to help. If you suspect that your friend may have a problem with her eating, you may want to encourage her to talk to you about it. Keep a helpful attitude, but if she seems to be getting worse, tell a trusted adult about the problem right away. While it's important to know that an eating disorder doesn't always follow a specific set of guidelines, there are certain signs that you can be on the lookout for.

What Is an Eating Disorder?

An eating disorder can be a very serious and often life-threatening condition. It usually occurs in women of any age but can start as early as eight years old. There are two common types of eating disorders: one is **bulimia** and the other is **anorexia.**

Bulimia is also referred to as "bingeing and purging," because the sufferer will eat very large quantities of food (bingeing), then quickly get rid of it by using laxatives or making herself vomit (purging).

With anorexia, the person will simply stop eating or barely eat enough to sustain her body. The statistics show that as many as 1 in 100 girls between the ages of twelve and eighteen have some form of anorexia.

There has not been a direct cause pinpointed for eating disorders, but some doctors believe that when an individual feels that her worth is dependent on having a particular (usually low) weight, certain triggers are set off in the brain. These chemical triggers may be responsible for the increasingly destructive behavior.

What to Look For . . .

If you suspect that a friend has an eating disorder, you can look for these signs, but remember that they are simply a place to start:

- Does she regularly eat large amounts of food at most meals, but without gaining any weight?

- Does she excuse herself just after finishing her food to go to the bathroom?

- Have you noticed any signs that she may have thrown up after a meal?

- Are there laxatives lying around? Diet pills? *Ipecac syrup* (to induce vomiting)?

- Does she seem to be unnaturally concerned that she is "too fat," even though she seems to be getting too skinny?

- Does she exercise too much? So much that nothing else is as important as the exercise?

How Are Eating Disorders Treated?

Non-drug treatments

National organizations like Eating Disorders Awareness and Prevention, Inc., have a toll-free number to call for information and referrals. This isn't a counseling service, but rather a non-threatening and confidential resource for addressing questions about eating disorders and obtaining local referrals. Trained EDAP staff answer questions about eating disorders, offer support for addressing food and body-image issues, and provide treatment and counseling referrals by mail or fax. That number is 1-800-931-2237. The hot line is currently staffed from eight A.M. until noon Pacific daylight time, and callers can leave voice-mail twenty-four hours a day, seven days a week. Most requests for information or referrals can be filled within forty-eight hours. They also sponsor a Web site at www.edap.org.

OTC treatments

Eating disorders are a serious medical concern and shouldn't be self-treated.

The Drug Lady Recommends . . .

If you or someone close to you has an eating disorder, it can be a very scary thing. If you are the one fighting this problem, it can seem like things have spun completely out of control without you even realizing it. If you have a friend going through this, she may seem very different from the person you once knew—but don't give up. Your friend is still in there; she's just sick right now. Help isn't far away. See "Resources" on page 368 for other places to go for help for yourself or a friend who may have an eating disorder.

Prescription treatments

Eating disorders are best treated by a doctor who is experienced in both the physical and mental sides of this disease. Because an eating disorder may be seen as a symptom of a deeper problem—stress, anxiety over appearance, fear, or depression—treatment with prescription medications is often successful. Antidepressants (like **Prozac** or **Zoloft**) can sometimes help by changing the chemical balance in the brain, and counseling with regular follow-up visits is a very important part of the treatment.

Sweating

(See Chapter 5, page 148.)

Underweight

Q. *I have a problem being too skinny. I eat lots, but I can't seem to gain any weight. Gym class is a pain because I look like I have sticks for arms and legs. What can I do to gain more weight?*

A. Being skinny is tough! When you're in middle school or high school, you've got enough to worry about. I'll tell it to you straight, though—it will get better as you get older. It's all part of that puberty mess again. Your body is growing at different speeds in different areas. I know that's not much consolation right now, so in the meantime here's what you can do to ensure that you're gaining as much weight as you should be.

What Controls Weight Gain?

For every pound that you want to put on, you have to take in 3,500 more calories than you burn. That's right—3,500 calories for one pound! A typical teenager eats about 2,200 calories a day, so you must add the extra calories to that over a period of time for weight gain to occur. Your metabolism also plays a part. If you're active and burning lots of calories, it takes more effort to put on weight.

How Is Weight Gain Accomplished?

Non-drug treatments

So how do you gain weight? you ask. EAT! Eating well-balanced meals with lots of carbohydrates, proteins, and even some good old fat is a good start. Snacks that have lots of calories (like ice cream or nuts) can add an extra boost to your calorie count.

Also, remember that muscle tissue weighs more than fat. Start a workout program with emphasis on the major muscle groups. After a couple of weeks, you should notice a weight gain AND you'll look buffed!

OTC treatments

Nutritional supplements like **Boost** or **Ensure** are vitamin-fortified and make quick and high-calorie snacks when you're on the go. Just grab a can and you're set to add more calories.

In your sports-nutrition store you may see special powders that are advertised as "weight gainers." Take a close look at these, because many are just made from lots of high-calorie ingredients like sugar (fructose) and fats (soybean oil). Save your money and make a milkshake at home with an extra spoonful of honey in it for flavor. You'll get the same benefit calorie for calorie, and it will probably taste lots better too!

The Drug Lady Recommends . . .

For serious weight gain, try the *Scandishake* line of products from the Scandipharm company. Each vanilla, chocolate, or strawberry packet (which you mix with whole milk) contains a whopping 440 calories. Add a couple of these into your regular diet every week and those extra 3,500 calories add up very fast!

Prescription treatments

While most teenagers will gain weight as they mature, there are times when a medical problem may be the reason for being underweight. Talk to your doctor about having a physical to rule out any other problems. Everything is probably just fine—but it'll make you feel better to know for sure.

THIRTEEN

Women's Health:
Direct from the Planet Venus

Breast Cancer ▓ Breast Enhancement ▓ Contraception and Condoms ▓

Depression ▓ Excessive Hair Growth (see Chapter 5) ▓ Hot Flashes ▓

Menstrual Cramps ▓ Stretch Marks ▓ Urinary-Tract Infections ▓

Vaginal Yeast Infections ▓ Weight Gain ▓ Wrinkles

T'S GREAT TO be a woman in the twenty-first century! We have come a long way in the last hundred years, and the opportunities are endless. We work harder at our jobs, we work harder with our families. It can certainly also take a lot out of us. Being a woman does come with its fair share of problems that are unique to being female. Women need to understand their bodies, listen to their bodies, and take care of their bodies. It's a woman's prerogative! Let's look at some of the female conditions that we hear about most often.

Breast Cancer

Q. *My mother was diagnosed with breast cancer last year and, as you would expect, things have been a little crazy. She is very concerned about my risk for breast cancer. Is there anything I can do to be proactive?*

A. First, you are to be commended for taking the time now to learn about your own health risks and all the options available. Having a family member diagnosed with cancer can be a stressful and traumatic experience, but one of the greatest gifts you can give your mother is to look after your own good health. Please take the time to sit down with your own doctor and talk about your options.

Best of health to you and your mother!

What Is Breast Cancer?

Cancer of the breast is not only one of the most common forms of cancer among women, but also is one of the most curable when detected early. The first sign you may notice is a small, hard, nodular lump as you do your monthly breast self-exam. A **mammogram** will show the existence of these lumps much earlier. While the majority of breast lumps are non-cancerous (benign), it is best to have anything suspicious or unusual checked out by a doctor right away.

How Is Breast Cancer Treated?

Non-drug treatments

A good place to start thinking about breast cancer is with the risk factors in your life. A risk factor is anything that increases your chance of getting a disease. Different cancers have different risk factors. For example, unprotected exposure to strong sunlight is a risk factor for skin cancer. But having a risk factor, or even several, does not necessarily mean that you will get the disease. Some women with one or more breast-cancer risk factors never develop the disease, while many women with breast cancer have

How to Do a Breast Self-Exam

Breast tumors may appear anywhere within the breast, but over half are found in the upper-outer quarter closest to your underarm. While you're there, feel around the nodular lymph nodes deep in and around your underarm. Check your breasts about a week after your menstrual period—this is when there are the fewest changes in breast tissue due to differences in hormone levels. After menopause, when hormonal fluctuations cease, any day of the month is fine.

1. First, stand facing a mirror with your hands at your sides. Look for any unusual bumpiness, puckering, or dimpling.

2. Check the nipples for discharge by gently squeezing them.

3. Lift your left arm and rest your hand on the top of your head. Look for any unusual bulges and changes in skin texture. Using three or four fingers and moving gently in small circles, probe the breast. Start from the outside and move toward the nipple. Repeat this procedure on the right side.

4. Lie flat on your back on the floor with a pillow or small towel supporting your head and shoulders. This helps stretch and flatten the breast and makes changes easier to detect. Put your left arm behind your head. Again, move your fingers in slow circles around the entire breast and armpit area. Repeat on the right side.

If you do notice a lump, there is a very good chance that is it benign (harmless), but don't take any chances. Call your doctor right away for a follow-up examination. Remember that your best chance of beating cancer is early detection.

no apparent risk factors. That may sound a little like double-talk, but unfortunately, cancer isn't that predictable. Here are some different kinds of risk factors.

- For breast cancer, simply being a woman is the main risk factor. Breast cancer can affect men, but this disease is about one hundred times more common among women than among men.

- A woman's risk of developing breast cancer increases with age. About 77 percent of women with breast cancer are over age fifty at the time of diagnosis. Women aged twenty to twenty-nine account for only 0.3 percent of breast-cancer cases.

▨ Recent studies have shown that only 5 to 10 percent of breast-cancer cases are hereditary. But if your mother or a first-degree relative (mother, sister, or daughter) has had the disease, it approximately doubles your risk. And having TWO first-degree relatives increases your risk fivefold!

What should you do if you are aware that you are at a higher risk for breast cancer? At present there is no certain way to prevent breast cancer. Because most breast cancers have several gene mutations that are not inherited, but instead develop during a woman's lifetime, it would appear that environmental factors come into play. You may want to reduce lifestyle risk factors like alcohol consumption, a high-fat diet, and excessive weight if any of these apply. Antioxidants like *coenzyme Q-10, vitamin C, vitamin A,* and *vitamin E* may help protect cells from the damaging free radicals thought to contribute to cancer.

The Drug Lady Recommends...

You should be having yearly **mammograms** from the age of forty on. If you have a family history of breast cancer, then move that age up to twenty-five or thirty. Even talk-show host Rosie O'Donnell has gotten on the bandwagon for this important exam. Mammograms use low levels of X rays to look through breast tissue. For women over fifty, having a mammogram every one to two years can decrease your chance of dying from breast cancer by 35 percent!

OTC treatments

Soy isoflavones, available as the brand name ***Estroven*** and by many other manufacturers, contain plant estrogens called phytoestrogens. Phytoestrogens may be helpful in blocking the absorption of estrogen produced in the body. This is important for breast cancers that appear to be estrogen- or hormone-sensitive. These phytoestrogens are a close match to the estrogen receptors in the breast tissue and fit where human estrogen normally would. This is important because human estrogen in those receptors speeds the cancer growth.

On the other side of the coin, there is the possibility that phytoestrogens increase the growth rate of breast cells, which may increase the chance for developing breast cancer. I generally don't recommend that anyone who has a family history of breast cancer use soy supplements, but for others it may be beneficial.

Prescription treatments

For women at high risk for breast cancer, one possible drug choice is **Nolvadex** (*tamoxifen*). Results from the Breast Cancer Prevention Trial (BCPT) have shown that women at high risk for breast cancer are less likely to develop the disease if they take this anti-estrogen drug. After an average of four years of taking tamoxifen, these women had 45 percent fewer breast cancers than women with the same risk factors who did not take it did. However, there is a very slight risk of developing endometrial or uterine cancer.

Another drug, **Evista** (*raloxifene*), was found, in a study of almost 8,000 women, to reduce the incidence of breast cancer in postmenopausal women by as much as 70 percent. That's really good news! And the results indicated the drug did NOT increase the incidence of endometrial or uterine cancer. Raloxifene, like tamoxifen, is a selective estrogen-receptor modulator (SERM), which blocks the negative actions of estrogen in some tissues, such as the breast, and mimics estrogen's benefits in other areas of the body (like in the bones, where it helps to maintain bone mass). Side effects may include hot flashes or sudden feelings of warmth, especially during the first six months of use as your body gets used to the change in estrogen levels.

The prescription treatments discussed here are for prevention of breast cancer either in high-risk patients or for those who have undergone treatment to put the cancer into remission. The treatment options for women diagnosed with breast cancer are increasing every day and should be discussed in detail with your physician.

Breast Enhancement

Q. *Are there any products I can use to increase my breast size? I've seen all types of things advertised and I wonder which ones really work.*

A. Well, the very short answer is that some people really want to increase their breast size and some companies are more than happy to supply a product just for that purpose, whether it works or not. There are many different supplements, creams, drops, and even exercises that advertise the ability to increase or enhance breast size. However, these products have not been shown to be safe or effective in scientific studies. I have yet to talk to even one individual who has used any of the products successfully, but I'll keep an open mind and let you know what's available.

What Determines Breast Size?

Breast size in women, like penis size in men (see "Penis Enlargement," chapter 9, page 231), is determined by your genetic makeup. The genes that were passed on to you, and your own levels of the female hormone estrogen, determine the size of your breasts.

How Can Breast Size Be Increased?

Non-drug treatments

Most breast-size increasers are herbal in nature. **Herbal Grobust** capsules contain eight ingredients: *saw palmetto, damiana, dong quai, dandelion root, blessed thistle, kava kava, wild yam,* and *mother's wort.* **Wonder Cream** has *wild yam* and *aloe vera* as ingredients. **Erdic Breast Growth** contains extracts from *wheat, barley, hops, rye, malt, buckwheat, black oats,* and *maize.* Other than the claims made by the companies selling these products, I haven't found any good scientific studies backing them up.

OTC treatments

Some products on the market (like **Athena II**) claim that using them will increase your bra-cup size in ninety days if you do certain exercises. There is a little more validity in these products than with the herbal supplements because they work by strengthening and building the chest muscles under the breast. The breast itself doesn't actually get larger, but the muscles underneath do.

Prescription treatments

For women who feel that a larger breast size increase is a must, there is hope. Through surgery you can have implants put into your breasts or have fat injected from other areas of your body. Surgical alteration is a more permanent way to achieve larger breasts, but there are risks. Infections, rejection of the implants, and even implants that leak have been reported. This is a decision to make VERY carefully.

Contraception and Condoms

Q. *My boyfriend and I are concerned about birth control. We want something that is both safe and effective. What are our options?*

A. You have quite a few choices with birth control today—from prescription birth-control pills to diaphragms, from hormone implants to condoms (male and female), to spermicides and sponges. It's great that you're looking at this responsibly, because you'll not only prevent pregnancy but may also protect yourselves from sexually transmitted diseases (STDs). (See "Sexually Transmitted Diseases," chapter 9, page 236.)

What Is Contraception?

"Contraception" means any process, device, or method that prevents pregnancy (i.e., conception). The risk of pregnancy increases with the greater number of partners you have, and the less consistently you use effective birth control.

- Birth-control pills work by adding enough hormones to your body to fool it into skipping ovulation and making the mucus that is normally in the vagina very thick and harder for sperm to make their way through.

- Diaphragms and sponges provide a physical barrier inside a woman to prevent sperm from reaching and fertilizing the egg.

They are used with spermicides, like *nonoxynol-9,* which work by killing live sperm.

▓ Contraceptive implants are a convenient way to deliver the same hormones found in birth-control pills in a constant dosage. Inserted under the skin (usually the arm), these implants provide protection against pregnancy for up to five years, but not against sexually transmitted disease, unless a condom is also used.

▓ A condom is a thin rubber sheath. The male condom slips on and snugly covers the erect penis, while the female condom is inserted into the vagina and party covers the labia. The condom catches sperm during ejaculation and prevents them from entering the vagina. It also prevents some skin-to-skin contact. Only condoms provide significant protection against pregnancy, sexually transmitted diseases, and HIV/AIDS. Some condoms even have a spermicidal lubricant to further increase effectiveness.

Non-drug contraceptives

While not recommended for anyone looking to protect themselves from sexually transmitted diseases or pregnancy, there ARE natural methods of birth control. The "rhythm method" depends on predicting ovulation to figure out exactly when you are fertile, and avoiding sex during those times. This method has resulted in many "surprise" bundles of joy and does NOT protect against sexually transmitted diseases (STDs).

The "withdrawal method" depends on removing the penis just before ejaculation. This is especially dangerous because often there are live sperm in the pre-ejaculatory fluid and they can still reach and fertilize an egg. As with the rhythm method, withdrawal also provides NO protection against STDs.

OTC contraceptives

The rate for avoiding pregnancy with condoms is about 90 percent, but for protection against sexually transmitted diseases (STDs) the rate goes up to nearly 100 percent. However, latex condoms are the ONLY type considered protective against both bacterial and viral transmission. Some individuals who suffer from latex allergies (see "Latex Allergies," chapter 2, page 47) find that they get protection and allergy relief by using a lambskin condom under the latex one. Please, PLEASE don't use a lambskin condom alone—there are tiny microscopic holes in the condom's material that allow viruses to pass through easily.

The female condom, **Reality**, is a soft, loose-fitting plastic pouch that lines the vagina. It has a soft ring at each end. The ring at the closed end is used to put the device inside the vagina and holds it in place against the cervix. The other ring stays outside the vagina and partly covers the labia.

With condoms there is the possibility of an allergic reaction to the latex rubber in the condom or to the spermicide (*nonoxynol-9*) added to the condom. The symptoms of this type of allergy include a burning sensation of the vagina or penis. There may also be redness and irritation whenever the condom is used. If the allergy is mild, simply switching brands may be effective. For more serious allergies, it may be necessary to find an alternate form of birth control.

It's important to be aware that condoms with spermicide in them have actual expiration dates. Because a stored condom can break down in warm conditions (like a purse or wallet), it is a good idea to throw out those that have been around a while and purchase a new set of insurance policies!

The contraceptive sponge is a birth-control device that's inserted deep into the vagina before intercourse. It contains the spermicide *nonoxynol-9*, which slows down and kills sperm and helps prevent them from fertilizing the female egg. The sponge protects against pregnancy for up to twenty-four hours, no matter how many times you have intercourse. You must leave it in place for at least six hours—but no longer than twenty-four hours—after intercourse.

Spermicides like **Semicid** and **Ortho Options Conceptrol Contracep-**

The Drug Lady Recommends . . .

To increase your rate of avoiding pregnancy, use condoms with the spermicide *nonoxynol-9*. Some condoms even advertise the spermicide as a lubricant. You may also use lubricants made especially for condoms, like **K-Y Jelly**, but other lubricants should be avoided because they may weaken the latex.

tive Gel contain the powerful sperm-killer nonoxynol-9. These are typically applied or inserted no more than one hour before intercourse. Side effects may include sensitivity or a rash from a mild allergic reaction to the spermicide.

Prescription contraceptives

With birth-control pills, you have several choices. However, the only difference is the type and percentages of the hormones *estrogen* and *progestin*. Combination pills have both estrogen and progestin. "Mini-pills" contain progestin only; these are best for women who can't tolerate estrogen. Multiphasics (including biphasics and triphasics) mimic the actual hormonal changes your body goes through every month. You'll even hear birth-control pills advertised as "acne fighters." High levels of testosterone cause acne, and birth control pills contain the hormone estrogen, which decreases testosterone levels. *Ortho Tri-Cyclin* was the first pill to get FDA approval for this use, but theoretically any birth-control pill with estrogen can do this. Unfortunately, birth-control pills come with some side effects.

Drugs That May Decrease the Effectiveness of Birth-Control Pills

It is thought that certain levels of specific bacteria help move the hormones in birth-control pills between the GI (gastrointestinal) tract and the bloodstream. When these bacteria are reduced in number, the hormones may not be moved and the pills' effectiveness may be reduced. With other drugs, like anti-seizure medicines, we simply aren't sure why they make the pills less effective—though it may be related to liver-enzyme metabolism. However it happens, using a backup contraceptive (like condoms) is recommended whenever you are taking any of these medicines with birth-control pills.

These are the medications to be aware of:

- PENICILLINS—*amoxicillin, ampicillin, dicloxacillin,* and *penicillin*
- TETRACYCLINES—*doxycycline, minocycline,* and *tetracycline*
- ANTIFUNGALS—*fluconazole, griseofulvin, itraconazole,* and *ketoconazole*
- ANTI-SEIZURE DRUGS—*carbamazepine, phenobarbital*

The Drug Lady Recommends . . .

Keep a copy of your birth-control pill package insert handy. This information sheet contains a wealth of knowledge, including side effects and what to do if you miss a pill during the month.

The estrogen component of birth-control pills can cause bloating (fluid retention), nausea, and breast tenderness. If these continue for over one month, let your doctor know so that he or she can decrease your estrogen dosage as needed. If you notice that your pills don't quite stop your period and small amounts of blood appear during the rest of the month (called breakthrough bleeding or spotting), you probably aren't getting enough estrogen. Progestin can also be responsible for breakthrough bleeding, weight gain, acne, and mood changes.

Implants, like the **Norplant System,** contain implantable *levonorgestrel,* a progestinlike hormone. The implant is used for long-term birth control. It is inserted into the upper arm by your doctor. The six one-inch-long capsules within the implant slowly release the drug into your body, where

The "Morning-After" Pill

The "morning-after" pill, or emergency contraception pill (ECP), is available by prescription from your doctor or pharmacist. It can prevent pregnancy after you've had unprotected sex or when accidents occur, such as a condom breaking during sex. It is not designed to be a method of birth control.

Two types of ECPs are available. One is *Preven;* like regular birth control pills, it contains the hormones *estrogen* and *progestin,* but in higher doses. The other is called *Plan B;* it contains only progestin. You need to take the first dose of ECP within seventy-two hours of intercourse, with a second dose twelve hours later.

If you would like more information about ECPs, call your doctor, pharmacist, or the toll-free Emergency Contraceptive Hotline at 1-888-NOT-2-LATE. This twenty-four-hour hotline can also give you a list of providers nearest you who prescribe ECPs.

An old country doctor went out to the country to deliver a baby, so far out that there was no electricity. When the doctor arrived, no one was home except for the laboring mother and her five-year-old child. The doctor instructed the child to hold a lantern up high so he could see while he helped the woman deliver the baby. The child did so, the mother pushed, and after a little while, the doctor lifted the newborn baby by the feet and spanked him on the bottom to get him to take his first breath.

"Hit him again," the five-year-old said indignantly. "He shouldn't have crawled up there in the first place!"

it remains active for up to five years. It works by inhibiting ovulation and regulating the menstrual cycle.

If you don't react well to the hormones of birth-control pills, ask your doctor about the possibility of having a diaphragm fitted. A diaphragm is a cuplike device, used with a spermicide, that fits over the cervix inside the vagina. It prevents sperm from entering the uterus. This barrier form of contraception has fewer side effects than with the estrogen- and progestin-based hormonal contraceptives.

Depression

Q. *I've been feeling a little down and blue lately. Some days I feel so alone and isolated—I think I might be depressed. Is there something available over-the-counter that I can take? What can I ask my doctor to prescribe that won't make me sleep all day?*

A. It is wonderful that you're taking the first step in recognizing that there may be a problem. It's important to know that everyone feels sad or blue occasionally, especially when great changes are going on in your life. With more severe depression, the common tasks of daily life can become so difficult that normal functioning is almost impossible.

The good news is that depression is very treatable and may even be traced to something physical like a hormonal imbalance or thyroid disorder. See your doctor FIRST before self-treating this condition. Having your smile back is very important!

What Is Depression?

The three most common types of depression are major clinical depression, dysthymia, and bipolar disorder. Major clinical depression involves disabling episodes that interrupt sleeping, eating, and the ability to enjoy life. Dysthymia is a less serious, but longer-term, condition, with similar but less severe symptoms that nevertheless still prevent a person from experiencing life to its fullest potential. Bipolar disorder (once known as manic depression) is characterized by cycles of extreme highs (mania) and lows (depression) that create serious internal conflict for the individual trying to function normally in society. Unfortunately, bipolar disorder is often a chronic condition that tends to recur cyclically unless treated medically.

There are cases in which you may feel all of the symptoms of a major depressive episode but are not actually suffering from depression. If you have recently experienced significant losses (death, divorce, or a difficult move), had an injury to the brain, or have been diagnosed with another form of mental illness, your symptoms can mimic those of clinical depression. Your doctor will be able to determine the best course of treatment under those conditions.

Depression is not just one symptom, but a persistent and recurring problem. Since depression is such a widespread and debilitating condition, many physicians are getting special training to keep abreast of the ever-changing treatment options; they may also work in close collaboration with psychologists or psychiatrists for a whole-body approach.

Depression occurs almost twice as often in women as in men, with the average age ranging from twenty-five to forty-five. Depression is a very real disease, and trying to talk yourself out of it can be impossible. It is important to realize that you're not alone and that there is a great deal of help available.

Signs and Symptoms of Depression

If you've experienced five or more of these symptoms nearly every day during the past two weeks, there is a good chance you are clinically depressed.

- a loss of interest in things you used to enjoy

- feelings of sadness, unhappiness, or being blue

- a change of appetite, and either gaining or losing weight as a result

- trouble sleeping (too little or too much)

- lowered energy levels or sluggishness

- restlessness or feelings of moving too slowly (as if in slow motion)

- feelings of worthlessness or guilt

- problems concentrating, remembering, or making decisions

- persistent thoughts of death or suicide, or actually trying to kill yourself

(If you checked this last one, PLEASE seek help immediately!)

The National Mental Illness Screening Project has suggested that if you have even just one or two of these symptoms, it may be a good idea to talk with your health-care provider—I agree heartily. Many of the millions of adults suffering from depression in America deny the existence of the disease, even though there are very effective treatments available. Those who care about you will recognize the change—and so will you!

How Is Depression Treated?

The good news is that over 80 percent of people suffering from clinical depression show improvement with treatment by the end of one year. The key here is treatment. If you don't seek treatment, depression can rob you and those who care about you of many happy moments. Many types of treatment are available, from medications to psychotherapy (either private sessions or with a group). DON'T give up!

Non-drug treatments

I just can't emphasize enough how important it is to have depression diagnosed and treated by your doctor BEFORE attempting to treat it yourself. While there are herbal medicines (like *St. John's wort* and *SAM-e*) that are showing great promise for mild depression, you should discuss this in detail with your doctor.

Studies have shown that St. John's wort, in a standardized dosage of 300 mg (*0.3% hypericin*) taken three times daily, may alter brain chemistry slightly to relieve symptoms of mild depression. This should NOT be taken along with prescription antidepression medicines.

SAM-e (*s-adenosyl-L-methione*) is an amino acid that has shown great promise in the treatment of mild depression. The dosage is 400 mg taken three times a day, then maintained at 300 mg daily. We aren't exactly sure how it works, but it certainly seems to do the job in some individuals. There are few side effects, but the worst seems to be stomach upset.

OTC treatments

Depression isn't a condition that lends itself to self-treatment from the OTC shelf. Talk to your doctor about possible treatment options. Remember, if you have a question about your depression medications, you can always ask your pharmacist. He or she is accessible and concerned about your condition. Also, the pharmacist may be able to point you toward other referrals in your area: Mental-health clinics, support groups, and hot lines may provide a respite until further help can be found.

Prescription treatments

Medication therapies for depression have come a very long way in recent years. Selective serotonin reuptake inhibitors (SSRIs) are drugs that alter the way certain chemicals are channeled in the brain; some examples are **Prozac** (*fluoxetine hydrochloride*), **Serzone** (*nefazodone*), and **Zoloft** (*sertraline*). These drugs have had amazing success in treating depressive disorders. One serious caution to keep in mind, however, is that these drugs should not be used in combination with another class of antidepressants, called MAO inhibitors (e.g., **Nardil, Parnate,** and **Marplan**). In fact, the manufacturers of most SSRIs recommend that you not start taking their drugs until fourteen days after you have stopped a MAO inhibitor, or that you allow up to five weeks to pass before starting the SSRIs after taking an MAO inhibitor. Side effects that may occur include confusion, restlessness, high blood pressure, and convulsions.

The tricyclic antidepressants, like **Sinequan** and **Adapin** (*doxepin*), **Elavil** (*amitriptyline*), and **Pamelor** (*nortriptyline*), also work by altering the chemistry of the brain. It may take a few weeks before the full effect is felt, but the past track record with these medications has been good. Some individuals may experience mild drowsiness with the tricyclic family, but that often fades with regular use. Strict warnings about combining tricyclics with MAO inhibitors also apply: Serious side effects—and even death—have occurred when the two were combined.

For bipolar disorder (formerly called manic depression), *lithium carbonate* is still the drug of choice. It is used both to treat the manic episodes and, at lower dosages, to prevent the disorder's recurrence. It sometimes takes awhile before the amount of drug in the bloodstream reaches a therapeutic level. Dosage is VERY important in the treatment of this disease, so you should not suddenly stop taking lithium; it is important to keep constant levels of lithium in your blood for the effects to be felt. Also, you need to drink plenty of water while taking lithium and have your blood lithium levels checked by the doctor every two months.

Excessive Hair Growth

(See Chapter 5, page 137.)

Hot Flashes

Q. *I feel like I'm in an oven—and it's November! What can I do about these hot flashes?*

A. Sometime between the ages of forty-five and sixty-five, our bodies begin the process known as menopause. Our normal monthly periods begin to slow, then cease altogether. With this phase of life come many other body changes and symptoms, one of the more unpleasant of which are hot flashes. You are not alone, either. It is estimated that over 80 percent of all women going through menopause will experience hot flashes at one time or another.

What Causes Hot Flashes?

Hot flashes, or the unbearable inability to cool down, may cause a drenching sweat or extreme flushing of the face and neck, and there may be a feeling of chills immediately after one of the flashes has passed. Hot flashes are often associated with night sweats (extreme sweating, flushing, and a rapidly pounding heart); both are caused by the same hormonal fluctuations. Hot flashes generally last from two to three minutes, but may continue for up to five minutes, especially during the first years of menopause. They are the body's attempt to regulate internal temperature when estrogen levels are fluctuating rapidly. The blood vessels dilate, skin temperature rises, and redness and flushing occur. The key to stopping these symptoms is to treat what's causing it—those falling estrogen levels.

How Are Hot Flashes Treated?

Non-drug treatments

Soy, soy, soy! There has been a tremendous amount of literature touting the beneficial effects of *soy* products for the symptoms of menopause, especially hot flashes. Soy products have mild estrogenic activity, but do not seem to be associated with any of the side effects of prescription *estrogen* replacement. Soy can be found naturally in soy flour, soybeans, and soy sprouts, as well as in soy products such as tofu. The active part of the soy seems to be the *isoflavone,* and 200 mg of soy isoflavones daily has been shown to relieve hot flashes in many women.

Red clover and *dong quai* also have high levels of the phytoestrogen (plant estrogen) isoflavones, thought to benefit hot-flash sufferers. A daily dosage of 40 mg of red clover for several weeks has been shown to have good results in decreasing hot flashes, as well as in making other symptoms of menopause more bearable. A typical dosage for dong quai is three to fifteen grams a day—again, for at least three weeks to get the maximum effect.

The Drug Lady Recommends...

Studies have also shown that exercise increases the production of chemicals called endorphins, which greatly decrease the severity and frequency of hot flashes. The amount of exercise needed seems to be approximately three and a half hours each week. Any less than that, and women seemed to experience longer and more severe hot flashes.

Wild yam (a natural progesterone), applied to the skin in cream form, also has been shown to help ease hot flashes and night sweats for some women. As with most natural products, some studies claim that all of these work well and other studies claim they don't work at all. I generally recommend that they be given a three- to four-week trial, and then you choose for yourself.

OTC treatments

Products like **Promensil** (with *red clover*) and **Rejuvex** (with *dong quai*) are over-the-counter products specifically designed to make the transition through menopause as easy as possible.

Prescription treatments

Thankfully, it takes only a small dosage of *estrogen* to slow down hot flashes. **Premarin** (conjugated *estrogen*) is one of the most commonly prescribed medicines in the United States today. Some side effects of estrogen are headaches, nausea, breast tenderness, and slight mood swings; there is also an increased risk for long-term side effects like breast or endometrial cancer. Taking **Provera** (*medroxyprogesterone*) with estrogen can almost eliminate the risk of endometrial cancer.

Menstrual Cramps

Q. *Every month, just like clockwork, I'm in bed with awful cramps during my period. What can I do to avoid them, or at least make them more bearable?*

A. Monthly periods are just one of those things that we, as women, must endure, but we needn't suffer with painful periods. There are very effective treatments for lessening the pain and even ways to prevent cramps from being quite so severe.

What Is a Menstrual Cramp?

The official name for menstrual cramps is **dysmenorrhea,** which means "painful menstruation." Nearly every woman who has had a monthly period has experienced the abdominal cramping and uterine muscle contractions and spasms that typically occur just before the period and as it starts.

Severe cramps may produce pain that radiates down the legs and back, along with nausea, vomiting, headache, fever, and diarrhea. Menstrual-cramp sufferers seem to have unusually high levels of prostaglandin hormones. Prostaglandins cause inflammation and make the nerves more sensitive to pain. These hormones may also decrease the amount of oxygen delivered to the lining of the uterus; muscles without oxygen contract more painfully than those receiving more oxygen. Women who have had children, and those who are more physically fit, seem to have less painful cramps than those who are childless and overweight.

How Are Menstrual Cramps Treated?

Non-drug treatments

A heating pad and gentle stretches are wonderful natural treatments for the pain of menstrual cramps. Getting enough exercise is also important, as is keeping off excess weight.

A mineral to look for in cramp treatment is *magnesium.* A dosage of 100 mg three times daily for the week before and up to your period may relax the uterine muscles and prevent cramps from occurring.

The herb *dong quai* has been used for centuries to increase muscle tone of the uterus; with the increase in muscle tone comes a subsequent relaxation of the muscles in the uterus. A fluid extract of 1 ml taken three times daily during the menstrual period may make this time of the month more bearable.

Evening primrose oil (EPO) has prostaglandin-lowering properties, in a dosage of 500 to 1,000 mg twice daily. However, it may take up to three months for the body to build up sufficient stores to decrease inflammation, so additional treatment may be required for a few months until EPO begins its effect.

OTC treatments

Most women turn to the OTC shelf for help with monthly cramps. Non-steroidal anti-inflammatory medicines, like *ibuprofen, ketoprofen,* and *naproxen,* actually help decrease prostaglandins in the body. Lower levels of prostaglandins decrease the intensity of uterine contractions and make the body less sensitive to pain impulses. Because they may take up to an hour to work, it is a good idea to take them at the first twinge of pain. Also, be sure to take these drugs with food to avoid irritating your stomach.

Prescription treatments

One prescription prostaglandin-inhibitor is called **Ponstel** (*mefenamic acid*). This medicine may take several hours to reach its maximum effect, so take it early, before the pain becomes severe.

Some doctors will prescribe combination birth-control pills to help severe menstrual cramps. The idea is to stop ovulation from occurring, thereby averting any cramps at all. Also, the body doesn't slough off the uterine lining, so fewer prostaglandins are produced.

Stretch Marks

Q. *I've some really awful stretch marks after the birth of my two children. What can I do to get rid of them or at least make them less noticeable?*

A. Well, I don't know if you'll be able to put on that bikini by summer, but there may be some hope. Stretch marks can be tough to fade completely due to the damage done to the layers of skin.

What Are Stretch Marks?

Stretch marks occur in the middle layer of the skin, or the dermis. This is the skin's elastic layer, with collagen fibers that allow the skin to stretch. When the layer is continuously stretched over a long period of time (during pregnancy or weight gain), its elasticity breaks down. The skin tries to make itself stronger by increasing the amount of collagen in the tissue, resulting in the silvery scars we call stretch marks.

How Are Stretch Marks Treated?

Non-drug treatments

While *vitamin E* and *cocoa butter* are excellent for keeping the skin moist and pliable, they do nothing to reverse the damage done by stretch marks. These products, best in cream or oil forms, are most effective in the prevention of scar tissue. Use them every day while pregnant to keep that skin soft and supple.

OTC treatments

Unfortunately, stretch marks are difficult to treat. With time, some stretch marks will slowly improve. Many creams or ointments that are applied to the skin are available, but few have been shown to improve stretch marks quickly.

The Drug Lady Recommends . . .

One product that has received a great deal of attention recently is *Mederma*. Its unique combination of onion extract and *allantoin* (a uric acid product that promotes wound healing) in a gel base may help reduce stretch mark (or scar) formation. It is advertised to help damaged skin appear softer and smoother. It is important to start treatment as early as possible with this product as newly damaged skin responds better than older injuries. Mederma is massaged into the skin three to four times daily. Package instructions label this product as safe for all members of the family, so nursing mothers can get started on those stretch marks right away.

Prescription treatments

There seems to be a very distinct decrease in stretch marks found in those using **Renova** (*tretinoin*). In fact, one study showed fifteen out of sixteen patients with stretch marks had some benefit from using Renova. Although side effects are relatively minor, some patients report red, peeling, or dry skin, and others experience burning or stinging. Pregnant women should not use Renova because of risks to the unborn child. It should also not be used by people with a recent sunburn, or by people with eczema or other chronic skin conditions. A number of drugs, including several commonly used antibiotics, will interact with the cream to make the skin very sensitive to sunlight. Be sure to cover those bikini areas if you're using this treatment.

Urinary-Tract Infections

Q. *This can't be happening! I feel a urinary-tract infection coming on and I'm going on vacation in a few days. What can I do to get the fastest cure possible?*

A. This is an easy one. Because bacteria cause a urinary-tract infection, your first step is to get on the phone for an appointment with your doctor ASAP. Your doctor can prescribe an antibiotic that will get rid of it fast. So, what about relief before you can see the doctor? And how can you prevent this from happening again? Read on.

What Causes Urinary-Tract Infections?

A urinary-tract infection (UTI) occurs when bacteria find their way into the urethra (the tube through which urine leaves the body). The bacteria make their way up the urethra into the bladder and the (ureters) canals that connect to the kidneys. Symptoms include burning upon urination; dark, foul-smelling, bloody, or cloudy urine; and having a frequent feeling that you need to urinate, but only being able to go a small amount. It may progress to a feeling of tiredness, fever, and generally being very uncomfortable. Urinary-tract infections may also be referred to as "cystitis." UTIs tend to recur with irritation (from sexual intercourse, restrictive clothing, dyes in some toilet paper, bubble baths, or diaphragms).

How Are Urinary-Tract Infections Treated?

Non-drug treatments

Drinking lots of water is VERY important when treating UTIs. This flushes out your system and prevents bacteria from easily finding a home in the urinary tract.

Cranberry, in the form of juice or dried capsules, works for UTIs by preventing bacteria from sticking to the inside of the urinary tract. To prevent infections, it is necessary to drink three ounces or more of cranberry-juice cocktail daily, which is equal to about six capsules of dried cranberries. Once you have an infection, you need to drink 12 to 32 ounces of cranberry-juice cocktail a day to treat UTIs. A pure cranberry-extract product is also available, under the name ***AZO Cranberry Supplement Tablets.*** Cranberry should not be substituted for prescription antibiotics when treating an infection, but you may use it in combination with antibiotics or as a preventive measure.

OTC treatments

While over-the-counter medicines shouldn't be used to treat a UTI, they can provide pain relief until you can get into the doctor for an antibiotic. "Urinary analgesics" are medicines that make urination less painful. **Azo-Standard** and **Uristat** contain the active ingredient *phenazopyridine*, which works in the bladder to relieve pain; the strength is 95 mg, about half that of prescription products. It will turn urine, tears, and sweat a bright orange-red color. This medicine can also stain contact lenses.

The Drug Lady Recommends . . .

Call the doctor when you first feel the UTI coming on. If the symptoms occur while you're away on vacation or during the weekend, you might try *Cystex*. Cystex contains the antibacterial *methenamine,* as well as *sodium salicylate* as a pain reliever.

Anti-inflammatory medicines like *ibuprofen, ketoprofen,* or *naproxen sodium* work well to relieve pain while the antibiotics work.

Prescription treatments

One of the most common and effective prescription treatments for a UTI are the sulfa-based antibiotics **Bactrim** or **Septra** (*sulfamethoxizole* and *trimethoprim*). It is generally given in a twice-daily dosage for ten days, but may be prescribed for a shorter duration for less serious infections, usually only three days for a mild UTI. Another popular antibiotic your doctor may prescribe is **Macrobid** (*nitrofurantoin*). It is taken twice daily for up to ten days.

Often, a urinary analgesic like **Pyridium** (*phenazopyridine*) is prescribed at the same time (it has the same active ingredient as similar OTC products). This relieves the burning and pain until the antibiotic kicks in, but has the same side effect of turning your sweat, tears, and urine bright orange. Watch out for those stains on your contact lenses!

Prevention of Urinary-Tract Infections

▦ Keep the genital area clean, and wipe from front to back after a bowel movement.

▦ Wash the genital area each time you bathe or shower. Use soap only on the outside of your vagina, because the chemicals in soap may cause additional irritation.

▦ Never alternate anal and vaginal intercourse because this can introduce harmful bacteria into the urinary tract.

▦ Wear cotton underwear, which allows better air circulation than nylon. Wear pantyhose that have a cotton crotch.

▦ Avoid clothes that fit tightly over the genital area, such as control-top pantyhose or tight jeans.

▦ Don't wear a wet bathing suit for long periods of time.

▦ Drink plenty of cranberry juice to help keep bacteria from sticking to the bladder wall.

▦ If you use a diaphragm, consider other forms of contraception. Studies show that diaphragms can increase your risk for UTIs from the added pressure on the urethra.

Pill Humor

Click. "Welcome to the Psychiatric Hot Line."

- "If you are obsessive-compulsive, please press 1 repeatedly."

- "If you are codependent, please ask someone to press 2."

- "If you have multiple personalities, please press 3, 4, 5, and 6."

- "If you are paranoid-delusional, we know who you are and what you want—just stay on the line so we can trace the call."

- "If you are schizophrenic, listen carefully and a little voice will tell you which number to press."

- "If you are manic-depressive, it doesn't matter which number you press—no one will answer."

Vaginal Yeast Infections

Q. *I have another yeast infection! What will work the fastest and will be the MOST effective?*

A. "Another yeast infection" is a term most women dread. The itching, burning, and painful urination followed by thick, cottage cheese–like discharge make this condition particularly unpleasant. The organism that causes this is with us all the time; however, only under certain circumstances can it gain a strong-enough foothold to cause problems.

What Is a Vaginal Yeast Infection?

You may also see a vaginal yeast infection referred to as "candidiasis." This infection is caused when the fungal yeast *Candida albicans* begins to overgrow in the moist vaginal area. It can do this whenever the immune system is weakened—like when you are taking antibiotics for an infection. Antibiotics generally aren't selective as to "good" bacteria versus "bad" bacteria—they wipe out everything. This gives the *Candida* yeast free rein to grow, and grow quickly. Other possible causes for this condition are: taking corticosteroids (like *prednisone*), pregnancy, the use of spermicides, and even wearing tight clothing (like pantyhose) that can trap moisture for long periods of time. This fungus is especially fond of high levels of sugar in the body, so diabetics are especially at risk of contracting a vaginal yeast infection.

The first symptoms generally begin with a burning or itching in the vaginal area, followed by a discharge that is white, sticky, and like cottage cheese in consistency. The discharge typically has a mild yeasty odor. There may also be pain when urinating and having sex.

Luckily, this type of condition can be taken care of quickly once it is correctly diagnosed.

How Is a Vaginal Yeast Infection Treated?

Non-drug treatments

Herbs for chronic yeast infections include *barberry* (*Berberis vulgaris*) and *goldenseal.* Try these in a tea form, and drink it three times a day when you first feel the symptoms begin.

Also, cut down on high-carbohydrate foods as well as those with a high yeast or sugar content; these seem to predispose some women to yeast infections.

Stress can decrease the naturally friendly bacteria that keep *Candida* at bay—so try to relax! Massage, aromatherapy, and yoga help give the body the best chance of fighting infections.

Garlic has antifungal properties, as well as being a wonderful extra addition to your pasta sauce! Garlic in odorless form, like **Kwai Odor-Free Tablets,** is a good choice for those who must go out in public while fighting a yeast infection. Another food that helps the body fight yeast infections is yogurt. Yogurt has active cultures of the "good" bacteria, in the *lactobacillus* family. Look for yogurt with "active" cultures.

The Drug Lady Recommends . . .

When your natural levels of "good" bacteria are low, replace them with **probiotics** like *lactobacillus acidophilus* or *Bifidobacterium bifidum*. I generally recommend that any woman who has a history of vaginal yeast infections take one of these probiotics supplements (friendly-bacteria replacers) whenever she fills a prescription for an antibiotic. This helps to ensure that the *Candida* yeast has a tougher time finding a home in the body. If you take an antibiotic and a probiotic, be sure to separate the doses by at least two hours.

OTC treatments

Since many women experience yeast infections rather frequently, it's a good idea to know what's available over-the-counter. You have quite a few choices: 1-day treatments, 3-day treatments, 7-day treatments . . . tablets . . . creams with applicators. All of these contain antifungal medications; names to look for are **Monistat** (*miconazole*), **Mycelex** and **Gyn-Lotrimin** (*clotrimazole*), and **Femstat** (*butoconazole*). One-day and three-day treatments are more convenient, but some yeast infections don't respond as well to this short-term therapy.

While all of these seem to have relatively high rates of effectiveness, a product that I especially like is the **Monistat 7 Combination Pack.** It contains a seven-day supply of miconazole vaginal suppositories that melt the medicine into the vagina, as well as a miconazole cream to treat external vulvar itching. It does double-duty on the yeast infection!

Prescription treatments

While it's okay to treat a vaginal yeast infection with OTC medicines, it's important that you contact your doctor the first time you have these symptoms to verify that a yeast infection is indeed the problem. It's also important to contact your doctor anytime you have these symptoms along with stomach pain, fever, or a foul-smelling vaginal discharge, since this may mean you have a bacterial infection and stronger antibiotics may be required.

One prescription treatment for vaginal yeast infections is a onetime dose of the antifungal **Diflucan** (*fluconazole*); it may be repeated in one week if necessary. Often this medicine is given as a prescription at the same time an antibiotic prescription is written, especially if a woman has a long history of yeast infections.

An older antifungal medicine that is still being used is *nystatin*. It's available as a vaginal-tablet insert with an applicator, and is used once a day for seven days.

Weight Loss

Q. *What is the best diet pill? Are they safe for everyone to use? Sorry for all of the questions, but I need to lose weight fast!*

A. These days, it seems that more and more people are becoming pre-occupied with their weight. It is a diet-drug frenzy out there! With the introduction of both federal legend (prescription required) and over-the-counter drugs to combat weight gain, it is no wonder you have these questions. At one time the prescription drug Redux (which has since been removed from the market) was averaging 85,000 prescriptions a week!

There are lots of choices in the weight-loss market. Prescription medicines are available for those who have a weight problem that endangers their health. Then there are the numerous herbal and over-the-counter products—they claim to do everything from killing cravings to boosting your metabolism. But are they really effective and, more important, are they safe?

What Causes Weight Gain?

There is a very easy answer to this question, but we just don't want to hear it. Unless our weight gain is attributed to a medical disorder like a thyroid condition, being overweight is a result of taking in more calories than you burn. So the best way to lose weight is to consume fewer calories than you burn.

Okay, but what about that magic pill that is advertised to help you lose weight? All those magic diet pills generally have an ingredient (or two) that helps suppress the appetite center in your brain—that wonderful area that tells us it's time to grab a candy bar or have "just a slice more" of that chocolate cake in the refrigerator.

For every pound that we want to lose, we must burn 3,500 more calories than we consume. This doesn't have to be done in one day. Just by cutting back a little on what we eat, changing our eating habits away from the high fats (which have more calories), and getting up and exercising more, we will find that those 3,500 calories burn up quickly. Also remember that muscle mass is a great calorie burner; higher-density muscles in your body (from walking instead of driving) burn calories much more efficiently than fat does.

How Is Weight Loss Accomplished?

Non-drug treatments

One of the big players in the OTC market is the herbal combination containing *ephedra* (*ma huang*). You may have seen it advertised as "herbal Phen/Fen." Ephedra is a plant that contains the active ingredient *ephedrine*, a central-nervous-system (CNS) stimulant. Like all CNS stimulants, ephedrine stimulates the heart and causes blood vessels to narrow, increasing blood pressure and heart rate.

Side effects and drug interactions of this herb should be taken VERY seriously. Ephedra may decrease the effectiveness of blood-pressure medications. When combined with some of the older antidepressant drugs, ephedra can cause a dramatic rise in blood pressure, increasing the risk of stroke. It also enhances the effects of other stimulant drugs (like *caffeine* and *pseudoephedrine*). Other common side effects are nervousness, headaches, insomnia, and heart palpitations. Scary, huh? It is so scary that the FDA has posted warnings on the sale of products in this combination. The FDA considers this an unapproved drug form.

Another natural product with fewer side effects is *L-carnitine* (*levocarnitine*), a form of the amino acid *carnitine*. It supposedly assists in the metabolism of fats, particularly during physiological stresses such as a prolonged fast. Excess fat is flushed out through the kidneys. Actual weight-loss results have been sketchy with use of this product.

The Drug Lady Recommends...

There is no escaping the simple truth that diet and exercise are the keys to attaining and maintaining a healthy weight. To lose weight you must burn more calories than your body takes in. Start with simple walking. Add some weekend bike-riding or swimming; tennis is also fun. ACTIVITY is the key. Stay away from couch-potato time in front of the TV and video games for a bit and see what's outside. Just say no to Chee-Tos!

Chromium picolinate is a trace element that promotes the activity of insulin and is a critical component of normal glucose metabolism at a dosage of 200 mcg daily. This element stimulates insulin activity, which helps metabolize glucose and fat. However, one study found that chromium picolinate supplements resulted in significant weight *gain* in subjects who did not exercise.

OTC treatments

For many years, the staple of the over-the-counter diet industry has been *phenylpropanolamine* (PPA). This ingredient was also found in some cough, cold, and allergy products. Recently, however, the FDA issued a public health warning on the possible increased risk of hemorrhagic stroke in women aged eighteen to forty-nine with use of PPA. While this is a relatively rare condition among young women, it is still of *very* serious concern. The FDA is taking steps to remove PPA from drug products and is asking drug companies to discontinue products with PPA in them.

There are other weight-loss products that work in a different way. ***Chitosan*** is a diet aid made from the crushed shells of shrimp, crab, and lobster. It purportedly works by binding with the fats that you eat and helping them out of your body before they have time to be absorbed. Unfortunately, this does nothing for the already-stored fat in your body. Those with a shellfish allergy, and pregnant or nursing women, should avoid this product. Side effects may include diarrhea and stomach cramps. Because this diet aid encourages fats and fat-soluble vitamins (like vitamins A, D, E, and K) out of the body before they have a chance to be absorbed, taking a multivitamin at least four hours before Chitosan is a good idea.

Prescription treatments

The older prescription medicines for weight loss generally focus on the appetite center of the brain, in the hypothalamus; with short-term use, they decrease the desire to eat. You take in fewer calories—the weight comes off. It is a gradual process, but effective for those whose increased weight can be detrimental to their health. Generally, weight-loss medications should only be prescribed for individuals who are clinically obese—that is, at least 30 percent over their recommended body weight, or 20 percent over their recommended body weight along with life-threatening conditions like high blood pressure, high cholesterol, or diabetes. Some names of drugs to discuss with your doctor are *Adipex-P* or *Ionamin* (*phentermine*), *Tenuate Dospan* (*diethylproprion*), and *Plegine, Bontril,* or *Adipost* (*phendimetrazine*).

Two of the newer prescription medications for weight loss are *Meridia* (*sibutramine*) and *Xenical* (*orlistat*). Meridia was approved in November of 1997 and belongs to a relatively new class of antiobesity drugs called neurotransmitter reuptake inhibitors. That's a lot of words, but what it means is that Meridia works by preventing the reabsorption (reuptake) of *serotonin* and *norepinephrine,* two brain chemicals involved in appetite control. Selective serotonin reuptake inhibitors (SSRIs), like the antidepressant *Prozac,* have been used effectively for years. Meridia is the only drug in this class used for obesity.

Xenical (*orlistat*) is the newest diet medication, approved in April of 1999. It is the first in a new class of drugs called lipase inhibitors. These prevent digestive enzymes from breaking down some dietary fat as it passes through the body. It can decrease fat absorption from food by 30 percent, but still won't affect the fat that is already present in your body. Before this drug, weight-loss medicines were focused only on decreasing appetite, but now this "magic pill" lets you eat terribly and still lose weight. Combining Xenical with diet modification and exercise, individuals lost an average of 5 to 10 percent of their body weight in one year. Would they have lost the same on diet modification and exercise alone? Probably.

Unfortunately, this drug also comes with some pretty unpleasant side effects. Because Xenical prevents fats from being absorbed, they must come out of the body. Side effects include oily spotting; flatulence accompanied by discharge; fatty and and oily stools; and an increased need and urgency to defecate. These side effects were reported in as many as 27 percent of test subjects, who typically experienced them from one to four weeks, although some were reported for as long as six months. Something else to remember—if you're taking Xenical, add a multivitamin with the oil-soluble *vitamins A, D, E, beta carotene,* and *K* to replace those that your body can't absorb from the fats that are quickly eliminated from the body.

Wrinkles

Q. *My friend has the most amazing skin! No wrinkles at all. She says she has a secret wrinkle cream that helps erase her laugh lines. What is this and could this be what I've been waiting for all my life?*

A. The fountain of youth in a tube? Not exactly, but the Food and Drug Administration has approved a medication to help reduce certain kinds of skin damage, such as fine wrinkles, spotty discolorations, and rough skin. There are also lots of choices on the OTC and natural medicine shelves, too. So keep on smiling, you've now got ammunition for those laugh lines!

What Causes Wrinkles?

Wrinkles are caused by a breakdown of collagen and elastin, the proteins that keep the skin smooth and soft. Some of the main causes of wrinkles are exposure to the sun (bad, bad!) and environmental pollutants like cigarette smoke or smog. Just getting older is another reason for those annoying wrinkles.

How Are Wrinkles Treated?

Non-drug treatments

Natural *vitamin A* (*retinol*) in cream form is speculated to have some of the same keratolytic (skin-sloughing) effects as its prescription counterpart, **Retin-A,** but studies aren't showing this to be true. While there is some decrease in wrinkle appearance with this natural treatment, it seems to be the moisturizing effect of the cream base that is helping and not the retinol.

Topical *vitamin C* has a double benefit of protecting the skin from damage as an **antioxidant** and promoting new collagen to help keep skin firm. Apply daily with your sunscreen *before* going out in the sun and alone on days when it's rainy outside.

OTC treatments

To give your skin a new start, look to the *alpha-hydroxy* acid creams, like **Alpha Hydrox.** These acids work by removing the top layer of skin in a keratolytic action. Once this skin is removed, the fresh, unwrinkled skin is exposed. You need to be aware that this skin is now very vulnerable to the sun and any other irritants. Keep it covered and well protected.

The Drug Lady Recommends . . .

Moisturize! Moisturize! Moisturize! There have even been stories of wrinkle-free ladies who use hemorrhoidal creams as their secret weapon against wrinkles. Well, there haven't been any studies on this, but the mineral oil and cocoa butter ointment base certainly make sense as good moisturizers. Moisturizers, like these and the OTC *Lubriderm,* are effective for hiding wrinkles. The effect is a "plumping up" of the skin and diminished lines.

Prescription treatments

The drug **Renova** (*tretinoin*) was the first to get the government's okay as a "wrinkle eraser." Renova works by preventing the breakdown of collagen and elastin. The active ingredient, *tretinoin,* is a *vitamin A* derivative. You'll also see *tretinoin* in the popular product **Retin-A.** Many people have been using Retin-A as a wrinkle remover, but the FDA doesn't approve of it for that use. Renova is a prescription cream that should be applied at night and washed off again in the morning. You should notice some effect in three to four months, with the most noticeable effects at about six months.

There are some side effects such as skin irritation, although some patients report red, peeling, or dry skin, while others notice a burning or stinging feeling. Renova can't be used by pregnant women, by those with a recent sunburn, or by individuals with eczema and other chronic skin conditions. A number of drugs, including several commonly used antibiotics (like *tetracycline*), can interact with the cream to make the skin supersensitive to sunlight. This is a condition called **photosensitivity.** Extreme burns can result in a very short amount of time. Keep it covered!

Renova doesn't remove deep wrinkles, and it's not a license to abuse your skin by exposing it to the sun's harmful UV rays. Still, for many men and women, Renova is proving successful in bringing back the look of "lost youth."

Appendix A

Family First-Aid Kit

NOW, FOR EVERY "Oh NO!," "Ouch!," or "Ow-WEE!," there is something to put on it. Antibiotic ointments for those bike mishaps, anti-itch creams for when the gardener finds a new ant nest, *aloe* with *lidocaine* to numb a burn from grabbing a hot pot without thinking. Every home has its share of accidents, and with the "Family First-Aid Kit" you'll always be prepared "just in case."

Mishaps don't always occur when it is convenient to make a trip to the drugstore to pick up those extra **Band-Aids.** Be prepared. I know the Boy Scouts already have that motto, but it's a good one: Be prepared—a few minutes spent putting this kit together and storing it in a safe place will be well rewarded once you hear that dreaded *"Owwwww!!!"*

Bottom-shelf products (or those to keep very close by)

- thermometer
- tweezers
- **Band-Aids** (all shapes and sizes)
- antibiotic cream or ointment (like **Polysporin**)
- anti-itch cream (like *hydrocortisone*)
- burn-relief gels or sprays (like *aloe* with *lidocaine*)
- **Robitussin DM** (dextromethorphan and guaifenesin) for coughs
- **Tylenol** (*acetominophen*) for aches and pains

Middle-shelf products (not always needed for everyday use)

▦ elastic or "Ace" bandage

▦ hot/cold packs

▦ insect repellent

▦ sunscreen

▦ laxative or stool softener (*docusate sodium*)

▦ antihistamine (like **Benadryl**)

▦ decongestant (like *pseudoephedrine*)

▦ anti-diarrheal medicine (like **Imodium-AD**)

▦ day and night cough/cold/flu medicine (like **Dayquil** and **Nyquil**)

▦ anti-nausea (like **Emetrol**)

▦ antacid (like **Tums** or **Mylanta**)

Top-shelf products (hopefully these will just collect dust)

▦ rolls of gauze bandages and pads

▦ first-aid tape

▦ scissors

▦ sling

▦ splint

▦ first-aid guide

▦ moleskin

▦ alcohol pads

Appendix B

New Baby First-Aid Kit

YOU'RE GETTING READY—checking everything twice, then going back and checking it again. Be sure to have the "New Baby First-Aid Kit" together for those "just in cases." Keeping these items on hand ensures that your new little one will be taken care of. Also, now Dad will have a **Band-Aid** handy when he nicks his finger preparing a bottle for a 3 A.M. feeding.

- acetaminophen infant suppositories (like **FeverAll**) for fevers
- **Infants' Tylenol Drops** (*acetaminophen*) for fevers and pain
- ipecac syrup
- infant dosing syringes
- rectal or ear thermometer
- **Vaseline** for rectal thermometer
- bulb syringe
- **A & D ointment** (for diaper rash)
- **Infants' Mylican Drops** (for gas)
- alcohol pads
- antibiotic ointment (like **Polysporin**)
- baby **Band-Aids**
- three-by-five index cards with emergency numbers (these are great to give new grandparents, too): Poison Control Center, baby's pediatrician, taxi, emergency contacts, etc.

These make great baby-shower gifts, too. Just tuck all of these items in a cute basket and include a copy of this book—the book part is absolutely necessary. Be prepared for oohs and ahs from the mom-to-be, because you'll have brought the BEST present!

Glossary

Making Sense of "Pharmacy-Speak"

acupressure—The stimulation of the body's nerve pathways by use of pressure on certain meridian areas.

allergen—The culprit behind an allergic reaction; it can be dust, animal dander, or pollen.

allergic conjunctivitis—Itching or redness of the eye, caused by allergies. The eyes become inflamed, teary, and red.

allergic rhinitis—Also known as hay fever, allergic rhinitis is an inflammation of the nasal passages.

allergy—The body's reaction to an allergen or substance that it perceives to be a threat. Symptoms may include sneezes, hives, watery eyes, and runny nose.

alopecia—The absence or loss of hair on the body, especially on the head.

anaphylactic shock—A serious or life-threatening allergic reaction.

angioedema—Similar to hives; typically affects larger areas of the body.

anorexia—A loss of appetite, or the eating disorder anorexia nervosa, when a person refuses to eat based on their body image.

antihistamine—A substance that blocks the body's allergic reaction to histamine; it drys up the drips.

antioxidants—Agents that protect the body against the damaging effects of free radicals, including lutein, vitamin C, grape seed, and vitamin E.

antiperspirant—Slows down the production of perspiration.

antipyretic—Medication that lowers a fever; includes *acetaminophen* and aspirin.

aphthous ulcer—Canker sore.

apocrine glands—Sweat glands that open into hair follicles in the groin area and under the arms; these appear after puberty.

aromatherapy—The use of fragrant oils or other liquids to affect or alter moods.

astringent—An agent that constricts and drys up tissues.

atherosclerosis—A type of hardening of the arteries (arteriosclerosis) due to the buildup of fatty plaques.

atopic dermatitis—A skin rash of unknown origin; it may be traced to allergic, hereditary, or emotional reactions.

attention-deficit disorder (ADD)—A condition that is characterized by an unusually short attention span.

attention-deficit/hyperactivity disorder (ADHD)—Attention-deficit disorder accompanied by inappropriate hyperactivity.

bilirubin—A yellowish bile pigment formed from the breakdown of hemoglobin in red blood cells. Normally processed and eliminated by the liver, high levels of this in the blood are an indicator for jaundice.

bulimia—An eating disorder characterized by overeating, followed by forced vomiting; also referred to as "binge and purge."

cataracts—A foggy, opaque area on the lens or capsule of the eye.

cerumen—Earwax.

chronic fatigue syndrome—A condition whose cause is unknown; typical symptoms include weakness and extreme fatigue.

chronic obstructive pulmonary disease—A progressive condition in which the lungs lose their ability to function normally.

cluster headache—A recurring headache where the pain is clustered around the eye and radiates down the jaw and chin.

cold—An infection by the rhinovirus, resulting in possible fever, sore throat, runny nose, stuffed nose, or cough.

conjunctivitis—Infection or inflammation of the membrane covering the eyeball surface.

cough suppressant—A medication that controls the cough reflex, like dextromethorphan or codeine; used for dry coughs or those that are disruptive to sleep or other activities.

decongestant—The substance that narrows blood vessels to decrease inflammation during an allergy or a cold; it unstuffs stuffed noses.

dental fluorosis—A mottling, or white spots, on tooth enamel caused by too much fluoride.

dermabrasion—The process of removing scars or wrinkles by taking off the top layers of skin with a sandpaperlike device.

dermatitis—Itching and inflammation of the skin caused by an irritant.

diabetic retinopathy—Damage to the retina of the eye brought on as a complication of diabetes.

earwax—Also called **cerumen**—an accumulation of brown, waxy secretions found in the external ear canal.

eccrine glands—Sweat glands located all over the skin surface; these are responsible for regulating proper body temperature.

electrocardiogram (EKG)—Records the electrical activity of the heart; important for diagnosis of heart conditions.

electroencephalogram (EEG)—Records the electrical activity of the brain; important for diagnosis of strokes or other brain disorders.

embolic stroke—A hemorrhage of a blood vessel in the brain due to a blockage by a blood clot or foreign substance that travels from another part of the body.

eustachian tubes—The 3–4 cm tube that connects the middle ear to the pharynx. A swelling or blockage of this tube is the culprit for most ear infections.

expectorant—A mucus-thinning agent, like guaifenesin or water; helps make coughs more productive.

flu (influenza)—A respiratory infection caused by a strain of the influenza virus; symptoms generally include fever, aches, chills, headache, cough, and sore throat.

glaucoma—A condition of increased pressure within the eye that causes damage to the optic nerve.

glomerulonephritis—An inflammation of the kidneys that can appear secondary to a strep infection.

halitosis—Bad breath.

hemorrhagic stroke—A burst blood vessel in the brain, possibly due to high blood pressure, infection, or the use of stimulant drugs.

hirsutism—Excessive hair growth.

histamine—The agent responsible for many different types of allergic reactions.

hives—A skin allergy, caused by many different things including insect bites and stress.

homeopathy—A type of therapy that is thought to be effective in treating certain disorders. The disorder is treated with very small doses of substances that simulate the actual symptoms of the disorder.

hyperhidrosis—Excessive sweating.

hyperopia—Farsightedness.

Kegel exercises—Used to strengthen the perineal muscles in women, which help control incontinence, and are used in childbirth and as an aid for greater sexual enjoyment.

keloids—Thick, raised scar formations after skin trauma that are unusually large for the area damaged.

keratoconjunctivitis sicca—Dry eyes due to blocked or malfunctioning tear ducts.

lactose intolerance—The inability of the body to process lactose, found in dairy products.

latex allergy—A severe allergic reaction to the proteins found in latex products.

macula—A spot or small colored area about $\frac{1}{16}$ of an inch in diameter located in the center of the retina. This area controls the central point of vision.

mammogram—A low-grade X ray of the breast, used for early detection of cancer or precancerous conditions.

migraine headache—A common type of headache caused by an abnormal sensitivity of the surrounding arteries.

motion sickness—a feeling of nausea (it may or may not be accompanied by vomiting) that is directly related to and caused by irregular movements, such as on a boat or on a plane.

myopia—Nearsightedness.

nebulizer—A device used to administer various medications via the nose. The nebulizer produces a mist of medication for easy inhalation.

neurologist—A specialist in diseases of the nervous system.

non-productive cough—A dry, hacking cough that is not accompanied by mucus.

non-steroidal anti-inflammatory drugs (NSAIDS)—Treatment used to treat mild to moderate pain and inflammation; medications include *ibuprofen, ketoprofen, naproxen,* and *diclofenac.*

onychomycosis—Disease of the nail caused by a fungus.

osteoarthritis—A degenerative disease of the joints, characterized by a decrease in cartilage.

otitis externa—Also known as **swimmer's ear**—characterized by inflammation, infection, and itching within the outer (external) ear canal that leads from the outside to the eardrum.

otitis media—Infection associated with an inflammation of the middle ear.

overflow incontinence—Spillage that occurs when the body produces more urine than the bladder can hold.

peak-flow meter—A handheld device that can be used by asthmatic patients to measure their air flow.

pessary—A device inserted into the vagina to serve as support for the uterus.

photosensitivity—Unusual sensitivity to the sun, resulting in burns or inflammation.

phototherapy—Also known as bililights; a treatment using blue lights to help break down **bilirubin** so that the body can more easily process it.

phytoestrogens—Plant-based products, like soy and black cohosh, that have mild estrogenic activity.

pink eye—Bacterial conjunctivitis, also the infection or inflammation of the membrane covering the eyeball.

post-herpetic neuralgia (PHN)—Pain along the path of a nerve; often located in an area where shingles has occurred.

presbyopia—Vision loss of near objects that typically occurs with aging. This condition may require reading glasses to see small print or details.

probiotics—"Good" bacteria replacements.

prostaglandins—Very active chemicals in the body that (among other duties) influence the body's response to pain and inflammation.

Reye's syndrome—A life-threatening condition involving the brain and liver of children between the ages of 4 and 15 and typically appearing suddenly after a viral infection like the flu or chickenpox. Has been closely related to aspirin given during that infection.

rheumatic fever—An inflammatory disease with fever that is caused by a prior infection by Group A strep.

rheumatoid arthritis—An inflammatory autoimmune disease that usually affects the joints.

rhinitis medicamentosa—An acute inflammation of the nasal passages brought on by overuse of nasal decongestants.

sclerotherapy—The injection of an irritating liquid into a vein, causing it to collapse; this forces the other veins to compensate. Commonly used to treat varicose veins.

seborrheic dermatitis—A condition where there is a flaking or scaling of the skin. It can affect many parts of the body; if it affects the scalp of an infant, it is called "cradle cap."

shock—Occurs when there is a problem with, or lack of, blood flow through the body. The reduced blood flow can cause low blood pressure or other serious conditions.

sinus headache—Headache that is caused by the swelling or inflammation of the sinus cavities behind the eyes.

sinusitis—Inflammation or infection of the sinus cavities.

sitz bath—A basin that holds just enough water to cover the hips up to the middle of the abdomen. Sitting in this bath increases blood flow to the pelvic areas and eases inflammation or discomfort.

SLE (systemic lupus erythematosus)—From the Latin word for wolf—lupus is a chronic inflammatory disease that involves the joints, skin, mucus, membranes, and nervous system.

sprain—Injury around a joint, usually attributed to damage or injury of the muscles, tendons, or ligaments.

strain—Muscular damage, usually resulting from excess physical activity.

strep throat—Bacterial infection of the throat caused by the red-blood-cell–destroying *streptococcus* strain.

stress incontinence—The inability to hold urine, with or without an urge to go; most commonly seen while laughing or engaging in strenuous activity.

sweatproof—Refers to products, like sunscreens, that adhere to the skin and block the action of pores.

swimmer's ear—See **otitis externa.**

tension headache—Headache caused by tightening muscles in the head area.

thrombolytic stroke—Rupture of a blood vessel in the brain by the obstruction of a stationary clot or a thrombus.

urge incontinence—A sudden need to urinate without sufficient time to make it to the bathroom.

urticaria—See **hives.**

urushiol—Irritant oil found in poison ivy, oak, and sumac that adheres to the skin and causes an allergic reaction.

waterproof—Refers to products, like sunscreens and bug sprays, that adhere to skin even after eighty minutes in the water.

water-resistant—Refers to products, like sunscreens and bug sprays, that adhere to skin for up to forty minutes in the water.

xerophthalmia—An eye condition in which a deficiency of vitamin A or chronic eye irritation causes dryness and a hardening of the skin around the eye.

Resources

Where to Go for Additional Information

Aches and Pains

National Headache Foundation
428 West St. James Place
Chicago, IL 60614-2750
1-888-643-5552
www.headaches.org

Arthritis Foundation
1-800-283-7800
www.arthritis.org

American Chronic Pain Association
PO Box 850
Rocklin, CA 95677
1-916-632-0922
www.theacpa.org

Allergies and Asthma

Asthma and Allergy Foundation of America
1-800-7ASTHMA (1-800-727-8462)
www.aafa.org

Allergy and Asthma Network / Mothers of Asthmatics, Inc
2751 Prosperity Ave., Suite 150
Fairfax, VA 22031
1-800-878-4403
www.aanma.org

Children's Health

Children and Adults with Attention-Deficit/Hyperactivity Disorder
8181 Professional Place, Suite 201
Landover, MD 20785
1-800-233-4050
www.chadd.org

Aging

Administration on Aging
330 Independence Avenue SW
Washington, DC 20201
800-438-4380 (information about
  Alzheimer's disease); 800-222-
  2225 (information about other
  publications); 202-619-7501
  (National Aging Information
  Center); 202-401-7575 (TDD)
www.aoa.gov

**American Association of Retired
People**
601 E Street NW
Washington, DC 20049
800-424-3410; 202-434-2277
www.aarp.org

National Council of Senior Citizens
8403 Colesville Road, Suite 1200
Silver Spring, MD 20910-3314
301-578-8800
www.ncscinc.org

National Council on the Aging
409 Third Street SW
Washington, DC 20024
800-867-2755; 202-479-1200;
  202-479-6674 (TDD)
e-mail: info@ncoa.org
www.ncoa.org

National Institute on Aging
Public Information Office
Building 31, Room 5C27
31 Center Drive, MSC 2992
Bethesda, MD 20892-2292
800-222-2225; 800-222-4225
  (TTY); 301-496-1752
www.nih.gov/nia

Older Women's League
666 11th Street NW, Suite 700
Washington, DC 20001
800-825-3695; 202-783-6686

AIDS

AIDS Action Council
1875 Connecticut Avenue NW, 700
Washington, DC 20009
202-986-1300

**The American Foundation for AIDS
Research**
120 Wall Street, 13th Floor
New York, NY 10005
212-806-1600
www.amfar.org

CDC National AIDS/HIV Hotline
800-342-AIDS (800-342-2437)

Gay Men's Health Crisis
119 West 24th Street
New York, NY 10011
212-367-1111 (Development);
  212-367-1030 (Volunteer)
noah.cuny.edu/providers/
  gmhc.html

National Association for People with Aids
1413 K Street NW, 7th Floor
Washington, DC 20005
202-898-0414
www.napwa.org

Universal Fellowship of Metropolitan Community Churches AIDS Ministry
5300 Santa Monica Boulevard,
 Suite 304
Los Angeles, CA 90029
213-464-5100
e-mail: ufmcchq@aol.com

Women Alive
1566 Burnside Avenue
Los Angeles, CA 90019
323-965-1564
e-mail: info@women-alive.org
www.women-alive.org

Alcoholism

Al-Anon Family Group Headquarters
1600 Corporate Landing Parkway
Virginia Beach, VA 23454-5617
888-4AL-ANON (888-425-4666)
www.al-anon.alateen.org

Alcoholics Anonymous
475 Riverside Drive
New York, NY 10015
212-870-3400
www.alcoholics-anonymous.org

Allergy and Asthma

Allergy and Asthma Network/ Mothers of Asthmatics, Inc.
2751 Prosperity Avenue, Suite 150
Fairfax, VA 22031
800-878-4403; 703-641-9595
www.aanma.org

Asthma and Allergy Foundation of America
1233 20th Street NW, Suite 402
Washington, DC 20036
800-7ASTHMA (800-727-8462);
 202-466-7643
e-mail: info@aafa.org
www.aafa.org

Alzheimer's Disease

Alzheimer's Disease and Related Disorders
919 North Michigan Avenue,
 Suite 1000
Chicago, IL 60611-1676
800-272-3900; 312-335-8700
www.alz.org

Alzheimer's Disease Education and Referral Center
PO Box 8250
Silver Spring, MD 20907-8250
800-438-4380
e-mail: adear@alzheimers.org
www.alzheimers.org

Amyotrophic Lateral Sclerosis

The ALS Association
National Office
27001 Agoura Road, Suite 150
Calabasas Hills, CA 91301-5104
800-782-4747 (patients only);
  818-880-9007
www.alsa.org

Ankylosing Spondylitis

Spondylitis Association of America
PO Box 5872
Sherman Oaks, CA 91413
800-777-8189
www.spondylitis.org

Arthritis

Arthritis Foundation
1330 West Peachtree Street
Atlanta, GA 30309
800-283-7800; 404-872-7100
www.arthritis.org

Attention Deficit Disorder

Children and Adults with Attention-Deficit/Hyperactivity Disorder
8181 Professional Place, Suite 201
Landover, MD 20785
800-233-4050; 301-306-7070
www.chadd.org

Learning Disabilities Association
4156 Library Road
Pittsburgh, PA 15234-1349
412-341-1515
www.ldanatl.org

National Attention Deficit Disorder Association
1788 Second Street, Suite 200
Highland Park, IL 60035
847-432-ADDA (847-432-2332)
e-mail: mail@add.org
www.add.org

Autism

Autism Society of America
7910 Woodmont Avenue, Suite 300
Bethesda, MD 20814-3015
800-3AUTISM (800-328-8476),
  x150; 301-657-0881
www.autism-society.org

National Autism Hotline/Autism Services Center
605 Ninth Street
Pritchard Building
PO Box 507
Huntington, WV 25710-0507
304-525-8014

Balding

National Alopecia Areata
Foundation
710 C Street, Suite 11
San Rafael, CA 94901
415-456-4644
e-mail: naaf@compuserve.com

Birth Defects

Association of Birth Defect Children
930 Woodcock Road, Suite 225
Orlando, FL 32803
800-313-ABDC (800-313-2232);
   407-245-7035
e-mail: abdc@birthdefects.org
www.birthdefects.org

Federation for Children with Special
Needs
1135 Tremont Street, Suite 420
Boston, MA 02120
800-331-0688 (in MA);
   617-236-7210
e-mail: fcsninfo@fcsn.org
www.fcsn.org

March of Dimes/Birth Defects
Foundation
1275 Mamaroneck Avenue
White Plains, NY 10605
888-663-4637; 914-428-7100
e-mail: resources@modimes.org
http://www.modimes.org

Blindness and Vision Problems

American Association of the Deaf-
Blind
814 Thayer Avenue
Silver Springs, MD 20910
800-735-2258; 301-588-6545
  (TTY)

American Council of the Blind
1155 15th Street NW, Suite 1004
Washington, DC 20005
800-424-8666; 202-467-5081
www.acb.org

American Foundation for the Blind
11 Penn Plaza, Suite 300
New York, NY 10001
800-232-5463; 212-502-7600
e-mail: afbinfo@afb.net
www.igc.org/afb

Association for the Education and
Rehabilitation of the Blind and
Visually Impaired
4600 Duke Streeet, Suite 430
PO Box 22397
Alexandria, VA 22304
703-823-9690
www.aerbvi.org

Association for Macular Diseases
210 East 64th Street
New York, NY 10021
212-605-3719

The Foundation Fighting Blindness
Executive Plaza 1, Suite 800
11350 McCormick Road
Hunt Valley, MD 21031-1014
1-888-FYI-EYES (888-394-3937);
    800-683-5551 (TTD); 410-785-
    1414; 410-785-9687 (TTD)
www.blindness.org

Glaucoma Research Foundation
200 Pine Street, Suite 200
San Francisco, CA 94104
800-826-6693; 415-986-3163
www.glaucoma.org

**National Association for Visually
Handicapped**
22 West 21st Street, 6th Floor
New York, NY 10010
212-889-3141
www.navh.org

**National Family Association for
Deaf-Blind**
111 Middle Neck Road
Sands Point, NY 11050
800-255-0411, ext. 275; 516-944-
    8637 (TTY)

Prevent Blindness America
500 East Remington Road
Schaumburg, IL 60173
800-331-2020; 847-843-2020
e-mail: info@preventblindness.org
www.preventblindness.org

Blood Disorders

Cooley's Anemia Foundation
129-09 26th Avenue
Flushing, NY 11354
800-522-7222; 718-321-CURE
    (718-321-2873)
www.thalassemia.org

Leukemia Society of America
600 Third Avenue
New York, NY 10016
800-955-4LSA (800-955-4572);
    212-573-8484
www.leukemia.org

**Sickle Cell Disease Association of
America**
200 Corporate Pointe, Suite 495
Culver City, CA 90230-8727
800-421-8453; 310-216-6363
www.SickleCellDisease.org

National Hemophilia Foundation
116 West 32nd Street, 11th Floor
New York, NY 10001
800-424-2634; 212-328-3700
www.infonhf.org

Brain Cancer

American Brain Tumor Association
2720 River Road
Des Plains, IL 60018
800-886-2282; 847-827-9910
e-mail: info@abta.org
www.abta.org

**Brain Tumor Foundation
for Children**
2231 Perimeter Park Drive, Suite 9
Atlanta, GA 30341
770-458-5554

Brain Tumor Hotline
University of Chicago
5841 South Maryland Avenue,
    Room J331
Chicago, IL 60637-1470
800-824-0040; 773-834-3000

Brain Tumor Society
124 Watertown Street, Suite 3-H
Watertown, MA 02472
800-770-8287; 617-924-9997
e-mail: info@tbts.org
www.tbts.org

**The Children's Brain Tumor
Foundation**
274 Madison Avenue, Suite 1301
New York, NY 10016
212-448-9494

National Brain Tumor Foundation
414 Thirteenth Street, Suite 700
Oakland, CA 94612-2603
785 Market Street, Suite 1600
San Francisco, CA 94103
800-934-CURE (800-934-2873);
    510-839-9777
e-mail: nbtf@braintumor.org
www.braintumor.org

**Pituitary Tumor Network
Association**
PO Box 1958
Thousand Oaks, CA 91358
800-642-9211; 805-499-2262
www.pituitary.com

Breast Cancer

**National Alliance of Breast Cancer
Organizations**
9 East 37th Street, 10th Floor
New York, NY 10016
800-719-9154; 212-889-0606
www.nabco.org

**The Susan G. Komen Breast Cancer
Foundation**
National Headquarters
5005 LBJ Freeway, Suite 370
Dallas, TX 75244
800-I'M AWARE (800-462-9273);
    972-855-1600
www.komen.org

**Y-ME National Breast Cancer
Organization**
212 West Van Buren Street
Chicago, IL 60607-3908
800-221-2141; 800-986-9505
    (Spanish)
e-mail: help@y-me.org
www.y-me.org

Cancer General

American Cancer Society
1599 Clifton Road NE
Atlanta, GA 30329-4251
800-227-2345; 404-320-3333
www.cancer.org

Cancer Care, Inc.
275 7th Avenue
New York, NY 10001
800-813-HOPE (800-813-4673);
    212-302-2400
e-mail: info@cancercare.org
www.cancercareinc.org

National Cancer Institute
NCI Public Inquiries Office
Building 31, Room 10A03
31 Center Drive, MSC 2580
Bethesda, MD 20892-2580
800-4-CANCER (800-422-6237);
    800-332-8615 (TTY); 301-435-
    3848
www.nci.nih.gov

**National Coalition for Cancer
Survivorship**
1010 Wayne Avenue, Suite 505
Silver Spring, MD 20910-5600
877-622-7937
www.cansearch.org

**Patient Advocates for Advanced
Cancer Treatments**
PO Box 141695
Grand Rapids, MI 49514-1695
616-453-1477

Cardiovascular Disorders (heart, lungs, and blood vessels)

American Heart Association
7272 Greenville Avenue
Dallas, TX 75231-4596
800-AHA-USA1 (800-242-8721);
    888-MY-HEART (888-694-3278,
    for women's health information)
www.americanheart.org

Coronary Club
9500 Euclid Avenue, A42
Cleveland, OH 44195
800-478-4255; 216-444-3690

**National Heart, Lung, and Blood
Institute**
PO Box 30105
Bethesda, MD 20824-0105
800-575-WELL (800-575-9355);
    301-592-8573 (information cen-
    ter)
www.nhlbi.nih.gov

Cerebral Palsy

**United Cerebral Palsy Associations,
Inc.**
1660 L Street NW, Suite 700
Washington, DC 20036
800-872-5827; 202-776-0406;
    202-973-7197 (TTY)
e-mail: ucpnatl@ucpa.org
www.ucpa.org

Childbirth/Pregnancy

America's Crisis Pregnancy Helpline
2121 Valley View Lane
Dallas, TX 75234
888-4OPTIONS (888-467-8466);
  972-241-2229
e-mail: acph@dallas.net
www.thehelpline.org

Maternity Center Association
281 Park Avenue South, 5th Floor
New York, NY 10010
212-777-5000
www.maternity.org

**The National Coalition for Birthing
Alternatives**
4755 West Avenue, L-13
Quartz Hill, CA 93536
e-mail: troy@mmcable.com
home.mmcable.com/birthingop-
  tions/

Cleft Palate

**American Cleft Palate-Craniofacial
Assocation and Cleft Palate
Foundation**
104 South Estes Drive, Suite 204
Chapel Hill, NC 27514
800-24-CLEFT (800-242-5338);
  919-933-9044
e-mail: cleftline@aol.com
www.cleft.com

Wide Smiles
PO Box 5153
Stockton, CA 95205-0153
209-942-2812
e-mail: info@widesmiles.org
www.widesmiles.org

Cystic Fibrosis

National Cystic Fibrosis Foundation
6931 Arlington Road
Bethesda, MD 20814
800-344-4823; 301-951-4422
www.cff.org

Deafness and Hearing Disorders

**Alexander Graham Bell Association
for the Deaf and Hard of Hearing**
3417 Volta Place NW
Washington, DC 20007-2778
800-432-7543; 202-337-5220
  (Voice); 202-337-5221 (TTY)
e-mail: agbell2@aol.com
www.agbell.org

**American Association of the Deaf-
Blind**
814 Thayer Avenue, Suite 302
Silver Spring, MD 20910
800-735-2258; 301-588-6545
  (TTY)

American Society for Deaf Children
PO Box 3355
Gettysburg, PA 17325
800-942-ASDC (800-942-2732);
   717-334-7922 (Voice/TTY)
e-mail: asdc l@aol.com
www.deafchildren.org

American Tinnitus Association
PO Box 5
Portland, OR 97207-0005
800-634-8978
e-mail: tinnitus@ata.org
www.ata.org

**Helen Keller National Center for
Deaf-Blind Youths and Adults**
111 Middle Neck Road
Sands Point, NY 11050
800-255-0411; 516-944-8900;
   516-944-8637 (TTY)
www.helenkeller.org

National Association of the Deaf
814 Thayer Avenue
Silver Spring, MD 20910
301-587-1788; 301-587-1789 (TTY)
www.nad.org

**National Deaf Education Network
and Clearinghouse**
Gallaudet University
800 Florida Avenue NE
Washington, DC 20002-3695
202-651-5051; 202-651-5052 (TTY)
e-mail: Clearinghouse.Infotogo@
   gallaudet.edu
www.gallaudet.edu/~nicd

Death and Bereavement

**AMEND (Aiding a Mother
Experiencing Neonatal Death)**
4324 Berrywick Terrace
St. Louis, MO 63128
314-487-7582; 203-746-6518

Choice in Dying
1035 30th Street NW
Washington, DC 20007
800-989-9455; 202-338-9790
e-mail: cid@choices.org
www.choices.org

**Compassionate Friends, National
Headquarters**
PO Box 3696
Oak Brook, IL 60522-3696
630-990-0010
www.compassionatefriends.org

Compassion in Dying Federation
PMB 415, 6312 SW Capitol High-
   way
Portland, Oregon 97201
503-221-9556
e-mail: info@compassionindying.
   org
www.compassionindying.org

Death with Dignity National Center
1818 N Street NW, Suite 450
Washington, DC 20036
202-530-2900
e-mail: info@deathwithdignity.org
www.deathwithdignity.org

Dying Well Network
PO Box 880
Spokane, WA 99210-0880
509-926-2457
e-mail: Rob.Neils@on-ramp.
  ior.com
www.ior.com/~jeffw/homepage.
  htm

Hemlock Society
PO Box 101810
Denver CO 80250-1810
800-247-7421
e-mail: hemlock@privatei.com
www.hemlock.org

Hospice Education Institute
190 Westbrook Road
Essex, CT 06426-1510
800-331-1620; 860-767-1620
e-mail: hospiceall@aol.com
www.hospiceworld.org

National Hospice and Palliative Care Organization
1700 Diagonal Road, Suite 300
Alexandria, VA 22314
703-243-5900
www.nho.org

Depression

National Depressive and Manic-Depressive Association
730 North Franklin Street, Suite
  501
Chicago, IL 60610-3526
800-826-3632; 312-642-0049
e-mail: nbunch@ndmda.org
www.ndmda.org

Recovery, Inc.
802 North Dearborn Street
Chicago, IL 60610
312-337-5661
www.recovery-inc.com

Diabetes

American Diabetes Association
1701 North Beauregard Street
Alexandria, VA 22311
800-DIABETES (800-232-3472);
  800-342-2383
www.diabetes.org

Juvenile Diabetes Foundation International
120 Wall Street
New York, NY 10005
800-533-2873; 212-785-9500
www.jdf.org

National Diabetes Information Clearinghouse
National Institute of Diabetes and
 Digestive and Kidney Diseases
One Information Way
Bethesda, MD 20892-3560
301-654-3327
e-mail: ndic@info.niddk.nih.gov
www.niddk.nih.gov/health/dia-
 betes/ndic.htm

Digestive Disorders

Crohn's and Colitis Foundation of America
386 Park Avenue South, 17th Floor
New York, NY 10016-8804
800-932-2423; 212-685-3440
e-mail: info@ccfa.org
www.ccfa.org

Digestive Disease National Coalition
507 Capitol Court NE, Suite 200
Washington, DC 20002
202-544-7497

Intestinal Disease Foundation
1323 Forbes Avenue, Suite 200
Pittsburgh, PA 15219
412-261-5888

National Digestive Diseases Information Clearinghouse
National Institute of Diabetes and
 Digestive and Kidney Diseases
Two Information Way
Bethesda, MD 20892-3570
301-654-3810
e-mail: nddic@info.niddk.nih.gov
www.niddk.nih.gov/health/di-
 gest/nddic.htm

United Ostomy Association
36 Executive Park, Suite 120
Irvine, CA 92612-2405
800-826-0826; 949-660-8624
e-mail: uoa@deltanet.com
www.uoa.org

Disabilities and Rehabilitation

Disabled American Veterans
National Headquarters
PO Box 14301
Cincinnati, OH 45250-0301
606-441-7300
www.dav.org

Fedcap Rehabilitation Services
211 West 14th Street
New York, NY 10011-7157
212-727-4200

National Easter Seal Society
230 West Monroe Street, Suite
   1800
Chicago, IL 60606
800-221-6827; 312-726-6200;
   312-726-4258 (TDD)
e-mail: info@easter-seals.org
www.easter-seals.org

National Organization on Disability
910 16th Street NW
Washington, DC 20006
202-293-5960; 202-293-5868
   (TDD)
e-mail: ability@nod.org
www.nod.org

**National Rehabilitation
Information Center**
1010 Wayne Avenue, Suite 800
Silver Spring, MD 20910
800-346-2742; 301-562-2400;
   301-495-5626 (TTY)
www.naric.com

National Rehabilitation Association
633 South Washington Street
Alexandria, VA 22314
703-836-0850; 703-836-0849
   (TDD)
www.nationalrehab.org

Paralyzed Veterans of America
801 18th Street NW
Washington, DC 20006
800-424-8200; 800-232-1782
   (hot line)
www.pva.org

**People-to-People Committee for the
Handicapped**
PO Box 18131
Washington, DC 20036
301-774-7446

Down Syndrome

**Association for Children with Down
Syndrome**
2616 Martin Avenue
Bellmore, NY 11710-3196
516-221-4700
www.acds.org

National Down Syndrome Congress
7000 Peachtree-Dunwoody Road
   NE
Lake Ridge 400 Office Park
Building 5, Suite 100
Atlanta, GA 30328
800-232-6372; 770-604-9500
e-mail: ndsccenter@aol.com
www.ndsccenter.org

National Down Syndrome Society
666 Broadway
New York, NY 10012
800-221-4602 (hot line);
   212-460-9330
www.ndss.org

**Parent Assistance Committee on
Down Syndrome**
208 Lafayette Avenue
Peekskill, NY 10566
914-739-4085

Drug Abuse

Cocaine Anonymous World Services
PO Box 2000
Los Angeles, CA 90049-8000
800-347-8998; 310-559-5833
e-mail: publicinfo@ca.org
www.ca.org

Substance Abuse and Mental Health Services Administration
Parklawn Building, Room 12-105
5600 Fishers Lane
Rockville, MD 20857
800-729-6686; 877-767-8432
   (Spanish); 301-443-4795
www.samhsa.gov

Hazelden Foundation
PO Box 11, CO 3
Center City, MN 55012-0011
800-257-7810; 651-213-4000
e-mail: info@hazelden.org
www.hazelden.org

Narcotics Anonymous World Services
PO Box 9999
Van Nuys, CA 91409
818-773-9999
www.na.org

Eating Disorders

The American Anorexia/Bulimia Association, Inc.
165 West 46th Street, Suite 1108
New York, NY 10036
212-575-6200
www.aabainc.org

Eating Disorders Awareness and Prevention, Inc.
603 Stewart Street, Suite 803
Seattle, WA 98101
206-382-3587; 800-931-2237
www.edap.org

Overeaters Anonymous
6075 Zenith Court NE
Rio Rancho, NM 87124
505-891-2664
www.OvereatersAnonymous.org

Endocrine Disorders

National Adrenal Diseases Foundation
505 Northern Boulevard
Great Neck, NY 11021
516-487-4992
e-mail: nadfmail@aol.com
www.medhelp.org/nadf

National Cushing's Association
4620½ Van Nuys Boulevard
Sherman Oaks, CA 91403
818-788-9235; 818-788-9239

Thyroid Foundation of America
Ruth Sleeper Hall, Room RSL 350
40 Parkman Street
Boston, MA 02114
800-832-8321; 617-726-8500
e-mail: tfa@clark.net
www.clark.net/pub/tfa

Epilepsy

Epilepsy Foundation of America
4351 Garden City Drive
Landover, MD 20785
800-332-1000; 301-459-3700
www.efa.org

Family Planning

**Association for Voluntary Surgical
Contraception (AVSC) International**
440 Ninth Avenue
New York, NY 10001
212-561-8000

**Planned Parenthood Federation of
America**
810 Seventh Avenue
New York, NY 10019
212-541-7800
www.plannedparenthood.org

Headache

**American Council for Headache
Education**
19 Mantua Road
Mt. Royal, NJ 08061
800-255-ACHE (800-255-2243);
  856-423-0258
e-mail: achehq@talley.com
www.achenet.org

National Headache Foundation
428 West St. James Place, 2nd Floor
Chicago, IL 60614-2750
888-643-5552; 312-388-6399
www.headaches.org

Hemochromatosis

Hemochromatosis Foundation, Inc.
PO Box 8569
Albany, NY 12208
518-489-0972

Iron Overload Diseases Association
433 Westwind Drive
North Palm Beach, FL 33408-5123
561-840-8512; 561-840-8513
e-mail: iod@ironoverload.org
www.ironoverload.org

Home Care

National Association for Home Care
228 Seventh Street SE
Washington, DC 20003
202-547-7424
www.nahc.org

Impotence

Impotents Anonymous
119 South Ruth Street
Maryville, TN 37803-5746
615-983-6092

Incontinence

National Assocation for Continence
PO Box 8310
2650 East Main Street
Spartanburg, SC 29305-8310
800-BLADDER (800-252-3337);
  864-579-7900
www.nafc.org

The Simon Foundation for Continence
PO Box 835
Wilmette, IL 60091
800-23-SIMON (800-237-4666);
  847-864-3913

Infertility

Ferre Institute, Inc.
258 Genesee Street, Suite 302
Utica, NY 13502
315-724-4348
e-mail: ferreinf@aol.com
www.ferre.org

Resolve
1310 Broadway
Somerville, MA 02144
617-623-0744 (National HelpLine)
e-mail: resolveinc@aol.com
www.resolve.org

Kidney Disorders

American Association of Kidney Patients
100 South Ashley Drive, Suite 280
Tampa, FL 33602
800-749-2257; 813-223-7099
e-mail: aakpnat@aol.com
www.aakp.org

American Kidney Fund
6110 Executive Boulevard,
  Suite 1010
Rockville, MD 20852
800-638-8299; 301-881-3052
ww.akfinc.org

National Kidney Foundation
30 East 33rd Street, Suite 1100
New York, NY 10016
800-622-9010; 212-889-2210
www.kidney.org

**National Kidney and Urologic
Diseases Information
Clearinghouse**
National Institute of Diabetes and
  Digestive and Kidney Diseases
Three Information Way
Bethesda, MD 20892-3560
301-654-4415
e-mail: nkudic@info.niddk.nih.gov
www.niddk.nih.gov/health/
  kidney/nkudic.htm

Learning Disabilities

**American Association on Mental
Retardation**
444 North Capitol Street NW,
  Suite 846
Washington, DC 20001-1512
800-424-3688; 202-387-1968
www.aamr.org

Learning Disabilities Association
4156 Library Road
Pittsburgh, PA 15234-1349
412-341-1515
e-mail: ldanatl@usaor.net
www.ldanatl.org

**National Center for Learning
Disabilities**
381 Park Ave South, Suite 1401
New York, NY 10016
888-575-7373; 212-545-7510
www.ncld.org

Liver Disorders

American Liver Foundation
75 Maiden Lane, Suite 603
New York, New York 10038
800-GO-LIVER (800-465-4837)
www.liverfoundation.org

Lupus

Lupus Foundation of America
1300 Piccard Drive, Suite 200
Rockville, MD 20850-4303
800-558-0121; 301-670-9292
www.lupus.org

Medic Alert

**MedicAlert Foundation
International**
2323 Colorado Avenue
Turlock, CA 95382-2018
800-432-5378
www.medicalert.org

Mental Retardation

**ARC (formerly Association for
Retarded Citizens of the United
States)**
500 East Border Street, Suite 300
Arlington, TX 76010
817-261-6003; 817-277-0553
  (TDD)
e-mail: info@thearc.org
thearc.org

FRAXA Research Foundation
45 Pleasant Street
Newburyport, MA 01950
978-462-1866
e-mail: info@fraxa.org
www.fraxa.org

Joseph P. Kennedy Foundation
1325 G Street NW, Suite 500
Washington, DC 20005-4709
202-393-1250

**National Association of
Developmental Disabilities Councils**
1234 Massachusetts Avenue NW,
   Suite 103
Washington, DC 20005
202-347-1234
www.igc.apc.org/naddc

Voice of the Retarded (VOR)
5005 Newport Drive, Suite 108
Rolling Meadows, IL 60008
847-253-6020

Multiple Sclerosis

National Multiple Sclerosis Society
733 Third Avenue
New York, NY 10017
800-344-4867; 212-986-3240
e-mail: info@nmss.org
www.nmss.org

Muscular Dystrophy

Muscular Dystrophy Association
National Headquarters
3300 East Sunrise Drive
Tucson, AZ 85718
800-572-1717
www.mdausa.org

Myasthenia Gravis

**Myasthenia Gravis Foundation of
America**
123 West Madison Street, Suite 800
Chicago, IL 60602
800-541-5454; 312-853-0522
e-mail: myasthenia@myasthenia.org
www.myasthenia.org

Nutrition

American Dietetic Association
216 West Jackson Boulevard
Chicago, IL 60606-6995
800-366-1655 (hot line); 800-877-
   1600; 312-899-0040
e-mail: infocenter@eatright.org
www.eatright.org

Osteoporosis

National Osteoporosis Foundation
1232 22nd Street NW
Washington, DC 20037-1292
202-223-2226
www.nof.org

Paget's Disease

The Paget Foundation
20 Wall Street, Suite 1602
New York, NY 10005
800-23-PAGET; 212-509-5335
e-mail: pagetfdn@aol.com
ww.paget.org

Pain Relief

American Chronic Pain Association
PO Box 850
Rocklin, CA 95677
916-632-0922
e-mail: acpa@pacbell.net
www.theacpa.org

**National Chronic Pain Outreach
Association**
7979 Old Georgetown Road, Suite
  100
Bethesda, MD 20814-2429
301-652-4948

Parkinson's Disease

**American Parkinson Disease
Association**
1250 Hylan Boulevard, Suite 4B
Staten Island, NY 10305-1946
800-223-2732; 718-981-8001
e-mail: info@apdaparkinson.com
www.apdaparkinson.com/

National Parkinson Foundation
1501 NW Ninth Avenue
Bob Hope Road
Miami, FL 33136-1494
800-327-4545; 305-547-6666
www.parkinson.org

Parkinson's Action Network
840 Third Street
Santa Rosa, CA 95404
800-850-4726; 707-544-1994
e-mail: info@parkinsonaction.org
www.parkinsonsaction.org

Parkinson's Disease Foundation
William Black Medical Building
710 West 168th Street
New York, NY 10032-9982
800-457-6676; 212-923-4700
e-mail: info@pdf.org
www.pdf.org

**Parkinson Support Groups of
America**
11376 Cherry Hill Road, 204
Beltsville, MD 20705
301-937-1545

United Parkinson Foundation
833 West Washington Boulevard
Chicago, IL 60607
312-733-1893

Prostate Cancer

US-TOO International
930 North York Road, Suite 50
Hinsdale, IL 60521-2993
800-80-US TOO (800-808-7866);
630-323-1002
www.ustoo.com

Prostatitis

Prostatitis Foundation
1063 30th Street, Box 8
Smithshire, IL 61478
888-891-4200
www.prostatitis.org

Psoriasis

National Psoriasis Foundation
6600 SW 92nd Avenue, Suite 300
Portland, OR 97223-7195
800-723-9166; 503-244-7404
e-mail: getinfo@npfusa.org
www.psoriasis.org

Psychiatric Disease

NAMI/NYC
432 Park Avenue South, Suite 710
New York, NY 10016-8806
800-950-6264; 212-684-3264
www.schizophrenia.com/ami

National Alliance for the Mentally Ill
200 North Glebe Road, Suite 1015
Arlington, VA 22203-3754
800-950-6264; 703-524-7600;
703-516-7227 (TDD)
ww.nami.org

National Institute of Mental Health
Public Inquiries
6001 Executive Boulevard, Room
8184, MSC 9663
Bethesda, MD 20892-9663
888-8-ANXIETY (888-826-9438,
for anxiety disorders); 800-421-
4211 (for depression); 800-64-
PANIC (800-647-2643, for panic
disorder); 301-443-4513
e-mail: nimhinfo@nih.gov
www.nimh.nih.gov

National Mental Health Association
1021 Prince Street
Alexandria, VA 22314-2971
800-969-NMHA (800-969-6644);
800-433-5959 (TTY); 703-684-
7722
www.nmha.org

Rare Disorders

National Organization for Rare Disorders
PO Box 8923
New Fairfield, CT 06812-8923
800-999-6673; 203-746-6518
e-mail: orphan@rarediseases.org
www.rarediseases.org

Respiratory (Lung) Disorders

American Lung Association
1740 Broadway
New York, NY 10019-4374
800-586-4872; 212-315-8700
e-mail: info@lungusa.org
www.lungusa.org

Asthma and Allergy Foundation of America
1233 20th Street NW, Suite 402
Washington, DC 20036
800-7ASTHMA (800-727-8462);
   202-466-7643
e-mail: info@aafa.org
www.aafa.org

Reye's Syndrome

National Reye's Syndrome Foundation
PO Box 829
Bryan, OH 43506-0829
800-233-7393; 419-636-2679
e-mail: reyessyn@mail.bright.net
www.bright.net/~reyessyn

Sexually Transmitted Diseases

CDC's National STD Hotline
800-227-8922

National Herpes Hotline
919-361-8488

Skin Cancer

Skin Cancer Foundation
PO Box 561
New York, NY 10156
800-754-6490
e-mail: info@skincancer.org
www.skincancer.org

Sleep Disorders

American Sleep Apnea Association
1424 K Street NW, Suite 302
Washington, DC 20005
202-293-3650
e-mail: asaa@sleepapnea.org
www.sleepapnea.org

American Academy of Sleep Medicine
6301 Bandel Road, Suite 101
Rochester, MN 55901
507-287-6006
e-mail: info@aasmnet.org
www.asda.org

Spina Bifida

Spina Bifida Association of America
4590 MacArthur Boulevard NW,
   Suite 250
Washington, DC 20007-4226
800-621-3141; 202-944-3285
e-mail: sbaa@sbaa.org
www.sbaa.org

Spinal Cord Injury

National Spinal Cord Injury Association
8701 Georgia Avenue, Suite 500
Silver Spring, MD 20910
800-962-9629; 301-588-6959
e-mail: nscia2@aol.com
www.spinalcord.org

Spinal Cord Injury Hotline
2200 Kernan Drive
Baltimore, MD 21207
800-526-3456
e-mail: scihotline@aol.com
www.SCHIHOTLINE.org

Strokes

National Stroke Association
96 Inverness Drive East, Suite 1
Englewood, CO 80112-5112
800-STROKES (800-787-6537);
  303-649-9299
e-mail: info@stroke.org
www.stroke.org

The Stroke Connection of the American Heart Association
7272 Greenville Avenue
Dallas, TX 75231
888-4STROKE
www.strokeassociation.org

Stuttering and Other Speech Disorders

National Aphasia Association
156 Fifth Avenue, Suite 707
New York, NY 10010
800-922-4622; 212-255-4329
e-mail: naa@aphasia.org
www.aphasia.org

National Stuttering Association
5100 East La Palma Avenue,
  Suite 208
Anaheim Hills, CA 92807
800-364-1677; 714-693-7554
e-mail: nspinfo@aol.com
www.nsastutter.org

Stuttering Foundation of America
PO Box 11749
3100 Walnut Grove Road, Suite
  603
Memphis, TN 38111-0749
800-992-9392; 901-452-7343
e-mail: stutter@vantek.net
www.stuttersfa.org

Sudden Infant Death Syndrome

National Sudden Infant Death Syndrome Resource Center
2070 Chain Bridge Road, Suite 450
Vienna, VA 22182
703-821-8955
e-mail: sids@circsol.com
www.circsol.com/SIDS

SIDS Network
PO Box 520
Ledyard, CT 06339
e-mail: sidsnet@sids-network.org
sids-network.org

Sudden Infant Death Syndrome Alliance
1314 Bedford Avenue, Suite 210
Baltimore, MD 21208
800-221-SIDS (800-221-7437);
    410-653-8226
e-mail: sidshq@charm.net
www.sidsalliance.org

Tay-Sachs Disease

National Tay-Sachs and Allied Diseases Association
2001 Beacon Street, Suite 204
Brighton, MA 02135
800-90-NTSAD (800-906-8723);
    617-277-4463

Women's Health

American College of Obstetricians and Gynecologists
Resource Center
PO Box 96920
409 12th Street SW
Washington, DC 20090-6920
202-863-2518
www.acog.org

National Women's Health Network
514 10th Street NW, Suite 400
Washington, DC 20004
202-628-7814; 202-347-1140
www.womenshealthnetwork.org

Information Services and Web Sites

General

The American Medical Association
515 North State Street
Chicago, IL 60610
312-464-5000
www.ama-assn.org

The Centers for Disease Control and Prevention
1600 Clifton Road NE
Atlanta, GA 30333
800-311-3435; 404-639-3534;
    404-639-3311
www.cdc.gov

The Merck Manual
Merck & Co., Inc.
PO Box 4
West Point, PA 19486
www.merck.com

National Institutes of Health
9000 Rockville Pike
Bethesda, MD 20892
301-496-4000
www.nih.gov

Parents of Chronically Ill Children
1527 Maryland Street
Springfield, IL 62702
217-522-6810

US Department of Health and Human Services
200 Independence Avenue SW
Washington, DC 20201
877-696-6775; 202-619-0257
www.os.dhhs.gov

US Food and Drug Administration
Office of Consumer Affairs Inquiry
   Information Line
888-INFO-FDA (888-463-6332)
www.fda.gov

Travel Medicine
Immunization Alert
PO Box 406
Storrs, CT 06268
800-584-1999

International Association for Medical Assistance to Travelers
417 Center Street
Lewiston, NY 14092
716-754-4883

International SOS Assistance
8 Neshaminy Interplex, Suite 207
Trevose, PA 19053-6956
800-523-8930; 215-245-4707
e-mail: info@travelcare.com

International Travelers Hotline
Centers for Disease Control and
   Prevention
National Center for Infectious Diseases
877-FYI-TRIP (877-394-8747)
www.cdc.gov/travel

Ask Your Pharmacist
www.webAYP.com

References

Non-drug treatments

Foster S., Tyler, V.E. *Tyler's Honest Herbal: A Sensible Guide to the Use of Herbs and Related Products.* The Hayworth Press, 1999.

Graedon, J., Graedon, T. *The People's Pharmacy Guide to Home and Herbal Remedies.* St. Martin's Press, 1999.

Herbal Medicinals: A Clinician's Guide. Pharmaceutical Products Press, 1998.

Kuhn, M.A. *Herbs, Drugs & the Body.* Medical Educational Services Inc., 1999.

Kuhn, M.A. *Herbs and Menopause.* Medical Educational Services Inc., 1997.

Lininger S., Wright, J., Brown, D. *The Natural Pharmacy.* Prima Health, 1998.

Miller, L.G. "Herbal Medicinals: Selected Clinical Considerations Focusing on Known or Potential Drug-Herb Interactions," *Archives of Internal Medicine*: 158 (1998).

Murray, M., Pizzorno, J. *Encyclopedia of Natural Medicine.* Prima Health, 1998.

Natural Prescriptions for Women, Rodale Press Inc., 1998.

The PDR Family Guide to Natural Medicines & Healing Therapies. Medical Economics Co., 1999.

PDR For Herbal Medicines. Medical Economics Co., 1998.

Peirce, A. *The American Pharmaceutical Association Practical Guide to Natural Medicines.* William Morrow & Co., 1999.

The Review of Natural Products. Facts and Comparisons, 1999.

Robbers, J.E., Tyler, V.E. *Tyler's Herbs of Choice: The Therapeutic Use of Phytomedicinals.* The Hayworth Press, 1999.

Silverman, H.M., Romano, J.A., Elmer, G. *The Vitamin Book: A No-Nonsense Consumer Guide.* Bantam Books, 1985.

Zand, J. Spreen A.N., LaValle, J.B. *Smart Medicine For Healthier Living.* Avery, 1999.

OTC treatments

Brodin, M.B. *The Over-The-Counter Drug Book.* Pocket Books, 1998.

Fudyma, J. *What Do I Take?—A Consumer's Guide to Non-Prescription Drugs.* HarperPerennial, 1997.

Garrison, R., Mannion M. *Pharmacist's Guide to Over-The-Counter and Natural Remedies.* Avery, 1999.

Handbook of Nonprescription Drugs. American Pharmaceutical Association, 2000.

Prescription treatments and clinical drug information

AHFS Drug Information 1999. American Society of Health-System Pharmacists Inc., 1999.

The American Psychiatric Press Textbook of Psychopharmacology. American Psychiatric Press Inc., 1998.

Applied Therapeutics: The Clinical Use of Drugs. Applied Therapeutics, 1995.

Briggs, G.G., Freeman, R.K., Yaffe, S.J. *Drugs in Pregnancy and Lactation.* Williams and Wilkins, 1998.

The Complete Book of Baby & Child Care. Tyndale, 1997.

Contraceptive Technology. Ardent Media, 1998.

Dickey, R.P. *Managing Contraceptive Pill Patients.* EMIS Inc., 1998.

Drug Facts and Comparisons. Facts and Comparisons, 1999.

Hansten, P.D., Horn, J.R. *Drug Interactions Analysis and Management.* Applied Therapeutics, 1999.

Harrison's Principles of Internal Medicine. McGraw-Hill Companies, 1998.

The Johns Hopkins Complete Home Encyclopedia of Drugs. Medletter Associates Inc., 1998.

Mayo Clinic Family Health Book. William Morrow & Co., 1996.

The Medical Advisor. Time-Life Books, 1997.

The Merck Manual of Medical Information: Home Edition. Merck & Co., 1997.

Micromedex Healthcare Series. Micromedex Inc., 1999.

Nathanson, L. *The Portable Pediatrician for Parents.* HarperCollins, 1994.

Pharmacotherapy: A Pathophysiologic Approach. Appleton & Lange, 1999.

USP-DI Advice for the Patient: Drug Information in Lay Language. Micromedex Inc., 1998.

Index